Community Nursing
and Primary Healthcare
in Twentieth-Century Britain

Routledge Studies in the Social History of Medicine

EDITED BY JOSEPH MELLING, *University of Exeter*
AND ANNE BORSAY, *University of Wales, Swansea, UK*

1. Nutrition in Britain
Science, Scientists and Politics in the Twentieth Century
Edited by David F. Smith

2. Migrants, Minorities and Health
Historical and Contemporary Studies
Edited by Lara Marks and Michael Worboys

3. From Idiocy to Mental Deficiency
Historical Perspectives on People with Learning Disabilities
Edited by David Wright and Anne Digby

4. Midwives, Society and Childbirth
Debates and Controversies in the Modern Period
Edited by Hilary Marland and Anne Marie Rafferty

5. Illness and Healing Alternatives in Western Europe
Edited by Marijke Gijswit-Hofstra, Hilary Maarland and Has de Waardt

6. Health Care and Poor Relief in Protestant Europe 1500–1700
Edited by Ole Peter Grell and Andrew Cunningham

7. The Locus of Care
Families, Communities, Institutions, and the Provision of Welfare since Antiquity
Edited by Peregrine Horden and Richard Smith

8. Race, Science and Medicine, 1700–1960
Edited by Waltraud Ernst and Bernard Harris

9. Insanity, Institutions and Society, 1800–1914
Edited by Bill Forsythe and Joseph Melling

10. Food, Science, Policy and Regulation in the Twentieth Century
International and Comparative Perspectives
Edited by David F. Smith and Jim Phillips

11. Sex, Sin and Suffering
Venereal Disease and European Society since 1870
Edited by Roger Davidson and Lesley A. Hall

12. The Spanish Influenza Pandemic of 1918–19
New Perspectives
Edited by Howard Phillips and David Killingray

13. Plural Medicine, Tradition and Modernity, 1800–2000
Edited by Waltraud Ernst

14. Innovations in Health and Medicine
Diffusion and Resistance in the Twentieth Century
Edited by Jenny Stanton

15. Contagion
Historical and Cultural Studies
Edited by Alison Bashford and Claire
Hooker

**16. Medicine, Health and the Public
Sphere in Britain, 1600–2000**
Edited by Steve Sturdy

17. Medicine and Colonial Identity
Edited by Mary P. Sutphen and Bridie
Andrews

**18. New Directions in Nursing
History**
Edited by Barbara E. Mortimer and
Susan McGann

**19. Medicine, the Market and Mass
Media**
Producing Health in the Twentieth
Century
Edited by Virginia Berridge and Kelly
Loughlin

20. The Politics of Madness
The State, Insanity and Society in
England, 1845–1914
Joseph Melling and Bill Forsythe

21. The Risks of Medical Innovation
Risk Perception and Assessment in
Historical Context
Edited by Thomas Schlich and Ulrich
Tröhler

**22. Mental Illness and Learning
Disability Since 1850**
Finding a Place for Mental Disorder in
the United Kingdom
Edited by Pamela Dale and Joseph
Melling

**23. Britain and the 1918–19
Influenza Pandemic**
A Dark Epilogue
Niall Johnson

24. Financing Medicine
The British Experience since 1750
Edited by Martin Gorsky and Sally
Sheard

**25. Social Histories of Disability and
Deformity**
Edited by David M. Turner and Kevin
Stagg

**26. Histories of the Normal and the
Abnormal**
Social and Cultural Histories of Norms
and Normativity
Edited by Waltraud Ernst

**27. Madness, Architecture and the
Built Environment**
Psychiatric Spaces in Historical
Context
Edited by Leslie Topp, James E. Moran
and Jonathan Andrews

**28. Lunatic Hospitals in Georgian
England, 1750–1830**
Leonard Smith

29. Women and Smoking Since 1890
Rosemary Elliot

**30. Community Nursing and Primary
Healthcare in Twentieth-Century
Britain**
Helen M. Sweet with Rona Dougall

**Also available in Routledge Studies
in the Social History of Medicine
series:**

Reassessing Foucault
Power, Medicine and the Body
Edited by Colin Jones and Roy Porter

Community Nursing
and Primary Healthcare
in Twentieth-Century Britain

Helen M. Sweet

with Rona Dougall

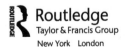

Routledge
Taylor & Francis Group
New York   London

First published 2008
by Routledge
711 Third Avenue, New York, NY 10017

Simultaneously published in the UK
by Routledge
2 Park Square, Milton Park, Abingdon, Oxon OX14 4RN

Routledge is an imprint of the Taylor & Francis Group, an informa business

First issued in paperback 2012

© 2008 Taylor & Francis

Typeset in Sabon by IBT Global

Library of Congress Cataloging in Publication Data
Sweet, Helen M.
Community nursing and primary healthcare in twentieth-century Britain / Helen M.
Sweet with Rona Dougall.
p. cm. —(Routledge studies in the social history of medicine ; 30)
Includes bibliographical references and index.
ISBN 978-0-415-95634-5 (hardback : alk. paper)
1. Community health nursing—Great Britain—History—20th century. 2. Primary health
care—Great Britain—History—20th century. I. Dougall, Rona. II. Title. III. Series.
[DNLM: 1. Community Health Nursing—history—Great Britain. 2. History, 20th
Century—Great Britain. 3. Primary Health Care—history—Great Britain.
WY 11 FA1 S974c 2007]

RT98.S94 2007
610.73'430941—dc22   2007015921

ISBN13: 978-0-415-95634-5 (hbk)
ISBN13: 978-0-415-54110-7 (pbk)
ISBN13: 978-0-203-93372-5 (ebk)

Contents

List of Figures   ix
Preface   xi
Acknowledgments   xiii
Glossary and Conventions   xv

Introduction   1

PART I
The History of District Nursing   15

1   Historical Trajectories: Background, c. 1850–1919   17

2   What Became of the Lady? The Interwar period, 1919–1939   35

3   War to Welfare State, 1939–1948   63

4   Changing Places, 1948–1979   81

PART II
Themes and Issues: The District Nurse and the
Changing World of Primary Health Care   105

5   Town Nurse, Country Nurse: District Nursing Landscape   107

6   Technology, Treatment, and TLC   135

7   Generalists and Generals: District Nursing
    Professionalisation   151

8   **Language of Caring: Care and Nurses' Lives**   165

9   **Portraits of a District Nurse**   187

10   **Discussion and Conclusion**   201

Endnotes   215
Sources and Bibliography   245
Index   261

List of Figures

Figure 1.1	Nurse Wolfe of Gotherington, Somerset.	25
Figure 1.2	Distribution graph of district nursing associations 1915 (England and Wales).	32
Figure 2.1	Cooperating in being: Health visitor meeting with district nurse.	41
Figure 2.2	District nurse (no date, but pre-1943).	45
Figure 2.3	Income sources of district nursing associations (England and Wales) 1915–1925.	52
Figure 3.1	Numbers of district nurses, England and Wales, 1919–1939.	65
Figure 3.2	Plymouth Queen's Nurses Cantrill and McCarthy picking their way over the debris from a bomb raid to the house of a patient.	68
Figure 5.1	1960s recruitment leaflet, front cover.	108
Figure 5.2	Superintendent and assistant superintendent and (Queen's) district nurses at the nurses' home in Cardiff (1926).	111
Figure 5.3	Maes-yr-Haf, opened Spring 1927.	129
Figure 6.1	District nurse preparing her bag for the day's visits.	136
Figure 6.2	Equipment required for a dressing and giving an insulin injection, c. 1948.	137
Figure 6.3	Equipment required for a dressing and giving an insulin injection after introduction of CSSD and disposables.	138
Figure 6.4	Mrs. Grey, rural village nurse-midwife, c. 1905.	143
Figure 6.5	Nurse Radburn on her motor scooter.	144

Figure 6.6   Nurses setting out.   145

Figure 6.7   Nurse's message slate, traditionally left outside her
               front door.   148

Figure 9.1   A Queen's district nurse, mid-twentieth century.   188

Figure 9.2   Cartoon of "The Workhouse Mrs. Gamp."   189

Figure 9.3   District nurse attending young child, c. 1920.   189

Figure 9.4   Advertisement for nurses' uniforms and bags.   192

Figure 9.5   Front cover of a 1948 textbook.   193

Figure 9.6   Film still from *Friend of the Family*: "The District
               Nurse visits one of her patients."   195

Preface

This book has been inspired in particular by several previous areas of research in which one or the other of the authors has worked. These included a study into the relatively recent creation and development of the new specialty of intensive therapy, as seen from the high-profile, technological end of the medical and nursing institutional spectrum.[1] This begged a question: What was happening at the other, essentially generalist and low-profile, domiciliary end of that spectrum that is arguably the oldest and most firmly established, professionally?

The second area of research that has particularly influenced this book included two studies of general practice medicine,[2,3] in which we had been involved in looking at the professional evolutionary development of the medical generalist. The interprofessional dimension of this raised a number of questions that could not be fully answered without an equally in-depth look at the other health professionals with whom the general practitioner came into increasing contact as the concept of the community care team emerged. In particular, this was the need to address issues of gender relationships central to a (nursing) profession largely composed of women (throughout the period of study) working alongside a (medical) profession largely composed of men. Central to this power play of institutional and occupational imperialism is an understanding of the effects of conflict and concord both intra- and interprofessionally on the development of district nursing, including extended professional roles, social and political professional issues, changing power bases, and the apparent conflict between a desire for recognised professional autonomy and accepted membership of a community health care team.

In addition, for one of us there was a third, more personal influence on the choice of subject, namely having trained as a nurse and midwife and practised for a short time as a district midwife, and having felt the privilege of working alongside several of the "old school" of district nurse-midwives who practised relatively autonomously from their homes rather than from group practices as a part of a team, and who lived within the community they served. We especially wish to thank those district nurses who gave us their personal memories during the oral histories that permeate this book.

Acknowledgments

We would like to extend our thanks to a number of people, without whom this book would not have been possible. First and foremost, our gratitude goes to the nurses to whom we spoke, who were without exception hospitable, friendly, and interesting. They were all remarkable in their own way by virtue of living through such a cultural shift in nursing in the community. Although they did not all find the many changes easy, nor always for the better, they adapted and remained committed to an ethos of good nursing care that, we feel, has not been lost on the present generation of district nurses. We hope we have represented them all fairly.

We would like to record our gratitude to Jo Melling for his unstinting support and his perceptive editorial comments, and to the editorial staff of Routledge (Taylor and Francis Group), for their support in bringing this book to completion.

Among the librarians and archivists who have generously provided their expertise in locating sources for this study, we would especially like to thank Shirley Dixon and Lesley Hall, archivists at the CMAC Wellcome Institute; Adrian Allan, Liverpool University archivist; the librarians of Oxford Brookes University; the Wellcome Unit Library, Oxford; the Radcliffe Science Library, Oxford; and the Wellcome Institute Library, London. Thanks to the staff at QNI Scotland (Castle Terrace, Edinburgh) and at QNI England and Wales (Albermarle Way, London) for their enthusiasm, for allowing access to their records, and for providing funding for a series of pilot interviews in the case of the Scottish work and providing free permission to use images from the Institute's journals and photographic collections. We owe gratitude to the Wellcome Trust for funding the initial collection of the Scottish nurses' oral histories, and Rona's supervisors in that task, Professor Willie Thompson and Professor Jean McIntosh. Thanks also to Dr. Chris Nottingham, Glasgow Caledonian University, who provided additional critical comments on the Scottish work.

Also we wish to express our particular thanks to Susan McGann for initially inviting Rona to undertake what became her contribution to this book and for her support and advice both as RCN Archivist and as a valued friend and colleague to us both. Susan and her staff have been incredibly patient with our many enquiries, and made our visits to the archives a real pleasure thanks to their unique combination of professional expertise and the warmth of friendship and support so generously given.

Likewise, numerous other friends and relations at home and work have been extremely supportive in a variety of ways and Helen would like to mention in particular colleagues in the History of Nursing Research Colloquium, the RCN History of Nursing Society, and the staff and fellow research students of the School of Humanities at Oxford Brookes University. She is also very grateful to Professor John Stewart and Elaine Ryder, who offered helpful advice and perceptive comments at an earlier stage of this work. More recently a big "thank you" goes to Professor Mark Harrison, Dr. Margaret Jones, Carol Brady, Belinda Michaelides, and research colleagues at the Wellcome Unit for History of Medicine, University of Oxford, who have so warmly supported and encouraged her throughout the publication process.

In particular, Helen also wishes to record an enormous debt of gratitude to Professor Anne Digby for her unstinting contributions of support and encouragement, advice and constructive criticism, steadfastness, and stimulation! Working with her guidance and friendship has added an especially enjoyable dimension to the experience.

Finally, we would both like to thank our families for their loving support and encouragement throughout our studies over the many years leading up to this publication, most of all John, Jennifer, Robert, and Wendy, and likewise Rona's family, all of whom have lived with the book from the earliest stages of PhD theses to its present state. They have unfailingly provided much moral and intellectual support, loving understanding, and encouragement throughout. We therefore dedicate this book to them.

Glossary and Conventions

BMA   British Medical Association: The doctors' professional organisation and independent trade union.

BMJ   *British Medical Journal*: Official journal of the BMA.

CMB   Central Midwives Board: British midwives' professional organisation.

CSSD   Central Sterile Supply Department: Area that centralises the sterile processing activities, in which reusable medical devices and surgical instruments and equipment (excluding the operating theatre procedures) are processed and issued for diagnostic and patient care procedures.

DN   [Journal of] *District Nursing* continued as *Journal of Community Nursing*.

DNA   District nursing association: For the purposes of this book, district nurses are defined as those nurses who provided community nursing care in patients' homes, working within clearly geographically defined districts or parishes. The district nursing association was a locally run and financed organisation, which pre-NHS employed the district nurse(s), originally to care for the "sick poor," although this qualification was later modified. These associations were often affiliated to the QNI (see later), which advised the DNA's executive committee and supervised the district nurse's professional practice.

GMC   General Medical Council: Official body that registers and regulates medical practitioners. Doctors must be registered with the GMC to practice medicine in the United Kingdom.

GNC   General Nursing Council: Three separate bodies (for England and Wales, Scotland, and Ireland) acted as official bodies to register and regulate nursing from 1923 until 1980. These became the United Kingdom Central Council, which in turn gave way to the Nursing and Midwifery Council (NMC) in 2002.

GP   General Practitioner: A medical doctor who provides primary, nonspecialised health care from a community-based "practice." Most of their work is carried out during consultations in surgery and during home visits.

HV   Health Visitor: A qualified and registered nurse or midwife who has undertaken further (post-registration) training to take particular responsibility for the promotion of health and the prevention of illness in all age groups.

MOH   Medical Officer of Health: A medical practitioner working for the local health authority with responsibility for administering public health policy and practice.

NHS   National Health Service: The publicly funded health care system of the United Kingdom, established by 1946 Act of Parliament that came into force in 1948.

QN   Queen's Nurse: Fully trained general nurses who had successfully completed a further training period in district nursing at a Queen's Institute training centre and had been admitted to the Queen's Institute Roll of Nurses.

QNI/QIDN   Queen's Nursing Institute, Queen's Institute of District Nursing, also QVJIN Queen Victoria's Jubilee Institute for Nurses: Professional organisation for Queen's Nurses and advisory body across the U.K. for district nursing associations having affiliation agreement with the QNI. It was established following Queen Victoria's Golden Jubilee in 1887. Separate Councils ran the national branches of England and Wales, Scotland, and Ireland.

QNI(S)   Queen's Nursing Institute for Scotland.

QNM   *Queen's Nurses' Magazine*: Official journal of the QNI.

RCN   Royal College of Nursing: Nurses' representative body, established 1916.

RGN   Registered General Nurse (also SRN)

SCM   State Certified Midwife

SEN   State Enrolled Nurse

SRN   State Registered Nurse

UKCC   United Kingdom Central Council for Nursing and Midwifery (*see* GNC earlier)

Introduction

A QUESTION FROM TODAY

As part of the World Health Organisation European policy for health across the 51 member states, since 2001 a scheme piloting the Family Health Nurse was introduced within the United Kingdom. In its first year this new nurse was described thus:

> The Family Health Nurse role combines caring for those who are ill with health assessment of the whole family together with public health activities along the "life course" . . . In some areas they will be the only health care practitioner or nurse, in others they will integrate into existing primary care teams.[1]

The scheme, which was first piloted in rural areas including the Highlands and the Western Isles, was said to be "exploring alternative community health models."[2] The proposal that a new model was required, coupled with the title Family Health Nurse, implied a need to strengthen the relationship between nurses in rural and island areas and the families they dealt with, as well as a recognition that this relationship, as it currently stood, was not providing optimal benefits to health. The Family Health Nurse scheme might be an "alternative" model employed to tackle this, but it is also distinctly reminiscent of the kinds of informal relationships that district nurses of the past claim to have had within their communities. This claim includes close involvement with their patients and, in many situations, a particularly close knowledge of the families in their district. Furthermore, this relationship is held to be one of the defining characteristics of past district nursing in both rural and urban areas. If this is the case and yet there is a recognised need to establish this relationship today, then somewhere along the line something must have changed. In this book we examine this notion of change. We trace the history of district nursing throughout the United Kingdom during the twentieth century and document nurses' experiences and what they felt were defining events of change.

DISTRICT NURSING AND
THE QUEEN'S NURSING INSTITUTE

A wonderful melange of providers fall into the category of community nursing throughout the period covered by this book. This included village nurses, "bible" or "mission" nurses, midwives, private nurses, nurse-midwives, triple-duty nurses, Queen's Nurses, health visitors, and most recently, a range of community specialist nurses as well as practice nurses. To provide a definition of what a district nurse was, is a difficult—if not impossible—task, as the role covered by "district" was (and still is) always evolving. When the term was first used in the mid-nineteenth century, it referred mainly to those women who provided care for a section of the community generally known as the "sick poor," living in their own homes. These women worked within clearly geographically defined districts. However, the role adopted by them continually changed to encompass patients from the working, middle, and even upper classes. As the type of care needed changed, so did the training and organisational requirements of the district nursing associations for which these nurses worked. As the twentieth century progressed, men were included among their ranks and districts became "GP attachments"—practices covered by general medical practitioners with which the district nurses had an increasing affiliation.

Until 1948 district nursing was organised in a voluntary system of local associations, many of which were affiliated to the Queen's Nursing Institute (QNI)[3] and adhered to their standards of practice and system of supervision. From its institution in 1889, the QNI remained the dominant force in district nursing in Britain until it ceased training district nurses in 1970. It is referred to repeatedly throughout this book for this reason, but also because it still retains contact with retired Queen's nurses to the present day.[4] This book makes no attempt to set out a comprehensive institutional history of the QNI;[5] rather, the QNI is significant here because it acted as a focal point for nurses who often felt isolated in their posts. Queen's nurses (as district nurses qualifying through the QNI called themselves) tended to express a sense of belonging to the QNI and enjoyed the benefits of ongoing training through their affiliation with the institute.[6]

A further subject that deserves clarification from the outset is the system by which district nursing associations were financed. Although this subject is dealt with in subsequent chapters, we should explain the concept of the Provident System that provided an extension to the welfare provision offered by Poor Law and National Health Insurance Acts until the National Health Act came into force in 1948.[7] Unemployment insurance was greatly extended in the first decade of the twentieth century through a series of welfare legislative acts culminating in the National Health Insurance Acts of 1911 and 1920, and a contributory pension scheme was introduced in 1925. Local authorities then accepted responsibility for the impoverished, a function previously undertaken by Boards of Guardians under the provisions of the Poor Laws. However, during the depression of the late 1920s and throughout the 1930s the National Insurance Fund became inadequate. Benefits, already meagre, were cut and the period of entitlement was also limited.

The Provident scheme was based on the methods developed by Friendly Societies formed to counteract the worst social effects of the Industrial Revolution under the ethos of self-help. These used regular contributions made to a society either by an employer or an individual to provide benefits such as an income in old age or insurance against sickness or inability to work, thereby enabling people to look after themselves. In the case of the district nursing associations, money would be collected weekly according to ability to pay, which would then provide nursing and midwifery care for whole families in time of need. The money would be used to run the association and pay the nurses. As one nurse remembered, for patients it was "twopence for the doctor, a penny for the nurse."[8]

HISTORIOGRAPHY

Current scholarship in the area of community nursing has tended to focus either on the earlier period leading up to the founding of the Queen's Institute for District Nursing (1897)[9] questioning the Dickensian image of the district nurse midwives as portrayed by Betsy Prigg and Sarah Gamp[10] or by considering the work of William Rathbone in Liverpool;[11] the "mission women" of Manchester, Salford, and London;[12] or examining the rationale behind Florence Nightingale's hostility toward hospital-based health care. Alternatively the emphasis has been focused either on the district nursing associations prior to the NHS Act (1948),[13] or on the contemporary rather than the historical aspects of recent community-care reorganisation following the 1993 Community Care Act with the emergence of GP fund-holding practices; changes in structure of work, pay, and conditions of district nurses; and the rise of the practice nurse.[14]

Other members of the community health team receiving recent attention from medical historians relating to this period include GPs,[15] health visitors,[16] and midwives,[17] and the historical development of the hospital nurse has also been widely researched.[18] By comparison, therefore, serious consideration of the district nurse through this period of the twentieth century was long overdue and should provide a better understanding of the evolving community care team by contextualising the developments in this field of nursing and by expanding the view of interprofessional relationships within community care. The tendency of nursing history has been to view nurses as if they were a homogenous group of professionals: even where they are divided into subgroups such as district nurses or health visitors, it is difficult to see them as individuals. The title of Allan and Jolley's book, *Nursing, Midwifery and Health Visiting Since 1900*, recognises individual nursing identifications and they are dealt with individually in separate chapters.[19] However, it also implies a commonality between the services: That the three, along with the sometimes omitted social worker, cannot be fully discussed without reference to each other is indubitable. This has particular significance for any discussion of district nursing in Scotland given the importance of triple-duty nursing, where the three roles were combined, in so many of its small towns and rural districts. Dingwall et al. introduced a significant historical difference between the hospital and home nurse. Of their relationship during the late nineteenth century they noted:

> [T]he boundary between medicine and nursing in the community appears to be rather different from that in the hospital. The hospital nurse is a subordinate craftsman. . . . Her counterpart in the community is much closer to the doctor, as a treatment assistant.[20]

Kratz reaffirmed the persistence of this hospital–home split in nursing by noting in 1982 that "all is not well" between district nurses and their hospital colleagues.[21] In much of the literature discussing nursing it is the case that the different responsibilities of nurses in the community are not brought into any analysis, thus contributing to an effective marginalisation of the district nurse and her community-based colleagues. Citing Ferguson and Fitzgerald, Dingwall et al. also pointed out that histories covering the period of World War II discuss several important aspects of nursing but include nothing on district nursing.[22] This is notable in nursing history but it also applies to works in other disciplines such as sociology. A prime example of this can be seen in the work of Walby et al. and Wicks.[23] These otherwise excellent discussions of the professional boundaries between doctor and nurse, the former dealing with the United Kingdom and the latter with Australia, focus exclusively on the ward nurse. By taking wound healing as an example of an unrecognised nursing skill usually controlled by the medical staff within hospitals and therefore "central to the practice of medicine," not nursing, Wicks effectively limited the discussion of nursing skills to the hospital situation:

> Here was an area of healing, that of wound dressing, which has always been recognised as being central to the practice of medicine and here was a nurse, quietly telling me that not only could she do the job better than many doctors, but that at least one specialist/Consultant recognised this and referred his most difficult patients to her.[24]

Wound dressing has always formed a considerable part of the district nurse's caseload and as such was a well-practised skill recognised by most GPs and evident in their patterns of referral. In its neglect of district nursing, the historical analysis of nurse–doctor relationships that Wicks entered into is therefore a contracted one. Walby et al. stated explicitly that district nursing is outside the scope of their discussion. However, nursing in general is a relatively new area of historical study that still struggles to identify itself as worthy of scholarly interest. In this context, the neglect of nursing in the community and its individual contribution to nursing history is perhaps not surprising. This book uses oral history and records of individual nurses in an attempt to rectify this and to address the different experiences of nursing in different regions and environments.

Maggs[25] criticised historians of nursing for writing very little about the actual history of nursing itself; he asserted that most scholarship in this field to date has focused either on nurses, nursing organisations, professionalisation of nursing, or nursing institutions and specialisms. In this book oral history will be shown to be particularly valuable in addressing this deficiency, not only in highlighting changes in perception of status and interprofessional relationships, but also in revealing what the nurse actually *did*, providing detail of the daily tasks, routine, workload, and personal experience. Together with some archival material from district nursing association records, the oral histories present a uniquely vivid picture of both regional variations and the shared experience of what it meant to be a district nurse. This makes it possible to suggest that being a district nurse in South Wales in the 1920s might have been quite different from being a district nurse in Lancashire in the 1970s or in Glasgow in the 1990s, yet nurses in each of these environments would recognise certain commonalities that were essential to their work as district nurses and that represent an "essence" of district nursing that transcends both time and region. This book differs from other works in the weight it gives to establishing and understanding the changing relationships between district nurses and other members of the emerging community health care team over the twentieth century. In particular it gives expression to the diversity of experience and role that existed within the developing sub-profession of district nursing throughout this time.

The first part of this book outlines the development of the district nurse that occurred in a time of considerable change in the nursing profession and community health provision generally. Early work suggested a number of interrelated themes and issues and it was anticipated that aspects of professionalisation and legislation would provide the central focus to the book. This entailed two main considerations. First, the transfer of Poor Law administration to local authorities in 1929 was coupled with the growth of voluntarily organised district nursing associations in the 1920s and 1930s. This raised questions relating to professional development and how it changed following the 1948 NHS Act and subsequent Health Service reorganisation. The second consideration was understanding the political complexities surrounding the establishment of district nurse training and education nationally, which were only resolved at the very end of this period.

This led us to question the extent to which local authorities adopted any form of national standard for district nurse training and whether there were rural, urban, or regional differences in training provision and requirements. Research into this aspect of district nursing's professional development was based to some extent on research led by Dr. Lisbeth Hockey[26] on behalf of the QNI in the 1960s and on the recommendations of subsequent parliamentary and professional reports.[27] It was supplemented by oral testimony, which included several discussions with Dr. Hockey herself.

As the research progressed, other considerations came to the fore, among them the need to determine the relative importance of intra- and interprofessional tensions and the concept of nursing as a sub-profession to medicine. This became a central theme running throughout the book and exposed a number of dichotomies:

- How accurate is the stereotypically perceived dominant, paternalistic role of GP as gatekeeper and curer, and subordinate role of district nurse as handmaiden and carer? How and why did these change over the period of study?
- How are these roles related to changes in perceived social status within the public and private spheres of the community as well as to professional status within the medical team (community and hospital), and to changes in training and job descriptions?
- Is it possible to assess changes either in public image and awareness of district nurses and in the self-images and perceived status of the district nurse during this period?
- Where does the idea of vocation fit in with professionalisation in the community context in which district nursing is located?

As a result, dilemmas of professionalisation within district nursing came to represent the major, if not overarching, preoccupation of this book. Specifically, these involve attainment and maintenance of an elusive professional status and public respect, control of standards through recognised and autonomous regulation, control and (to a large extent) internal accountability of district nurses, autonomy of practice, and influence over conditions of service. The major theme running throughout this book is that of a developing community-care team within which district nurses had to negotiate and secure their place while simultaneously fighting to develop an autonomous professional standing. We give considerable space to district nurses' inter- and intraprofessional relationships, particularly with GPs and health visitors, but also with their hospital colleagues. These can be seen as underpinning hegemonic, interprofessional influences producing a form of "occupational imperialism."[28] Located within a wider framework of -restricted, class-based citizenship, the nature of these relationships contributed to nurses' limited participation in influential bodies, such as NHS planning committees and post-NHS representative bodies, to be discussed in Chapters 5 and 6. Complementing this we consider the changing internal power bases as control of many aspects of district nurses' professional and private lives moved from "Lady Superintendents" to the "Committee of Ladies," often under the auspices of the QNI, and eventually the transfer of responsibility for employment, training, and regulation to local government.

A number of minor, but interrelated themes are also pursued, all of which can be directly linked with this precarious professional balancing act. One recurrent issue arising throughout this study is the emergence of technologies such as prepackaged sterile supplies, new materials, communications technologies, and developments in means of transport. Issues of gender and class are also raised, including the introduction of male nurses from 1947. Likewise, variations and changes in the district nursing experience including pay and conditions, workload, and mobility of practice are also related to geographical location of practice throughout this book, shown both through the urban–rural contrast and when comparing several regions across England and Wales.

Worldwide, changes in patronage, perception of the patient, perceptions of illness, and changing roles and tasks of the nurse and doctor as carer and medical investigator, respectively, have produced a series of changes both in interprofessional relationships and in perceptions of what it is to be a professional. We suggest this was especially true in the case of community health care provision with an increasing emphasis toward science and technologically based medicine. Until recently in Great Britain, this focused professional status heavily on those in the hospital—especially with the introduction of specialisation and reductionism—at the expense of the generalist practitioners.

Davies[29] and Witz[30] both argued that professionalisation, and the determinant factors that decide what is and what is not a profession, has its basis in gender- and class-influenced value judgments, to which Shula Marks[31] added race and ethnicity where these are relevant. Accordingly, the development of professions such as medicine and law appears to involve establishing a "male" (hierarchical and elitist) value system of control of entry, training, practice, and ethical codes of conduct. This value system then becomes established as orthodox and the benefits are increased status and professional power for those within, generally establishing a knowledge base and technological aspect on which the understanding of practice is based as an alternative to that of the layperson, diminishing status and power for the "fringe" practitioners outside that profession. Gamarnikow referred to the structure and working relationships that evolved between the gender-divided health care professions of nursing and medicine as "inscribing patriarchy in a particularly pristine way."[32] Taking this theoretical stance, district nursing as a subgroup of the nursing profession is viewed here over a period of sixty years during which it underwent a number of fundamental changes in organisational structure directly affecting the way in which its professional role and status evolved. This is achieved not only by looking at the changes that took place within district nursing bringing about transformations from within, but by viewing them as a part of a larger group of health care professionals working within the community and focusing on the inter-and intraprofessional tensions and rivalries as they affected district nursing's professional image and standing.

For many years histories of nursing were written by nurses and were often biographical. In 1980 Davies[33] cited Abel-Smith's *A History of the Nursing Profession*[34] as a turning point, noting that his questions for the history of nursing remained untackled. Davies presented a challenge to nursing historians characterising nursing history up to that point as a history of elites and progression, producing histories that are "the ratification if not the glorification of the present."[35] She called for a move away from the linear narrative account toward a greater awareness of the mechanisms of social change. Godden et al. reiterated this point in the early 1990s in relation to the tradition of insider histories of nursing written by nurses themselves, which they claimed, result in "a lack of critical analysis, a lack of socio-political and economic contextualisation, and the location of nursing history outside social history."[36] In terms of historical writing, taking up Davies's challenge entails a theoretical perspective affecting the selection of sources and the questions posed of them. The influence of this challenge has impacted subsequent histories of nursing and shaped the new history of nursing. The tenets of this new history were conveniently listed by Godden et al. and include as legitimate historical questions the meanings of nurse and nursing, conflicts of interest in nursing, and the social structure of nursing situations using a wide range of sources including oral history.[37]

Nursing historiography is now developing in line with this new history (witness, for example, the content of the influential *Nursing History Review* or the *International History of Nursing Journal*[38]) and Sioban Nelson more recently claimed that the trend of social history has "flowed over into nursing" with progress begun in the 1980s meaning that the "traditional nursing narrative [has] almost collapsed under the weight of critique."[39] However, Christopher Maggs also reminded us that "the study of the past of nursing must have something to say to nursing itself."[40] In this work we have tried to remain aware of the need for nursing history to avoid blind introspection and to identify areas where it can contribute to an understanding of wider nursing and social issues.

In current professional nursing literature, the experience of being a district nurse in the present day finds expression in the many vignettes, case studies, and testimonies used to exemplify the practices and attitudes of district nurses.[41] However, the experience and attitudes of district nurses of the past remains underrepresented. This book offers a perspective on district nursing of the past concerned with its nature and the experience of practice as told by district nurses. In this sense there is continuity in the approach of this study and current explorations of nursing practise. Although the content of current literature is not of a historical nature, much of it resonates with testimony of those interviewed for this book.

SOURCES

The primary and secondary sources used throughout this research deliberately encompass a broad range.

Primary Literature

1998 saw the launch of the Queen's Institute's Archive catalogued by the Contemporary Medical Archives Centre of the Wellcome Institute for the History of Medicine, making records such as registers and correspondence of affiliated branches of the Institute easily accessible.[42] Although some of this material was available to earlier researchers, the acquisition and detailed cataloguing of such a wide range of material in one repository enabled a more comprehensive study than was possible previously. During our research, the files of the Scottish branch of the QNI were transferred to the RCN Archive in Edinburgh, where we had the opportunity to consult them as they were catalogued.

It might be suggested that this gives an elitist view through an overemphasis on Queen's Nurses at the expense of non-Queen's nurses, but we would argue that a considerable amount of the material in these files related to both groups, and any bias has been partially offset by looking at other, non-Queen's sources. In particular, the detailed listings of district nursing associations published in Burdett's Hospital Directories and Yearbooks[43] were found to contain valuable and previously unexplored material relating to the district nursing associations of England and Wales. These suggested that a combined quantitative and qualitative analysis might prove particularly illuminating (see methodology later). This had its own problems, not the least of which was the sheer size of the lists and subtle changes of information provided in entries from year to year, and conversely, the failure of some associations to update their records regularly. Although there is no alternative means of checking the accuracy of the data, taking the information from so many associations served to minimise the impact of these problems on the overall picture.

In addition, the three editions of the *Handbook for Queen's Nurses*[44] plus contemporary (non-QNI) textbooks of nursing throughout the sixty-year period provided a glimpse of the profession's view of itself and of the changing role and daily work of the Queen's district nurse. The journals of the Queen's Institute, *Queen's Nurses' Magazine* [QNM],[45] *District Nursing* [DN],[46] and the *Queen's Nursing Journal* [QNJ],[47] provided valuable insight into the developing profession's self-image; priorities; and political, economic, and social outlook, while revealing regional differences. Again, these books and journals were produced for, and largely written by Queen's Nurses, and to gain a more balanced overview, other journals were also studied in as much depth as time allowed, including *Midwife, Health Visitor and Community Nurse*,[48] and *Nursing Mirror* and *Midwives' Journal*,[49] together with material gleaned from a number of other nursing, medical, and public health journals. It is, nevertheless, significant that the Queen's Institute represents the main producer of professional texts relating to district nursing for most of the period covered by this study as this serves to underline its crucial position as the mouthpiece for, and main force behind, district nursing throughout most of the twentieth century. This was a particularly important role bearing in mind the otherwise non-institutional nature of district nursing, as seen in its struggle for professional recognition set alongside its hospital counterpart. This theme is developed in Chapter 9.

Secondary Literature

Previously published histories of district nursing[50] and unpublished theses[51] were invaluable in providing an informed background to this book, and the notes[52] Mary Stocks made in the preparation of her book were most helpful in pointing to areas that she felt deserved attention, but were beyond the remit laid down to her by the Queen's Institute; in particular, the changing relationship between district nurses and their supervising authorities (viz. the Lady Superintendents and the ladies of the lay district nursing association committees) are examined in Chapters 3 and 4. On the other hand, the histories written by Stocks[53] and Baly[54] were both subject to the confines of being commissioned institutional histories for the QNI and therefore somewhat neglectful of the district nurses who were not Queen's trained. Also, neither provides more than a very limited insight into the changes in daily work and evolving role of the nurse at the grassroots level, nor into the relationships between district nurses and their professional colleagues within the community. This is particularly so where the wartime experiences of district nurses are concerned, as most secondary accounts are limited to brief references of heroic acts by midwives during the blitz, with the main focus centring on the QNI's battles with the Ministry of Health in the negotiations leading to the introduction of the NHS.

The ground-breaking thesis in this field by Fox,[55] although providing a well-researched administrative institutional history of district nursing presented "as a case-study of voluntarism",[56] concentrates on changes in social policy for the period leading up to the NHS Act (1948) with particular attention given to the relationship between statutory and voluntary agencies, and with an emphasis on the rural rather than urban community setting. Her source for material for this was mostly the (centrally located) official records of the QNI and of the Ministry of Health. In her conclusion, she noted that "local studies are the most productive means of extending knowledge of district nursing as a service,"[57] but that as this had not been within her remit, she had not chosen to follow that course or make use of oral history. Consequently, her thesis does not give prominence to professionalisation nor does it attempt to define the district nurse's tasks or changing role.

There is a considerable wealth of literature on gender and professionalisation and on labour issues, which has provided extremely helpful secondary evidence. However, even where this is directed specifically at nursing as a developing profession, most studies have focused on the institutionalisation of nursing with the hospital setting rather than taking the community as focus. This is largely because this area is well resourced with data such as pay and conditions, numbers of nurses employed, training and qualifications, and duties expected of the nurses. It has been interesting to test some of the findings of these studies for their applicability to the district nursing profession, and similarly to elucidate comparisons where the key texts in these fields have been based on women in professions other than nursing, such as the teaching or medical professions and secretarial work, or in industries such as textiles manufacturing. It highlights the Cinderella status of nursing's historiography that, at least until very recently, very little has been written about nursing as part of the labour market, particularly in the interwar period.

THE STUDY

The study has applied a prosopographical and institutional interdisciplinary approach to the history of district nursing and to a wider view of the history of professions combining social, gender, and political history with a more contemporary view of community health care. This methodology has enabled a longitudinal as well as a cross-sectional comparative study of the selected regions within Scotland, England, and Wales. As well as consulting orthodox material, we have undertaken more than 100 oral histories of district nurses and other members of the community health team. These have been deposited with the RCN's Oral History Project Archives and in the National Sound Archives Life-Story Collection, in line with legal and ethical requirements.

The time scale of the study period has been selected to reflect the fact that a small number of interviewees were still working in the service when interviewed in 1999 and as such were inevitably influenced by current events, attitudes, and practices in district nursing. However, the focus remains on the historical perspective held by individuals and so to some extent a rigorous adherence to a defined time period is illogical, if not impossible. The nature of memory, experience, and retelling is such that the past and the present converge. Although certain twentieth-century events or innovations have been recalled as important and are given most attention here, their impact and relative significance will no doubt be subject to future reappraisal in the light of contemporary cultural experience and historical thinking.

The book is divided into two parts: The first takes a chronological view of district nursing's history, and the second is largely thematic. Chapters 1 to 4 provide the reader with the historical context for the development of district nursing in Britain. This places district nursing within a wider framework of feminist and social welfare reform movements and sets the scene for later discussion of its role in professionalisation and changing concepts of professional identity addressed in Chapter 7. While focusing on the professional development (or otherwise) of district nursing, we consider the gradual disappearance of the "private nurse" from domiciliary nursing and how this might relate to the loss of private general practice medicine over the same time period. It views the nurse's position in the early development of the welfare state, and the profession's hopes and fears raised by government legislation in this area, particularly perceptions of contested professional territory between the trained, semitrained, and untrained district nurse, the health visitor, and the GP. We outline the change in remit from one where the (trained) district nurse's primary duty was to provide nursing care for the "sick poor and working classes in their own homes without distinction of creed," to a much wider remit through associations supported by subscription and public as well as private contribution and encompassing the middle classes as recipients of nursing care on a provident basis. We challenge previously held views that the interwar period was static as far as district nursing was concerned, showing it to have been a period of transition. The introduction of the NHS in 1948 resulted in changes in pay, conditions of employment, and employing authority, which combined to alter the relationship between nurse and patient in a number of ways. It was also a period during which roles were extended and workloads dramatically increased. We look at district nurse training through a wartime and immediate post-war culture of austerity and deference. Finally we evaluate the effect of the NHS on district nursing in postwar Britain, including examples of the problems of transferring from private to state service. We consider changing organisational structures, including the impact of GP attachments and health centres, and also describe a period of decline in the QNI with loss of control over district nurse training.

The second part of the book draws on the themes and issues emerging from the historical context in Part I. Part II considers the influence of the urban–rural situation on the kind of work the district nurse did. It examines the changing role and relationship between the local associations and the nurses they employed. In particular, it asks how the associations influenced the nurses' lives, answering this by drawing from the testimony of individuals through oral histories and autobiography combined with evidence contained within official QNI reports. A number of case studies bring this to life, vividly demonstrating the extent to which the role and experience of district nurses diverged as a result of demographic and cultural influences.

Using oral history, we explore the role of technology in influencing the changes experienced in the day-to-day work of the district nurse such as the advent of Central Sterile Supplies Departments (CSSD), a vastly expanding array of drugs and dressings, and widespread developments in means of transport and communication. We show the impact of changing nursing routines, technologies, and treatments through the testimony of those working in the community to understand how the NHS facilitated much of this change. The professionalisation of district nursing within general nursing is compared with those of general practice medicine and other members of the community nursing team, in particular the health visitors, midwives, social workers, practice nurses, and specialist community nurses. With the male nurse as a minority figure entering a woman's world, we are able to take an unusual view of gender, providing an interesting comparison with a reverse gender-biased situation in contemporary medicine through most of the same period. Oral histories from male district nurses and female GPs contribute their unique support to understanding the dynamics involved.

District nurses who began working in the 1940s and 1950s cite a different ethos of "nursing care" as a significant mark of difference between their practice and that of today's district nurses. After World War II, the working conditions of district nurses began to alter, significantly affected by changes in medicine, technology, organisation, and social attitudes, and this continued throughout the subsequent decades. With these changes, the concept of care became problematic and a new separation of nursing work and private life prevailed. Concepts of care with reference to religious belief, gendered attitudes, and the contemporary language of care are examined. The penultimate chapter looks at cultural representations of district nursing, including the portrayal of the district nurse in TV, film, and literature in comparison with images projected through textbooks and recruitment films and leaflets. Professional image and identity are shown to have changed according to a complex combination of internal and external influences.

The concluding chapter underlines the three key original contributions of this work: First, it contextualises the evolution of district nursing within the wider framework of an emerging community-care team. In doing so it transfers feminist theories relating to professionalisation from the institutional to the domestic sphere. Second, it looks at the changing working routine, variations in caseloads, personal experiences, and the changing role of district nurses from grassroots level, drawing on oral history and biography as well as quantitative analysis of data. This enables the study to achieve a unique view of nursing history that encompasses the nurses and the evolving nursing processes at all levels. The third major contribution is in presenting previously unresearched material, in particular the experiences of district nurses during World War II, the introduction of male nurses to district nursing practice, the effects of technical developments on the daily workload of the district nurse, and the region- and area-specific aspects of district nursing practice. In addition it aims to show how the understanding of district nursing's history provides the vital perspective necessary to understand in context current trends and issues, such as management of the long-term chronic sick, the development of the community matron, changes in workload and job description, and policy initiatives that affect the relationship between district nurses and GPs and other members of the primary care team.

Part I

The History of District Nursing

1 Historical Trajectories: Background, c. 1850–1919

Florence Nightingale, writing to Henry Bonham Carter in 1867, referred to nursing reform and its future through hospital and community nursing: "We were perfectly right to begin as we have done to have our aim defined . . . the reform of hospital nursing was essential as a beginning . . . But I would never look upon the reform of hospital nurses as an end—rather only as a beginning."[1]

WIDE OPEN VISTAS

At the time Nightingale made this observation, district and hospital nursing were each in their infancy as parts of an extremely diverse, rapidly developing profession. The last twenty years of the nineteenth century and first two decades of the twentieth century saw enormous strides in the development of nursing from a training and organisational viewpoint. Nevertheless, district nursing remained a service funded—and largely managed—by voluntarily run local associations, and staffed entirely by female nurses.[2] Hospital nursing developed skills directly linked to surgical and laboratory-based medicine and became the focus of professional nurse training. District nursing retained a more vocational image associated with the domestic environment, generalist bedside medicine, and a more altruistic raison d'etre. This chapter concentrates on the development of district nursing up to 1919, marked by the end of World War I and the hard-won introduction of nurse registration.

Although Dickens's gin-swilling caricature of the district nurse[3] is powerfully evocative and not without some foundation in reality, it represented only one image of the state of mid-nineteenth-century district nursing. Written as a caricature, this image persisted for many years and contributed to the marginalisation of district nursing within the profession. The nineteenth-century district nurse had a much more heterogeneous background, derived from a range of health care providers (varying from Bible nurses to corpse washers) whose history can be traced to well before the nineteenth century.[4]

Until the late eighteenth century, outside London there was a general reluctance to provide institutional nursing care[5] and the lay nurse fulfilled a range of roles including a formal or informal carer as in attendant, a handywoman, corpse washer, or village nurse or parochial nurse;[6] a private nurse or a member of the household; a midwife[7] or monthly nurse; or a herbalist or village wise woman.[8] Tasks undertaken by these women also varied considerably, from applying dressings and poultices based on a range of folk remedies, administering herbal infusions, or applying leeches. Some nurses even practised blistering or bleeding, although the latter intruded on the sphere of the local surgeon or medical practitioner. A nurse working in the community could have carried out any one or a combination of these roles either as a self-employed (often casually employed) independent practitioner, as member of a husband-and-wife team, or under contract to the voluntary hospitals and poor law relief committee. This wide range of duties has been described collectively as the "techniques of pre-industrial nursing."[9]

During this time, religious orders such as Elizabeth Fry's Protestant Sisters of Charity,[10] St. John's House,[11] or the Bible and Domestic Mission known as the Ranyard Sisterhood, supplied trainee and trained nurses to the provincial hospitals. On their return from these institutions to the community, these nurses provided nursing care to the sick poor in their own homes following the pattern established by French and German religious nursing organisations.[12]

In their communities these nurses came under supervision of the Lady Superintendent, in many cases earning their keep by caring for private patients, as was also the case in later secular schemes. For many years the Ranyard Bible Nursing Association was the largest district nursing association (DNA) in London, with 47 district nurses working in 1875 compared with most other associations whose numbers remained in single figures.[13] Ranyard Nurses continued to provide district nurses working in London into the second half of the twentieth century.[14] District nursing was also provided by the Church Army from 1887, and by the Nursing Sisters of the Poor, a nursing branch of the Little Sisters of the Assumption, but despite numbers of nurses being considerable, they were largely untrained. Although a few had midwifery certificates, most had received minimal, if any, hospital training.[15] Nevertheless, their duties, which might now be understood much more as a mix of health guidance, patient advocacy, and counselling, rather than nursing, brought a degree of expertise to the otherwise informal system of self-help that operated in poor communities. By merging the spiritual concerns of the order with the secular nature of medicine, social, and sanitary reform, they contributed to a more modern concept of nursing.[16,17] These nurses came under supervision of the Lady Superintendent, in many cases earning their keep by caring for private patients, as was also the case in later secular schemes. It is significant that the nurse-superintendent system represented a two-tiered, class-based, hierarchical system[18] that marked an important change from the independent but largely unqualified practitioner loosely described earlier as a nurse.

Ongoing changes in the Victorian economy, both in costs and standards of living, together with "a continued inability by the [medical] profession to restrict its own numbers," meant that the cost of medical treatment was prohibitive for most of the population.[19] At this time Britain operated an elementary welfare system that was enshrined in a succession of Poor Law Acts. Under this system, sick poor along with the destitute, known as paupers, were taken into their local parish workhouse where institutional support was provided. Crowther detailed the complexities of and variations in Poor Law provision during the mid-nineteenth century. Under this system, pauper nurses were often recruited from within the workhouse to care for the sick in the workhouse infirmary, as well as outside under the outdoor relief system.[20] In 1866 an official enquiry into nursing care provision in workhouses resulted in the Public Infirmaries Act and 1867 Metropolitan Poor Act.

Abel Smith described the workhouses at this time as "dumps" for the patients the voluntary hospitals had failed to cure or with types of illness they would not accept, and stated that "out of a total of 157,740 indoor paupers in 1869 about a third were sick";[21] that is, more than 50,000 patients compared with less than 20,000 in general and special hospitals recorded in the 1871 census figures. The result was a wide range of standards and duties carried out often just for token cash payments or special privileges such as improved rations and different dress, by nurses with minimal or no training under an equally variable range of supervision and management. They were frequently illiterate and often old and infirm, so there was little to distinguish them from their fellow pauper patients. These working-class nurses were generally hired by the Board of Guardians and supervised by a lady inspector.[22] Ten years later, the Poor Law Act (1879) provided for grants from boards of guardians "for the nursing of those in receipt of outdoor relief"[23] marked by the founding of the Workhouse Nurses' Association, which began the training of nurses for care of the sick poor in the same year.[24] This legislation clearly reflected some degree of public recognition of widespread developments in the organisation of nursing as a whole and more especially of district nursing in a number of urban areas.

At the other end of the spectrum where surgical intervention was inappropriate or where the application of principles of hygiene and sanitation were paramount, the trained nurse was arguably of greater significance to outcome and disease prevention than the doctor. During the 1849 cholera outbreak, one physician observed that "the nurse was then of more use to the patient than the doctor."[25] Although it is more likely that these trained nurses would have worked as private nurses, Ackland referred to the importance of nurses hired by the Oxford Guardians to care for the sick during the 1854 cholera epidemic.[26] Stocks recognised the valuable role played by trained and emergency-trained district nurses and the Lady Superintendents in the Liverpool epidemics of cholera in 1866 and relapsing fever in 1870 as forging a "closer link between the town's health authorities and the district nursing organisation" and particularly with the Liverpool Dispensary's doctors.[27]

TRAINED NURSES FOR NURSING THE SICK POOR IN THEIR OWN HOMES

It was the experience of care provided by a trained private nurse, Mrs. Mary Robinson, in the home of William Rathbone after his wife died of consumption in 1859, that provided the inspiration for his philanthropic establishment of district nurse training and provision for the sick poor of Liverpool. In 1862 Rathbone, a Quaker and wealthy ship-builder, established a training school and home for nurses attached to the Liverpool Royal Infirmary, and founded the Liverpool Queen Victoria District Nursing Association. These provided trained nurses for the infirmary, some private nurses, and district nurses for the poor who were supervised by a Lady Superintendent. At first the superintendent was a voluntary member of a "committee of ladies" who ran the DNA. With the exception of Liverpool, this situation changed by the end of the nineteenth century, by which time the Lady Superintendent was employed by the association and was, herself, a trained nurse.[28] In 1864, within two years of the Liverpool experiment, a similar association was set up in Manchester and Salford as the Sick Poor and Private Nursing Institute, with the Royal Derby and Derbyshire Nursing and Sanitary Association coming into being in 1865 and the Leicester District Nursing Association the following year. Similar associations followed in York and Birmingham in 1870 and Glasgow in 1875. By 1879 Liverpool had established a second association, the Woolton and District Nursing Society. The different titles suggest that a subtly different emphasis in roles existed between these early DNAs, with some including private nursing to boost the income of the association and others inclined more toward sanitary reform.

Dingwall et al.[29] suggested that the Manchester and Salford Ladies' Sanitary Association represents the direct development of the early role of district nurse and mission woman into the first health visitors (HVs). This is an oversimplification, as the two disciplines (health visiting and district nursing) remained quite independent of one another although they worked closely and were influenced by each other's working methods. The Ladies' Branch of the Manchester and Salford Sanitary Association, established in 1852, had more in common with the Ranyard Nursing Association, having a strong religious objective and using the same concept of the missing link between the ladies of the association and the working-class poor. These provided a role model and "mother's friend," and employed working-class mission women living within their working districts supervised by lady volunteers but with the mission women as sanitary visitors rather than trained bible nurses.[30] It must be acknowledged here that district nursing as a key part of a developing community health service is subject to the same critique as HVs so often characterised as public agents of moral and social reform. Like the HVs they were used to targeting the working-class mother and child to create and mould a particular type of family, thereby imposing middle-class Victorian values of health, hygiene and morality on the lower classes.[31] This was later extended to include control of the middle classes by gradually widening their area of responsibility along with other public health workers.[32]

Fundamental differences existed in the conception of district nursing organisations, for example, between the associations set up in the north of England based on the Rathbone concept of district nursing and some of those in London founded on Nightingale's principles. Rathbone's concept was based on provision of charity and philanthropy, often with religious overtones, and can be contrasted with Nightingale's emphasis on self-help and reform through education and example. There are marked similarities in this conceptual dichotomy with those discussed by Davies[33] on the battle confronted by the proponents of the Women Sanitary Inspectors' Association, and this is dealt with in more detail when considering the later development of professionalisation. Despite this issue proving divisive in the longer term, Rathbone and Nightingale agreed on the basic idea of employing hospital-trained nurses to care for the sick poor in their own homes, which became a key concept in district nursing organisation during the bid for the Women's Jubilee Offering for Queen Victoria's Golden Jubilee. With a few exceptions, from the end of the nineteenth century it was gradually accepted that, instead of the work being perceived as entirely benevolent, and any grants from public bodies or employers seen as acts of charity, the procurement of such nursing services should be paid for with due consideration for the patient's means. At the same time public authorities, such as boards of guardians and municipal and urban councils, were encouraged to take responsibility for the cost of nursing those under their jurisdiction.[34]

Apart from the religious societies mentioned earlier, there is some contention over the claim for the first district nursing organisation in London. The London Metropolitan and National Nursing Association was founded to a certain extent on the Liverpool model. It was supported by both Rathbone and Nightingale in line with the essential principles of providing hospital-trained and well-educated nurses to work in the district who regarded their nursing work as a profession "rather than as a *craft*."[35] This was established in 1874 with Miss Lees (who later became Mrs. Dacre Craven[36]) as its first superintendent. A report from 1864 entitled "The Organisation of Nursing in Liverpool" stated that "King's College Hospital has a large number of outpatients, and encouraged by the success of the missionary nursing, [. . .] the Lady Superintendent has established a system of out-nursing for the outpatients reported as requiring it by the medical men."[37] Similarly, the East London Nursing Society was founded in 1868,[38] employing district nurses trained at the London Hospital. However, Stocks described the confrontation between Florence Lees and the East London Society, noting that "the East London Nurses seemed to her 'nothing more than district visitors or mission women.'"[39]

Nevertheless, it can be seen that by the 1870s there was a perceived need for an increase in skill, competence and status of the district nurse. This was to be achieved through better training and qualification, even though there was some difference of opinion as to the level of training and class of woman needed. Taking the Nightingale stance, this also implied a need for organisation and regulation as well as an improved professional image and public status. By this time district nursing had made great progress toward professionalisation. Nursing leaders and the media were describing it in terms of holding a professional status that was readily adopted. A press comment on the founding of the National Association for the Sick Poor that failed to appreciate this fundamental concept stated, "It will open a new profession to the large and ever increasing number of women who require an employment of more interest than that of domestic servants, but who are not sufficiently well educated to become governesses."[40]

This was certainly not the intention of the founders of the Association, whose declared intention was actually to raise nursing standards and the social position of nurses. Lees recognised the need for a more comprehensive education and training to "make it a profession fit for women of cultivation."[41] To achieve this end, the training received by her nurses was designed to include an extremely tough one-month probationary trial period, followed by one year of hospital training, and finally three months of specialised district training. The latter combined practical training in the district with lectures in anatomy, physiology, and hygiene, sometimes including attendance at postmortems.

This opens up a second major area of debate: that of class. Reflecting serious tensions that would continue in nursing as a whole for many years, nursing leaders disagreed over the fundamental concept of whether nurses should be recruited from the same social class as the patients she was to nurse or whether sights should be raised to aim for the emerging professional class of women. This class tension underpinned the argument between the QNI in London and the Rathbone training association in Liverpool, but also between the different associations operating within London. This was to erupt in 1907 when the QNI was establishing the examination format to introduce tighter regulation and uniformity of training standards, but there is little doubt that it presented some degree of resentment before then.[42] Throughout the first half of the twentieth century the conceptual division remained unresolved. District nursing, like nursing in general at this time, retained a very diverse range of trained, semitrained and untrained nurses across the class spectrum. This ranged from Queen's Nurses, some holding multiple qualifications, through to Registered Nurses and village nurse-midwives, and finally to the unqualified village handiwomen.

It is significant that at this time a trickle of women were beginning to enter the medical profession, signifying a wider movement both toward reform in the education of women and women aspiring to work in the health professions. The following observation contrasted the poor remuneration of educated, trained nurses being employed in the homes of the wealthy as well as the poor compared with professional rates being charged by this minority group of female doctors:

> There is no reason why the rich should not obtain for money services which are freely bestowed upon the poor. Ladies will now take fees as doctors, but they will nurse only for charity . . . Invalids of the upper classes would soon feel the advantage of being tended by a lady of refinement and scientific training, and would be willing to remunerate her services at such a rate as would in time repay the expenses of her preparatory study . . .[43]

Similar views were expressed from The Metropolitan and National Nursing Association, the forerunner of the QNI. Notes from minutes recorded in 1875 relating to the perceived role of the district nurse state that, "Although it is intended that the Society's nurses should be mainly employed for the sick poor, the power should be reserved of sending those who have shown themselves to be specially meritorious (under certain restrictions) to the sick in the upper ranks of society."[44] In addition it was recommended that the nurses should be recruited not from the workhouses, but from the educated classes. Florence Nightingale is quoted in this same article as being in support of this ideal.

However, in a letter from Miss Nightingale to *The Times*, referring to the founding of the Metropolitan Nursing Association, Bloomsbury Square, this does not appear so clear-cut. Here she upholds the notion of the professionally trained nurse operating within a system aimed at providing for the poor. She did not see this as a charitable service per se, but one that would encourage responsibility among its users and ultimately the development of a system of financial contribution. Although directed at the sick poor, Nightingale's vision included the middle classes as contributing patients to finance an equitable service that would both provide and value skilled nursing to all in need.[45]

An alternative scenario might effectively have combined the ideals and organisation of district nursing with the more lucrative and potentially influential, private nursing. Such a hybridisation at that stage in nursing's professional evolution would be interesting to consider as counterfactual history. The most likely outcome would have been a two-tiered system of general practice nursing mirroring general practice medicine with far greater influence over health care policy and nurse registration rather than the fragmented forms that lingered into the twentieth century. Maggs's study of the first generation of hospital trained general nurses in England[46] (1881–1914), lends support to this thesis. He referred to the elite status and "supremacy of the General [trained] Nurse" as a form of "occupational imperialism"[47] and although this was particularly so within the new general hospitals, it was also the case in private practice nursing, where he suggested they presented a very real threat to the livelihoods of some general medical practitioners already fearing competition from midwives. To a lesser extent, district nurses presented the same threat. How much greater might this have been if the private and district nurses had been amalgamated under the QNI as their professional body?

Amy Hughes recognised the uniquely professional position of Queen's Nurses. Stating the case for the pro-registrationists as early as 1904, she wrote:

> Queen's Nurses should not forget they are the one body of nurses whose system of work includes a "register" the Roll of Queen's Nurses, in which their names, training and reports are entered, and from which they are liable to be removed if they forfeit the privilege of remaining Queen's Nurses. They are therefore specially able to weigh this question fairly, and to realise what such a register would mean to their fellow nurses, especially those who are working as private nurses, either in connection with institutions, or on their own account.[48]

THE FOUNDING OF THE QUEEN'S INSTITUTE: A PROFESSIONAL RATIONALE?

In 1874 the newly formed National Association for Providing Trained Nurses for the Sick Poor set up a Sub-Committee of Reference and Inquiry, to be chaired by Rathbone, and with Lees as Hon. Secretary. Lees travelled extensively around the United Kingdom to visit existing DNAs, and this was supplemented by a national questionnaire to all dioceses to establish where there were district nurses or whether one was felt to be needed. The Inquiry's Report was published in 1875 and reinforced the committee's belief in the need for an organised and regulated National Institution. The Queen Victoria Jubilee Institute for Nurses (later known as the QNI) was set up over the following decade with the London Metropolitan and National Association as its flagship, supported by the Queen's Jubilee Fund. Almost inevitably, a prominent ambassadorial role was played in the negotiations by a number of eminent men, particularly Sir Henry Ponsonby, the Duke of Westminster and Rathbone. It is also important to remember the parts taken in this by a number of eminent women, most notably Queen Victoria herself. Nightingale and Dacre Craven exerted considerable influence in an advisory capacity and Dr. Mary Scharlieb, herself a pioneer woman doctor, was appointed as one of the first lecturers to the trainee Queen's Nurses. The

QNI was granted a Royal Charter in 1889[49] and in 1890 Rosalind Paget, niece to Rathbone, was appointed as the first Inspector General. Further financial support was received at the Queen's Diamond Jubilee in 1897 and following her death in 1901 there was a sharp increase in numbers of DNAs established in the Jubilee year. In response, many of the local nursing associations[50] already in existence throughout the country became affiliated with the Institute, with Scotland having its own separate branch and council.

The Rural Nursing Association, which was founded in Gloucestershire in 1889 by Mrs. Elizabeth Malleson, established county nursing associations, with Hampshire founded in 1891 and Lincolnshire in 1894. Malleson was a "determined, radical and combative suffragist" and is quoted as saying "The work is more fitted to some of the excellent women I have known as nurses than to ladies."[51] A letter written in 1909 by a newly appointed County Superintendent of Somerset's County Nursing Association described cycling sixteen miles through heavy rain and mud to get to an inspection (carrying all her luggage for the week on her cycle), pacifying a discontented nurse and secretary, and finding an emergency replacement for a nurse who had been found drunk. She referred to the shortage of nurses saying, "We have to confer about 'Gamps' for country districts. This is C.C. [County Council of the QNI] work. Miss E. wrote to the C.C. asking where Gamps could be got and suggesting a scheme, and I have been asked by the C.C. to talk things over and draw up a scheme."[52]

By the end of the nineteenth century there were more than 900 trained QNs on the Institute's Roll. The stipulated training had been modified to include one year of hospital training, three months of midwifery, and three to six months of training in district work. The idea also spread throughout the Empire. The Canadian Victorian Order of Nurses was founded in

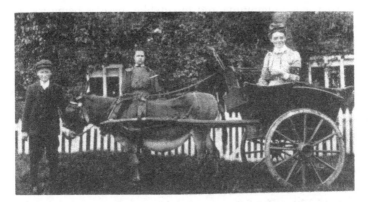

Figure 1.1 Nurse Wolfe of Gotherington, Somerset: A rural district nurse in the donkey-cart that she used to cover her district. From G. Ellice, "A Century of District Nursing," *The Countryman* 94:2 (Summer, 1989): 132. The authors and publishers of *The Countryman* made every effort to contact the holder of reproduction rights for this image but unfortunately without success.

1897, a Bush Nursing Service was inaugurated in Australia in 1910, and the King Edward VII District Nursing Service was founded in South Africa in 1912.[53]

By 1892 the Local Government Board had authorised the appointment of district nurses by all boards of guardians stipulating a minimum of one year of training, a good "moral character" and conditions of appointment similar to infirmary nurses.[54] This barred them from midwifery and placed them under the direction of the doctors who were to be instructed about the nurse's duties by the guardians. The (more expensive) alternative was to use nurses supplied by nursing associations or the QNI. In addition, particularly in more rural areas, cottage or village untrained nurses or handiwomen were employed by voluntary agencies as domiciliary nurses within the community, sometimes working under the supervision of trained nurses. The Royal Commission on the Poor Laws set up in 1905 noted in two separate reports published in 1909 that there was an inadequacy in the provision of nursing for the outdoor sick, particularly in remote rural areas, and set this as a high priority.[55] In particular, the report encouraged local boards of guardians to subscribe to DNAs where nursing care was provided to patients receiving poor relief in their own homes.

PUBLIC AND PROFESSIONAL PERCEPTION OF ROLES: A NEED FOR CLARIFICATION

What, then, was the relationship between general practice medicine and district nursing at the end of the nineteenth century and the beginning of the twentieth century? In 1874 Maria Grey, a nineteenth-century feminist and educationalist wrote, "Ladies who desire to study and practise medicine are told that it is unfeminine and unladylike, besides being too laborious for their sex, and are urged instead to become nurses . . . it is revolting to every feeling of womanly delicacy, for a woman to be a physician, but most feminine to be a nurse."[56]

The more advanced state of professionalisation within medicine (medical registration became mandatory from 1858 as part of the Medical Act[57]) gave doctors a dominant and paternalistic position. In hospital and in the community, they held authority over nurses and patients regarding patient management in areas such as admissions and discharges, expenditure, treatment, and even some nursing care decisions required medical orders such as bathing a patient.[58] This inevitably placed nursing, including district nursing, in a subordinate position to medicine at this time despite the QNI's royal charter and patronage.

Although appreciated by some doctors,[59] the emergence of the better qualified and professionally supported Queen's Nurses must have presented the less financially secure general medical practitioners, and especially those struggling to maintain a medical living in the poorer rural and urban areas,[60] with a perceived threat to their livelihood. This was especially so in the decade before the introduction of the National Health Insurance Act (NHI) in 1911 when GPs were feeling particularly insecure.[61] To some extent this might also be ascribed to a need for clarification of the functionally distinct roles. For example, a GP in 1899 expressed the concern that "to all intents and purposes [a nurse was becoming] a medical practitioner,"[62] and other doctors were anxious that the new, professionalised nurse might undertake medical tasks, causing the GPs to lose out on fees to the nurse, or that the nurse might undermine the GPs' authority or influence patients in their choice of doctor. Whether this was a momentary misunderstanding or more likely, a simmering mixture of resentment and aggravation held in check by a policy of conciliation recommended by the QNI, is unclear. This tension came to a head when the local medical associations a few years later fiercely defended the doctors' position. This was provoked by a case in 1908 in which a problem arose between Penwith Medical Union, Cornwall and the local DNA in which nurses were accused of attending patients without referring them to a medical practitioner.[63] It was felt that, "It was reversing the natural order of things that the nurse should send for the doctor; it should always be the other way around." Doctors even threatened to withhold their services altogether or not to attend if sent for by a nurse. The British Medical Association (BMA) took this up with the QNI, proposing a joint conference or conciliation board to discuss drawing up draft rules governing the work of district nurse-midwives in local DNAs. Among their suggestions were: the representation of medical profession on all local DNAs; confirmation of the position of district nurses working as auxiliaries to, and acting under instructions from, medical practitioners; clarification of the situation where district nurse-midwives act as a midwife without a doctor in attendance or attend private persons who could pay fees; and clarification of the situation where district nurses might leave the employment of the DNA and set up in private practice within the area in competition with the GP.

Replying to this and other suggestions a QNI committee member, himself a medical man, Dr. Arthur Shadwell commented that:

> to set up a formal or semi-formal tribunal (even if there were the power to do it) and accord the [BMA] Association a locus standing for intervention would be more likely to encourage than allay friction [. . .] it is no part of the Institute's functions to help bring it about. It should not be forgotten that the two bodies are not on the same plane in this matter. The sole object of the Institute is the welfare of the sick poor, whereas the aggrieved doctors are fighting for their own hand.[64]

At this time Cornwall had a well-established County Nursing Association. In 1910 it comprised sixty-three districts employing a total of seventy nurses, all but five of whom were certificated midwives and sixteen of whom were Queen's trained.[65] In the year 1909–1910 they nursed a total of 6,905 patients, and it is most likely that the midwifery cases were really at the centre of this controversy.[66] It is also significant that the Hon. Secretary of the Truro DNA was Miss Lillie Paul, who sat on a number of local committees, was a Poor Law Guardian, and was a prominent supporter of women's suffrage.[67]

It is significant that this and other examples of interprofessional rivalries took place just before the 1911 NHI Act, other instances arising later in the 1930s. Although the 1911 NHI Act made considerable changes to provision of medical care, and was supported in principle by the QNI, comparatively few of the district nurse's patients fell directly under its provision. Several contemporary written cameos of work in the district give an impression of the type of work performed and the range of patients visited. Although there is little doubt that they were modified or tempered to some degree for publication, they nevertheless provide valuable insight into work in the district at the time. In the first, the image of the Lady Superintendent as supervisor but physically remote from the actual duties of the more lowly district nurse, can be seen to be (at least in some cases) quite unjust. Hallowed cites one of Mrs. Dacre Craven's quarterly reports written while working as a superintendent in London in which:

> a vivid description is given of her tackling, along with the district nurse, an old woman who had not been washed for ten years and a room which had apparently not been turned out within the memory of man. Superintendent and nurse, after beating a retreat to the passage to overcome their nausea, dealt faithfully with this situation and did not leave until both room and patient had been, in Miss Lees' favourite phrase, "put in nursing order."[68]

Similarly, one patient's tribute, selected because it was "rather quaint," is quoted: "I didn't know there was nurses as got their living by it and weren't just missioners, or I'd have had some of you before and been thankful."[69] Another article written in 1922 quotes Miss Lees speaking at Committee in 1876 about elderly bedridden patients and describing the nursing care given:

> The nurse daily washes them and combs their hair (once a week baths them as far as a patient can be bathed in bed). She daily makes the bed, sweeps and dusts the room, shakes the bits of carpet, empties and washes the utensils, cleans up the hearth, sifts the cinders, and carries away the ashes. Such cases we term "cleaning cases," and according to the number of stairs the nurse has to run up and down for these purposes, so is the case a very heavy "cleaning" case or not. It must be remembered that the poor possess very few of the proper utensils for fetching and carrying. We have had to make several journeys to fill a heavy kettle, the only thing to fetch water in being a small tin can. Ashes and dust we often have to carry down in a newspaper, sometimes we

are obliged to borrow a brush for the floor, a broom with a long handle being unheard of. After we have borrowed this brush from a neighbour she will call when we have gone and see how them young persons have cleaned up.[70]

Likewise, an editorial written in 1924, looking back at the (anonymous) author's work as a district nurse in London in the late 1890s and first decade of the twentieth century, describes general "improvements in the surroundings and personal condition of the patients attended," stating that in 1897, "poverty and disease were rampant," and homes visited were "very scantily furnished" with virtually no household appliances and often "no towels, soap or basin for toilet use, and hot water hard to get [. . .] The difficulty of getting from case to case was great, the only vehicle available being a horse-bus or tram, and these were few and far between" so entailed a great deal of walking every day.[71] The author remembered that "with the coming of the universal use of gas cookers the work became much easier as regards hot water and sterilisation etc." and that the formation of Infant Welfare Centres (between 1903 and 1905) had been "the saving of many," as had been the Minor Ailment Treatment Centres for School Children, and finally claimed that notification of tuberculosis opened up "a wide field of work for nurses, more especially district nurses."

Martha Loane's *The Queen's Poor*[72] is claimed to have been largely based on the author's own firsthand experience of what she termed "the decent poor" as a district nurse and later a superintendent of district nurses, having worked in London, Buxton Derbyshire, and Portsmouth Hants. There is considerable anecdotal material,[73] much of which is presented as if it were oral evidence, but that has to be treated with considerable caution. Nevertheless, Cohen and Fleay defended this, noting Loane's (re)assurance that "every anecdote including the apocryphal ones to which she referred was genuine."[74] There is certainly much valuable sociohistorical testimony concerning health care, standards of living, and perceptions of health professionals and prevailing social attitudes. The role and professional and public images of a Queen's district nursing superintendent and district nurse are vividly revealed, and Loane's firsthand experience is evident in detailed descriptions of the considerable pressures, demands, and difficulties of working under the constraints of employment by a DNA committee in both urban and rural areas of extreme poverty. She exposed occasional abuses of the district nursing system aimed at providing nursing care specifically for the sick poor in their own homes and drew attention to serious failings of the Poor Law, revealing inadequacies and injustices in both institutional and outdoor relief. At the same time she strongly supported the ideas of the Eugenics movement,[75] believing many social problems were the result of uncontrolled population increase.

The description of a typical day in this early period takes district nurse and supervisor to a number of routine visits and emergency calls, from false alarms and the first-aid treatment of tending to a patient's injured thumb, to the trauma of a child's death, a terminally ill young man, and a victim of domestic violence. A case of pneumonia is described as "one of the few instances when a nurse can do anything more than alleviate pain," and when the nurse is asked if she has many male patients she replies, "Not nearly so many as women. In the first place, they have better health; and in the second place, when they are ill they are generally fit cases for a hospital, and no one would wish to nurse a man in his own house if there were any satisfactory alternative."[76] After the 1911 NHI Act and before the all-encompassing cradle-to-grave NHS Act of 1948, the disparity between those with access to medical and hospital treatment through the panel system (predominantly men) and those outside that safety net (predominantly women, children, and the elderly) accounts for this differentiation in the reliance on district nursing by the latter group. In addition, this was a period of high maternal and infant mortality and morbidity, and midwifery became an important aspect particularly of the rural district nurse's practice throughout the first half of the twentieth century.

CONDITIONS OF SERVICE UNDER WHICH THE DISTRICT NURSES WORKED

There were 2,100 Queen's Nurses in 1914 although the number had fallen to 1,989 by 1918 (largely as a result of nurses' contributions to wartime needs overseas and in military and civilian hospitals).[77,78] Mary Stocks's notes created in researching *A Hundred Years of District Nursing*[79] include an extract from the existing rules of Durham's DNA at the time of affiliation with the QNI in 1913. They paint a picture of considerable regimentation and hierarchical control, stating that "Nurses may not be out in the evenings without permission from the superintendent." Stocks suggested that "this condition for nurses was general all over the country," and that "at a later date latchkeys were provided for nurses."[80] In reality, these restrictions can only have applied to the urban district nurses living in nurses' homes, whereas the rural nurse would have had rather more personal freedom, living in rooms or a cottage.

Rates of pay and emoluments offered by DNAs varied very considerably throughout Britain, ranging from £10 to £90 per annum, but averaging around £38 with the upper wage limit being reached usually after three years of full-time employment and being an approximately £5 to £10 increase on the total annual income. The lower figure at first seems highly suspect, as the figures given in 1890 by the QNI[81] for the salary of a trained district nurse give a range between £25 and £50 per annum, although this might refer to a basic rate payment to a village nurse possibly supplemented through payments for additional nursing or midwifery services or private nursing. Lincolnshire Nursing Association conveniently provided a breakdown of their salaries, with Queen's Nurses being paid £90 to £100 per annum, nurses "with some hospital and district training" paid at £60 to £75, and "rural maternity nurses" at £50 to £65, indicating a considerable differential between the elite Queen's Nurse and the village nurse-midwife. Emoluments generally included board, lodging, and laundry and occasionally covered a uniform allowance that was between £4 and £10 annually. Uniforms had not been standardized, although the QNI was nearest to introducing this through recommending a style of dress to affiliated associations and providing a badge and brassard to be worn by all Queen's Nurses.[82] Also by this time, some associations were making a contribution toward the nurses' pension schemes; in particular, the Royal National Pension Fund for Nurses (RNPFN). One association recorded provision of an annuity for long service (stipulating a minimum of ten years), and two others offered sickness pay (one of these gives the rate as full pay for twelve weeks). It is reasonable to assume that others might have done the same but have omitted these details from their entry. Although most indicated that they provided nursing care for the sick poor, it is significant that there was no obvious standard policy concerning private nursing. Some associations quite openly supplemented their income through midwifery and maternity nursing or private nursing. Peckham DNA, for example, recorded "poor attended free, also attend middle class cases of sickness and operations." The high proportion of associations operating in London shown in Figure 1.2 included several religious organizations and entries for these suggest something more akin to sick visiting than nursing; for example, "sent at invitation of clergy" or "the Sisters visit the sick in their own homes, in hospitals and infirmaries."[83]

London was also unusual from an early stage both in the existence of the Central Council for District Nursing in London formed in 1915 and in the extent of collaboration between district nursing and the educational and public health services of the London City Council and Metropolitan Boroughs and some city hospitals.[84] This might in part reflect the early tradition of two-way cooperation that was required in the establishment of district nurse training. A significant number of the London associations were under royal patronage, in particular, that of Princesses Christian and Louise. The Duke and the Duchess of Westminster supported the Westminster Nursing Committee and the Chelsea, Pimlico, and Belgravia Nursing Associations, respectively. Only London and Liverpool associations note school nursing as a part of the nurses' regular work, with the London City Council financing this service through clinics and treatment centres. The West Midlands region had a surprisingly high number of associations whilst the South Midlands and less surprisingly the eastern region of Norfolk, Suffolk, and Essex had very few, probably due to the very rural and sparsely populated nature of that particular region. The remainder had between eleven and thirteen associations (eight or nine percent of the total) each.

Workload can be measured by looking at the number of cases (or patients) nursed over a set period, by recording the number of visits made to patients

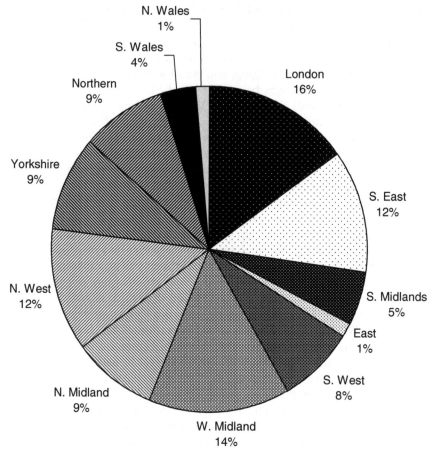

Figure 1.2 Distribution of district nursing associations 1915 (England and Wales).

over that time, or by both of these methods. For example, one case might only require one visit per week, whereas another might require twice-daily visits, but the first might take up more time or require greater nursing skills, so it is prudent to view both figures. Taking these figures for England and Wales as a whole, the average number of visits per nurse per year can be calculated as 3,356, each nurse attending an average of 160 cases per year. In reality this ranged from as few as 1,490 visits (or 138 cases) in rural Liskeard, Cornwall, to as many as 5,662 visits (or 183 cases) in the heavily populated city of Birmingham. In a few cases competence in maternity and fever nursing were specified as required skills, whereas others specified that duties would be "confined to district nursing." Subsequent chapters examine the changes that took place in the work and conditions of service under which the role of the district nurse evolved, and what effect these changes might have had on her role and professional image.

CONCLUSION

In this overview of the period leading up to 1919, we see that there were already several indicators of an existing professional self-image within district nursing that had been established to a large extent by the QNI and its founders. Through the rules of affiliation and through the hierarchy of its internal organisational structure, this legacy included a heavy emphasis on maintaining high standards of training, examination, a system of registration and self-regulation, pressure for standardization of pay, and the relative subordination of lay committees. Queen's trained nurses possessed a wide range of nursing skills and received a nationally standardized programme involving theoretical and practical training followed by written and practical examination, well in advance of other areas of nursing. Although there were many associations existing outside the QNI, several of which had been alienated by its elitist stance, it is clear that its influence was considerable and that it had set a standard, at a time when the rest of nursing was still struggling to achieve the goals of professionalisation. This is an issue that we return to in Part II. The relationship between the GP and the district nurse was an uneasy one throughout this period, with the latter being in some ways subservient to the former, yet representing a threat to the more vulnerable GPs, particularly before the NHI Act (1911). The development of this interprofessional relationship, the intraprofessional relationships between district nurses and their colleagues in the evolving field of community health care, as well as with their hospital counterparts, is therefore a central issue in the chapters that follow.

2 What Became of the Lady?
The Interwar Period, 1919–1939

Referring to the Nurses' Registration Act (1919), Dr. Addison, Minister of Health, emphasised in a speech to district nurses in London that it was:

> essential that "nurses should be adequately paid—the system which paid a nurse at the rate of a scullery maid was wrong" and he implored nurses to be "citizens first and nurses second," declaring as a professional man that, "the bane of professions was that their members were professionals first and citizens second."[1]

NURSES' REGISTRATION AND THE IMMEDIATE POSTWAR PERIOD

Having revealed the inadequacies in health care and welfare provision, World War I (1914–1918) accelerated governmental intervention in this area considerably. Under the direction of the newly formed Ministry of Health (1919), public health was emphatically promoted.[2] One aspect of this that had an important effect on district nursing was the Maternity and Child Welfare Act (1918), which shifted responsibility for the health of mothers and children from the Board of Education to local authorities and established a network of local clinics. As such, it was therefore also largely responsible for the promotion of health visiting, numbers of HVs having more than doubled during the war.[3] From 1919, the Ministry of Health also took over health responsibilities previously assigned to the Departments of Housing and Planning, thereby creating a larger and politically more powerful government department dealing with a broad range of local authority services including specialist areas such as tuberculosis and venereal disease treatment centres.[4]

The war also served as a catalyst for an increased awareness of the importance of professional status, and the need for unity among trained nurses.[5] Mrs. Fenwick, the leader of the Campaign for the Registration of Nurses since 1887, regarded the Nurses Registration Act (1919) as "comparable to the enfranchisement of women."[6] This comparison was not as overstated as it might now appear: nursing was a female occupation fighting for professional regulation in a male-dominated professional world. The power to sanction reform lay with the professions and a similarly male-dominated Parliament. However the two are more deeply correlated: The battle for enfranchisement that continued after the 1918 Representation of the People Act aimed to enfranchise those still disqualified from voting. Smith noted that these were typically young, educated, unmarried women, possibly those in a profession such as teaching that had a marriage bar, and would have meant they were working for insufficient pay to enable ownership of property.[7] The district nurse fitted this bill equally well: The changing attitude toward marriage in nursing as a whole has been described as "an unspoken prejudice against married women"[8] and this idea appears to be reinforced within district nursing. One of the most common reasons for the resignation of nurses noted in the QNI Registers was for marriage.[9] Rates of pay and conditions of service combined to make property ownership among district nurses very much the exception rather than the rule.

The wider intention of the campaign for suffrage was to "empower women to alter man-made institutions to reflect women's higher moral standards"[10] within society, rather than purely to attain equality with men. Public health issues such as hygiene, sanitation, improved housing, and health education were central to the overall ethos of the majority of the campaigners for women's suffrage and equal rights but also a considerable part of everyday district nursing. Although nurses have not traditionally been seen as active, effective feminists, as an organisation the College of Nursing (later to become the Royal College of Nursing [RCN]), formed in 1916, embraced the idea that women, and in this case nurses, could and should work toward social change. The RCN, on whose Council the QNI had a strong voice, regularly sent representatives to a range of women's associations and in doing so encouraged nurses to participate in active citizenship.[11]

Bearing this in mind, this chapter looks first at the development of district nursing from the organizational and institutional viewpoint and then at the inter- and intraprofessional difficulties encountered by these women. The title of district nurse might appear to have become clear-cut by 1919, but it was still applied to a wide range of skills and abilities. Variations in work experiences and practices as well as their terms and conditions of service, are the focus of the second half of the chapter.

ORGANISATIONAL AND INSTITUTIONAL
DEVELOPMENT OF DISTRICT NURSING

The Nurses' Registration Act of 1919 and subsequent formation of the General Nursing Council for England and Wales (GNC), imposed registration and regulation on the nursing profession as a whole, after many years of debate and division. There were three separate acts of Parliament enforcing nurse registration, one each for England and Wales, Scotland, and Ireland. From the outset, the unity that nurses had sought from legislation was obstructed through the formation of three separate councils, each with its own registers and educational standards. The process of registration enshrined in the Acts was phased in over several years, so that standards of training and practice continued to vary considerably throughout the country. State registration by examination qualification applied only to those completing their hospital training after the Act was introduced. In addition, the GNC failed to make the recommended training syllabus compulsory and made slow progress on setting an examination syllabus.[12] In effect, the term Registered Nurse encompassed a much more varied range of abilities than that of Queen's Nurse. Queen's Nurses had already established standardised entry qualifications and training throughout England, Wales, Scotland, and Ireland.

A further indication of the status of district nursing within nursing can be surmised from attitudes expressed through the College of Nursing. In line with government policy, the College of Nursing afforded community health care high priority at this time and appointed its own Public Health Advisory Committee in 1921. The College recognised recruitment to district nursing as being a matter of prime concern, and in its recommended scale of salaries of 1920 set £85 to £120 per annum for resident district nurses. Until that point there had been no standard rate, and although this was only a recommendation, it was seen as a step in the right direction and was promptly taken up by the QNI as a requirement for affiliated associations. At the annual conference of the Metropolitan and Southern Counties Association of Queen's Superintendents in 1922, a national standardisation of pay and conditions was suggested with a "salary immediately after training, [which] should start at £30 with uniform allowance of £8, in each county," and it was also recorded that a "minimum salary for village nurses immediately after their training is, as a general rule, £30, with uniform provided."[13]

The QNI was a well-established training institution that set high standards in district work. It was a requirement of all Queen's Nurses that they be trained general nurses and have completed one year attached to a QNI training home. Ironically, it was this insistence on professional quality that led the College of Nursing to turn its attention to another branch of community health care, that of health visiting. Many HVs had nursing experience, although this was not a requirement, and medical officers of health lent their support to the employment of nurses in this role, claiming that in such matters nursing knowledge was more relevant than medical knowledge and that their own professional skills as doctors would not be fully utilised in such work. However, HVs also lacked standardised training; a survey carried out in 1926 showed that 1,974 health visitors had between them twenty-two different kinds of certificates or varieties of experience, held in eighty-eight combinations, with some holding as many as five separate certificates.[14] Compared to district nursing, health visiting, as a nursing specialty, lacked professional direction and HVs were being canvassed by trade unions. In its efforts both to raise its own profile and to control nursing standards, the College of Nursing focused on health visiting to bring it into the sphere of professional nursing. In 1925 the College gained the required government approval to establish the first full-time health visiting course for nurses.

That the College of Nursing worked with the QNI rather than sought to absorb it in the way it did with health visiting is testament to the professional prowess of district nursing rather than its marginalisation. In terms of representation, a leading QNI figure always sat on the College of Nursing Council and the Council invariably supported the policies of the QNI and the expansion of district work. Although the QNI represented only Queen's Nurses, the College negotiated for improvements on behalf of all its members, including non-Queen's district nurses. The relationship between the QNI and the College of Nursing was one of professional cooperation. Only when the QNI ceased to provide training in 1969 did district nurses seek greater representation within the College of Nursing.

Despite the emphasis on health visiting in the 1920s, the 1922 White Paper outlined proposals for a National Health Service in which the only sector of nurses mentioned was the district nursing sector. It stated that "a full home nursing service must be one of the aims of the new organisation . . . all who need nursing attention in their own homes will be able to obtain it without charge."[15] This suggests a high point in the public image of organised district nursing, and more especially the recognition of its importance by the new Ministry of Health. A discussion also in 1922 concerning the introduction of a superannuated pension scheme noted that in England and Wales there were approximately 1,400 Queen's Nurses, a quarter of the total district nursing workforce.[16] A pamphlet produced by the Queen's Institute around 1925 noted that in England and Wales:

> there are over 5,800 nurses and midwives at work visiting over half-a-million patients annually and paying over 10,000,000 visits each year, but about 25% of the population of England and Wales live in an area where there are no District Nurses and for the other 75% the existing service is not yet adequate.[17]

By 1939 this situation had improved considerably, but in the 1920s some associations still experienced considerable difficulty in becoming affiliated to the QNI, not because of low standards or their inability to pay the salary demanded for a Queen's Nurse, but because they failed to comply with certain rules laid down by the Institute. In particular this included nonaffiliation to any religious organisation. Examples of this include the Ranyard Nurses and St. John's House, both of whom had been refused affiliation in 1891 on the grounds that they were sectarian organisations, whereas St. Helen's DNA in Lancashire was initially refused affiliation on the grounds that the religious element in the constitution was "too prominent," as was Stamford in Lincolnshire.[18] Despite this, there was some inconsistency among the inspectorate of the Institute; for example, another Lancashire DNA, Preston, was affiliated in 1925 despite the apparently damning, preliminary report that noted "a nurse has been supported for the last fifteen years by St. Silas Parish Church with that committee giving £100 p.a. to Preston District Nursing Association."[19] The report went on to request that the nurse be allowed to remain under the superintendence of the QNI "until she resigns of her own accord." It also recorded that the "Roman Catholic Church who number 40,000 [approximately one third of the town's population of 120,000 at that time] have 5 trained and 3 untrained nurses" and that "the doctors have been asking for some time for trained help—they are practically all in favour of the [Queen's Institute] scheme."

In England and Wales, all but East Anglia showed an increase in numbers of DNAs registered in hospital yearbooks[20] on a five-yearly basis from 1915 to 1931, with the biggest rise in relative terms being spread across the Midlands and South East of England, although it should be noted that in North and South Wales numbers of associations doubled. The largest increases in the sixteen-year period are reflected in 1931 coming after the Local Government Act (1929). A similar picture existed in Scotland where, by 1930, 465 associations had become affiliated with the Scottish Branch of the Institute.[21] Even in 1948, the year the service became the responsibility of local authorities, six Scottish associations still applied for affiliation, bringing the total number of DNAs affiliated at that time to 641.[22]

The percentage distribution of these DNAs reveals a decline in relative importance of London as the metropolitan focus of the organisation of the QNI (in England and Wales) and a move towards the formation of a number of regional strongholds. Of particular note in this decentralisation is the rapid expansion of the organisation throughout the West Midlands, and later still, a small but significant increase in numbers of associations in Wales and the South West of England. Effectively this reduced London from holding sixteen percent of the total number of associations in 1915, to just thirteen percent from 1925 onward and by 1931 the pattern of distribution appears much more evenly spread across England and Wales. The survey undertaken by the QNI and published in 1935 records the distribution of both QNI and non-QNI associations and of village nurse-midwives as well as Queen's Nurses, noting in its conclusion that in England ninety-six percent and in Wales eighty-seven percent of the country was already covered.[23] An editorial in the *Queen's Nurses' Magazine* (*QNM*) referred to the findings of this report, and in particular commented that in some large towns and cities the existing nursing service was inadequate to meet growing need. In rural and isolated areas the difficulty in service provision was connected more with geographical conditions.[24]

The difficulties encountered in rural areas were well illustrated by an example of a Dorset DNA in the immediate postwar period.[25] When the district nurse for the village of Alderholt died at the end of 1918 there was considerable concern expressed in the association's minutes about a serious lack of funds. The minimum amount the QNI Dorset County Association (with which Alderholt was affiliated) estimated as needed to employ a new nurse was £90, but the money raised from subscriptions only totalled £70. After a number of meetings and house-to-house visiting to raise new subscribers and donations, the required amount was raised, but the village remained without a nurse for a considerable length of time as a result. Fundraising was complicated by suggestions from the County Association that they should organize a "Nurse's Day" in the form of a garden fête to raise money for both local and county funds, and for "training nurses and increasing their salaries," but the response to the idea was not enthusiastic—the committee felt they would need all the money raised to support the local funds. Its future was only settled and a nurse employed when the association was amalgamated with two other villages. Although this provided a larger population from which to draw subscriptions, it also presented a wider geographical area for one nurse to cover.

As Poor Law institutions were transferred to local authorities in 1929, there was a promise that financial support would be more readily available. A marked increase in new DNAs and their affiliation agreements with the QNI suggests a response to this promise. This pattern was repeated with a second burst in 1936 following the Midwives Act. This required provision of midwives for the whole country and enabled DNAs to provide combined nursing and midwifery services, with financial support from local government.[26] The numbers of village nurse-midwives and other district nurses remained relatively unchanged, although there was a significant fall in the ratio of village district nurses to Queen's Nurses over this twenty-year period from almost 2:1 in 1920 to less than 1:1 after 1936.

INTER- AND INTRAPROFESSIONAL PROBLEMS

As the QNI developed its network of national organisation throughout the 1920s, it became increasingly concerned with the very recent epidemic of influenza[27] and other postwar public health concerns.[28] As far as Queen's Nurses were concerned, professional registration was not the new phenomenon it was for other nurses. Its main significance for them was that nurses coming for Queen's training should (theoretically) arrive with a more standardised level of training and level of competence; in practice this took rather longer to achieve. Nevertheless, concern was expressed in the pages of the *QNM* over the role of the district nurse within the new Ministry of Health, stating that, "on every side reform and reconstruction are in the air."[29] In particular these articles referred to the rising tide of bureaucracy encountered by district nurses and their patients and a confusing division of responsibilities among community health care providers. There were anticipated changes, therefore, in relationships with other health professionals working within the community. For example, an editorial as early as 1920 urged greater political awareness among district nurses, commenting that their "position . . . is by no means as secure as we would wish to see" and later referred to a perceived threat to their autonomy in organisation and administration: "It must not be possible for local inspection to be carried out over the work of fully trained nurses and midwives by Health Visitors, who themselves are neither one nor the other."[30] In some rural areas the district nurse was often midwife, HV, school nurse, and sometimes tubercular nurse as well. In the more remote areas of Scotland the triple-duty nurse remains in place at the time of writing.[31] A triple-duty nurse in rural Buckinghamshire in the 1930s commented, "It gave an excellent service to patients; the district nurse was known to everybody and understood every family. While washing grandpa she could do the health visiting. She wasted neither her own time nor the patients' who now have a multiplicity of callers."[32] However, the relationship with HVs remained an uneasy one (see Figure 2.1), becoming increasingly so in the postwar period, with their numbers more than doubling during the war period between 1914 and

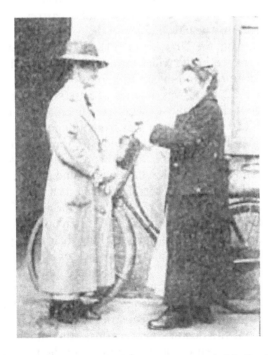

Figure 2.1 Cooperating in being: Health visitor meeting with district nurse. Photograph from "The Value of Co-operation" *QNM*, XVII:1(1920): 5–6. Reproduced by kind permission of the Queen's Nursing Institute. We are indebted to the Queen's Institute for granting copyright permission to publish this and all subsequent QNI-attributed images without charge.

1918.[33] At this stage the threat from this emerging profession was probably less well perceived than later, largely because contact between the two was minimal. Nevertheless, their expanding public health role into the field of maternal and child health and welfare was already threatening to infringe on that of the district nurse.

The district nurse's main professional contact was with the GPs, whose patients she nursed. This was by no means a regular contact in person, but more often an exchange of written notes or (increasingly from the 1930s) a telephone message. In Broughton (Vale of Glamorgan) a report of the presentation to Nurse Pritchard on her departure for midwifery training after six years in her post notes that over that time she had attended 1,500 cases, and had paid 18,900 visits and that she was "a willing, hard-working and painstaking nurse."[34] It then noted that the relationship between the two nurses working in that area and the GPs "with whom their nurses frequently came into contact" was a good one. How typical was this relationship?

Digby recognised 1920 as a "high point for the general practitioner" as a generalist before the growth of medical specialisation became a serious threat to general medical practice.[35] Compared with the generalist, the specialist was still perceived as having a rather narrow, less holistic, and impersonal approach. The introduction of the Panel system of medical practice that resulted from the NHI Act (1911), allayed GPs' earlier misgivings despite fears expressed in the wider medical field concerning the introduction of nurse registration and the creation of the GNC.

However, in 1932 there was a series of letters by doctors to the BMJ complaining about district nurses who were encroaching on their professional territory. The opening letter was from an anonymous Medical Officer of Health (MOH) working in an industrial area.[36] He described the local district nursing association as "long-established, flourishing" and "doing general and extensive midwifery work" and noted that his information was acquired through his HVs. This suggests a more positive contact between HV and district nurse. He described the local GPs as seriously underutilising the fully trained nursing staff, often not going, "beyond asking them to give an enema" and rarely seeking their help, yet "there being no professional hostility involved, nor any lack of appreciation of nursing services on the part of patients." Dr. Dill, from Galloway, replied the following week, commenting that this letter failed to appreciate the relative positions of doctor, nurse, and patient.[37] He pointed out that, although the doctor could recommend calling the district nurse, who would then, if she attended, carry out the doctor's instructions, "the onus of calling her, as also the meeting of expenses incurred, rests with the patient." This might be complicated by "the patient's omission to become a 'member' (annual subscriber) of the local association, and/or may even be found to be already in debt in respect of fees due to the association for previous nursing visits or confinements."

However, the correspondence then moved to concerns over competition and claims and counterclaims of malpractice that are very revealing. The first, from a Devonshire GP states:

> . . . the general practitioner has a hard job in these days to pay rents, rates and taxes, and school fees, if he can afford children. The District Nurse now takes most of his midwifery, does ante-natal and post-natal work, and, during these and other visits, is consulted on every ailment, which she diagnoses and treats. If she does not she is told they will not in future contribute their pence to the association. She is then up before her committee, who are themselves often her most exacting and troublesome patients: all use her to save a doctor's bill. She does minor surgery and sends patients to hospital for advice and treatment. . . . She has been known to diagnose and treat a pneumonia case. In other words, she is one of the general practitioner's most dangerous opponents, and therefore he treats her as such and prefers the old "Gamp," who is under his control. . . .[38]

Several GPs then wrote in defence of "their" nurses. One GP described the local district nurse as "valuable" in dealing "with minor ailments, and above all relieving me of routine midwifery" and "one of my staunchest allies."[39] Another declared that he was president of the two nursing associations in his area and that his district nurses "have always proved most willing and eager to do anything I have told them, and have shown themselves capable midwives. They save me many weary hours, and are always at hand to give an enema when required."[40]

In some areas district nurses clearly did not represent a threat to any doctor's medical living; for example, an interviewee brought up in a very poor area of London in the 1930s described her memories of a district nurse:

> If anybody got ill you didn't fetch a doctor—you didn't ask for a doctor to call, you went out to find Sister Brown who ran the Queen's District Nursing Home and she either came or she sent one of her nurses on a bicycle who would come. Now if they called the doctor—oh dear—you know—not much hope, but in the normal way she would come and say what she thought and what had got to be done and somebody was dispatched to the chemist for a bottle of what the chemist made up in various sort of forms.[41]

Clearly, these patients were too poor to afford a doctor's fee and the Queen's Nurse felt at liberty to diagnose, nurse, and treat them to the best of her ability, and to call for medical help only in the most difficult cases. This revealing correspondence also suggests that district nursing had in some ways reached a high point in professional autonomy. To the more vulnerable GPs they had become a threat through raised public perception combined with their range of skills, with midwifery being perceived as the biggest threat of all.

Some of the professional hostility from doctors can also be explained by the rather misleading term district nurse to cover several quite disparate groups: the two-tiered system of SRNs with or without district or midwifery training, and the village nurse-midwife with a midwifery qualification and just a few months of hospital nursing experience. This clearly created an impression of double standards or lack of standardisation, which is reflected in the inconsistency expressed in the experiences of doctors. Among these, a GP in Chichester offered examples of negligent midwifery practice and of nurses misdiagnosing a Colles fracture and a case of diphtheria without advising the patient to seek medical help.[42] Subsequent letters endorsed this: One calling himself "Country Practitioner" gave examples of nurses attempting to diagnose, prescribe, and treat with disastrous consequences. In support of his claim he cited the case of a child who died from meningitis having been treated by the nurse for five weeks for an "eruption of the face".[43]

However, these pockets of rivalry and distrust were not entirely one-sided. A Queen's Nurse wrote describing the 1918 Spanish influenza epidemic as experienced in "a very long, straggling and hilly district village in Yorkshire" served by two district nurses: "During November and the early part of December there were 116 influenza patients and in one week we paid 306 visits." The work was particularly onerous because several local GPs were away on active service and others found it difficult to get around to their own patients.[44] The writer described the resultant heavy demands on the district nurses, implying a degree of negligence on behalf of some of the doctors. In particular she cited a case of a mother who, together with two of her four children, became seriously ill. Her husband was serving in the army, but the doctor's attendance was not judged (by the nurse) to have been adequate to the severity of the case and, "as the child did not improve, the mother, after some persuasion, got another doctor to take on the case." She further noted that "There were a great many cases of a similar kind" and that "such difficulties as we have had, throw much responsibility on the nurses, and not only cause grave anxiety and thought, but call for the exercise of great tact during such times."

Oral histories reveal this "tact" in the form of significant "silences" that would often appear when nursing and medical professionals were asked about these tensions, and it seems reasonable to assume that much of the time the situation of professional tolerance would also have existed in this earlier period, with only occasional outbursts reaching the correspondence columns of the respective professional journals. In theory at least, it would seem that the relationship between doctor and nurse was more clearly defined than it had been a decade earlier in 1907 when the confrontation between BMA and QNI took place in Cornwall.[45] In a set of notes prepared by a county superintendent in 1922, for use in guiding a village group or neighbourhood wishing to set up a DNA, the author emphasised that the district nurse's role was not as a substitute for the doctor: "The nurse is *not* a doctor, but a worker who has been specially trained for three things." These three things were defined as carrying out the nursing treatment ordered by the doctors, assisting in emergencies until the doctor arrives, and teaching relatives how to provide help and comfort to the patient.[46] She insisted that if called in to attend an emergency, the Queen's Nurse should not continue to attend unless a doctor is called in to see the patient (see Figure 2.2).

RECRUITMENT AND THE HOSPITAL DILEMMA

What was the relationship between district and hospital nurses? That there appears to have been some failure in communication between the two is suggested in a speech made by the president of the Blackburn DNA, Lady Thom.[47] She urged closer cooperation between hospitals (particularly outpatient departments) and DNAs to avoid unnecessary patient inconvenience. Recruitment from training hospitals into the community clearly provided tensions from both sides, fuelled at times by a serious lack of trust and

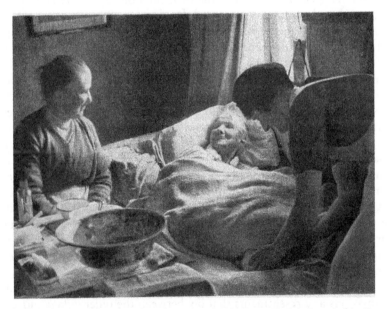

Figure 2.2 District nurse (no date but pre-1943). From E. M. Day (ed.), *Cassell's Modern Dictionary of Nursing and Medical Terms* (London: Cassell & Co. Ltd. 1939): 116. We acknowledge the author and Cassell Plc., a division of The Orion Publishing Group Ltd. (London), as the publishers; however, all our attempts at tracing the copyright holder of the image proved unsuccessful.

understanding between hospital and district. However, the recruitment situation resulted from a combination of factors, of which lack of cooperation from the hospital was just one. Many more professions were now open to women, providing alternatives to the long hours, hard work, and loneliness often felt as a district nurse. Nurses were also deterred by the additional training required, further examinations, and the contractual obligation to practise as a district nurse for one full year on completion of training, and all this with no integrated pension scheme as standard.[48]

In response to a QNI proposal that the probationer nurses in hospitals should receive a lecture about district nursing to inform them about the work and boost recruitment, many hospital matrons claimed that they were unaware of the possibilities of district work. A recruitment drive was proposed but many hospitals were unsupportive.[49] Furthermore, changes both in the way the GP worked and in the role of the hospital had a considerable effect on the caseload of the district nurse. With fewer surgeries taking place in the home by the 1930s, the emphasis in hospitals shifted from that of an acute facility toward one offering long-term care of chronic and terminal conditions not previously considered suitable for hospital care. Over time this contributed to an increase in status differential between hospital and district nurses.

There was a strong element of credibility in the concern voiced by the GPs and the hospital nurses over the variability of standards in district nursing practice, which further increased this division. For some time the training received by village nurses was felt to have been inferior and their support and supervision inadequate. At the annual conference of the Metropolitan and Southern Counties Association of Queen's Superintendents in 1922 a heated discussion followed a paper entitled "Status and Future of the Village Nurse."[50] In particular its author, B. M. Johnson, noted the difficulties for some districts in obtaining and also in paying for a Queen's Nurse. She admitted the main work was often midwifery and "what general work there was, the nurse-midwife was capable of undertaking." In outlining the main reasons why village nurses would not be able to undertake formal nurse training, she also suggested how a better structured and assessed, in-service training of eighteen months, with an agreed syllabus, assessed by practical and oral examinations, could be adopted as a standard.[51] It was agreed that the public were often confused as to the difference between the Queen's Nurse and the village nurse. One speaker urged that this distinction be made clear and suggested that better communication was the key to addressing many of the problems.

"A Page From an Assistant Superintendent's Diary" reveals the underlying divisions and resentments that lay between the older village nurses and the more professionally powerful and assertive Queen's Nurses:

> I ride along a riverside lane, cross the ferry, up a very steep hill, and arrive at Mrs. Gamp Number One. . . . She is over seventy and has poor

sight, but is still anxious to take cases; she shows me her bag "Her ladyship gave me with my certificate," and also says "I've had no cases since you was here, Miss; is it right? They all have the District Nurse now, a young thing like she; why, I was at it before she was born, and her mother afore her."[52]

The Superintendent visited five other women that day, all described either as "Mrs. Gamps" or "bona fides," recording several similar complaints of loss of midwifery engagements to the young district nurse, but considered, "as they are getting beyond the work, feel it is a blessing for the prospective mothers and infants that the nurse *has* arrived." One midwife quoted wanted to remain on the roll of practising midwives despite being eighty-seven. The attitudes expressed toward two of these cottage nurses were slightly different, however, and worth noting here. One was described as "about fifty, and anxious to do well," and was given a lesson on using a thermometer, although the tone was patronising and revealed serious professional misgivings on the part of the superintendent.

A more respectful description was given by a nurse who had worked with a village nurse-midwife trained in the 1920s:

> Hilda Curtis was one of the old village Midwives that had no general training but they were district trained—it was just when the Queen's Institute was beginning to—it was about 1924. Hilda Curtis was one of the people that had been trained as the village-nurse—she was part of the Nursing Association's growing up—the pre National Health. Hilda Curtis was a large lady with false teeth and she terrified me. . . . However, I learned a lot in the community from Hilda Curtis for all her teeth—or lack of them—she taught me quite a bit that I can see now that she was the rather rough and ready village midwife, trained by the Association in about 1924 or something like that.[53]

The difference in tone between the two accounts suggests a difference in relationship between the elite view of the superintendent (and by implication, of the QNI) and the non-elite view of personal experience. The latter had the benefit of a lifetime's experience at close quarters, whereas the former judged the cottage nurses by their educational shortfalls and betrayed a certain class prejudice. Nevertheless, it is mentioned that this was a "trained" village midwife, who would have received a token six months of general nursing training under the QNI in addition to midwifery training, unlike the elderly ladies encountered by the superintendent. The significance of these tensions is even more powerful when seen in the context of the maelstrom of contemporary debate over professional standards of nursing as a whole. By the mid-1920s, the professional status of nursing had become a political issue involving trade unions, class and social status, and gender concerns as well as relationships with the medical profession.

DISTRICT NURSES, THE ASSOCIATIONS,
COMMITTEES, AND THE "LADIES"

The professional organisation of salaried Queen's Superintendents predated the 1919 Registration Act by two years[54] and the disappearance of the voluntary Lady Superintendents was by then almost complete, as they were confined only to a few areas including Liverpool and Bournemouth. Stocks noted that in these districts, "non-professional voluntary workers still exercised supervisory functions."[55] The main restriction to district nurses' professional autonomy, however, probably came from their immediate employers, the local DNA, whose powers were potentially considerable. Had the lay "committee of ladies" superseded the lay Lady Superintendent? That many district nurses were from a lower, albeit educated class is suggested by the pay and conditions they accepted and their family backgrounds. If they had come from the higher educated middle classes, as had been the intention of Nightingale and Dacre Craven, would they not have been in a better position to withstand the threat from the doctors, described earlier, as well as from these influential ladies of the committee? Referring to what he termed a breach of professional etiquette by the nurse when she treated his private patients without his knowledge, a Somerset GP was not prepared to be removed from his preferred role as patients' gatekeeper. Despite this, he acknowledged the inherent dilemma for nurses: "The district nurse is between the devil and the deep sea. She must tout for subscribers and please the public, and she must beware of the doctor, upon whose field of work she generally encroaches so unprofessionally."[56]

The Committee of Ladies was the active core of most DNAs. Committee sizes varied considerably; for example, in 1925 Lytham St. Anne's had a committee of fifty plus an "executive of fourteen ladies," whereas Bradford had a committee of sixty and an (unspecified) executive of ladies.[57] In addition, the level of patronage was as formidable in 1925 as it had been in 1915, even though the names had changed. Many esteemed figures at the national or local level were formally linked to the DNAs including King Edward VII and Queen Alexandra; Princesses Louise, Beatrice, and Helena; and an impressive array of dukes and duchesses, counts and countesses, bishops, and mayors and mayoresses. In Scotland, in the Parish of Peterculter, the first meeting of the nursing association held in 1914 was presided over by landowner Theodore Crombie, and attended by paper mill owner James L. Geddes, with names in subsequent years including Mrs. Murison, wife of the county clerk; Mrs. Jessie Cormack, J. P.; and David Cossar, agent for the commercial bank.[58] The list of members of the Leith Jubilee Nurses' Association of 1933 includes an ex-provost as chairman, three medical doctors, two parish ministers, a knight of the realm, a member of the British Linen Bank, and several ladies who were doubtless locally prominent for their wealth and philanthropy.[59] Although it is unlikely that many of the patrons were involved in the running of the organizations at a local level, many were active at the county level, adding a degree of status to committee membership, and making the local committee a formidable employer. On the other hand, district nurses employed by nursing associations were usually women of a working or lower middle class background.[60] Class tension was inevitable and keenly felt by some nurses.

By the late 1930s it was estimated that there were 8,000 district nurses working in Great Britain, over half of whom were Queen's trained. At least forty percent of them were financially supported directly by the population they served. The process of fundraising and day-to-day administration was performed by voluntarily run local associations. By this time just over half the district nurses were Queen's trained (4,566 in 1939).[61] This represents a dramatic increase both in numbers of Queen's Nurses, and more generally, in all grades of district nurse throughout the interwar period. The relationship between district nurses and their committees was extremely varied, having to maintain a difficult balance between voluntary, lay employer, and, increasingly, the trained, professional employee. In the case of the QNI-affiliated societies, the intermediary figures of superintendent's and inspector's reports were intended to help facilitate this. A comment made at a conference held during the war (but equally pertinent to this interwar period) explained, "Members felt strongly that they were not sufficiently represented at their local Committees . . . Committees sometimes had little knowledge of the qualifications of their Nurses. It was pointed out by Miss Wilmshurst that there was a great art in tackling a Committee."[62] Although the number of serious instances of conflict reported in inspectors' reports were few, when they did occur, this communication gap generally featured problems not concerning actual nursing but the nurse's living arrangements, off-duty and holiday requests, or the availability of money for purchasing equipment such as a telephone or a new nursing bag. Personality clashes occurred inevitably from time to time and these were marked in minutes and QNI reports as "found not suitable." What the nurses viewed as patronising interference was the meddling by committee members in matters that revolved around the nurses' house and furniture. Nurses often had to guard their own privacy as well as patient confidentiality:

> All the district nurses, every area had a district nursing association. Now this is a very bad thing, I would have said. In one way it was good, others it was bad. Now it was usually the lady of the manor, and the lady of the manor would have . . . gone around collecting money, you know, for the district nurse, and give the patients a card, "Now if you need the nurse you'll have her services free." Now this was how it was done . . . You had to go for interview by this lady of the manor. And this lady of the manor and her committee thought they owned you, and they would have come to your house, you see, all nurses had a house supplied to them, they paid a rent, but, they would say, "Now what have you got nurse? Now I think you could be doing with a more comfortable chair.

Have you got a chair in your house Mrs. So and So?"—"Oh yes, I'll supply nurse." You see—charity. And, "Now, I noticed you were at Mrs. Smith's door. What's wrong with Mrs. Smith?" Now, that was none of their business. And, you see, a young nurse unless she was trained, sort of, to handle them, which you weren't, you know. You would come out of hospital and all this obedience and everything, you had to sort of, you know, be guided . . . Sometimes you had a doctor on the committee which didn't, wasn't always the right thing, you know, he's better, they're better not to know too much about the nurse and all that was going on.[63]

For district nursing as well as for the country's economy, the 1920s was a decade marked by financial struggle. This applied both to the local nursing associations and to the QNI as the main body for training and administration of district nurses nationally. Raising funds became a regular and increasingly creative task, with the QNI staging a range of events from victory balls to garden schemes and public appeals. Ironically, it was the greatly regretted death of Queen Alexandra that represented financial salvation for the QNI.[64] With Queen Mary as the new Patron, the name of the Institute became the Queen's Institute of District Nursing and in 1928 a Supplementary Charter was issued. In 1932 the QNI further benefited from a contribution from the National Birthday Trust, which enabled the acquisition of new premises for its headquarters in London. However, financial concerns were never far from the surface.

THE CHANGING ROLE AND
PUBLIC HEALTH RESPONSIBILITIES

As a result of the tight financial situation, widespread adoption and implementation of the Provident system of running and financing DNAs characterised the 1920s and 1930s as a period of change as well as consolidation. Although this was not a new system of generating income, its method of implementation and organisation changed significantly in the interwar period, coming to represent a rudimentary but more formal health care system than had existed before World War I.[65] This marked a move away from upper class philanthropic or charitable support for district nursing where the primary duty had been the care of the "sick poor and working classes in their own home without distinction of creed" that tended to focus on the working classes, elderly poor, and unemployed. The Provident system allowed much stronger links with the middle classes, both as patrons and recipients, supporting associations through regular subscription or contributions and functioning on a payment according to means basis.

Stocks saw this as "the Institute's readiness to exploit the growing familiarity of the British public, down to the lowest income groups, with the insurance principle, and their growing reliance on it."[66] In fact, income continued to be derived from a number of sources, principally subscriptions, direct payments, or a contributory scheme, but also donations, special events (bazaars, flag days, garden fetes, the National Gardens Scheme, etc.), insurance society and public authority grants,[67] legacies, and donations. Figure 2.3 presents the data provided for England and Wales for the years 1915, 1920, and 1925 showing the changes in source of income by the mid-1920s, suggesting a move from dependence on legacies and large donations to the provident system of subscription as well as an increase in diversity of service provision such as school nursing, midwifery and maternity care, and tuberculosis nursing.[68] Nurses were not generally involved in the fundraising process, but sometimes general collections were organised directly by the QNI and Queen's Nurses were asked to take part in these special collection days:

> Well, my sister once had to go in with a collecting bowl to a football match. For the Queen's, yes . . . And I remember being sent to a theatre in the Tollcross area, or somewhere, with my bowl and sitting at the back, and soliciting cash from the customers as they were going out. . . . In my uniform, oh yes, in my uniform. And the actor or the entertainer, whatever way you describe him, he put out a message, "There is a Queen's nurse at the back, and they do very valuable work, and we would be very pleased if you would find it in your means to make a little donation."[69]

However, Challis's notes on starting a DNA referred to earlier in this chapter give the object of district nursing as, "to provide a trained nurse for the benefit of the residents in a district, thus bringing the advantages of skilled nursing within the reach of people in their own homes."[70] She added that associations typically charge one penny per week or between five and eight shillings as a minimum subscription, collected on a quarterly or half-yearly basis with the exceptions being "persons in receipt of parish relief, also old age pensioners, and any necessitous cases," when nursing was free. Subscriptions covered expenses such as "nurse's salary, nurse's insurance, workman's liability insurance, general sickness insurance, equipment, . . . bicycle and upkeep, printing, postage, stationery, affiliation fees to QVJIN and County Nursing Association, holiday nurse, emergency nurse."[71]

Interwar industrial development and urban growth in conjunction with the providential system greatly increased the numbers of potential patients able to access district nursing care. We examine the county of Lancashire as an example. In 1930 a note from the DNA in Barrow on the contributory system for raising funds indicated that money was raised from "the works' employees enabling the nurses to make 22,127 home visits during to 854 patients in the previous year, to assist at 45 operations and to attend 72 Ministry of Health sessions."[72] In Rochdale the committee was particularly aware of the need to provide cars to cope with an increasing workload in

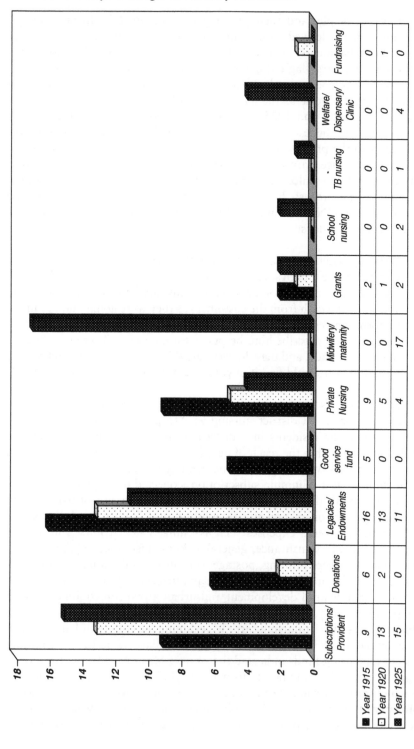

	Subscriptions/ Provident	Donations	Legacies/ Endowments	Good service fund	Private Nursing	Midwifery/ maternity	Grants	School nursing	TB nursing	Welfare/ Dispensary/ Clinic	Fundraising
Year 1915	9	6	16	5	9	0	2	0	0	0	0
Year 1920	13	2	13	0	5	0	1	0	0	0	1
Year 1925	15	0	11	0	4	17	2	2	1	4	0

Figure 2.3 Income sources of district nursing associations (England and Wales) 1915–1925.

"hitherto outlying districts, now densely populated" and it was reported that two cars had been provided as "generous gifts" and the DNA purchased a third.[73] In Birkenhead, need clearly outstripped supply and extension of the borough increased "the difficulty of finding nurses of the right type." In Blackburn, the following year, 800 cases were nursed including 200 cases of pneumonia, and 212 sick children under five years of age, together with the nurses having assisted at 94 operations, and attended to 174 "long chronic cases," totalling 14,000 visits.[74] For that year there were fifteen district nurses working for Blackburn DNA excluding superintendents, and care was "free to poor, others 3s per week, operations 5s–10s private: daily visiting [charged at a rate of] 9s to 12s 6d, per week, maternity, £2 per case."[75]

Between 1915 and 1925 the trend was noticeably toward fewer visits being paid per nurse each year but with an increase in the numbers of cases nursed (i.e. the take-up of the service). This increase in patient numbers by the early 1930s changed the working experience of the district nurse. An increase in caseload reduced the amount of time that nurses were able to spend with each patient, subtly changing relationships. With a wider class range of patients, some of whom might previously have employed a private nurse, expectations and attitudes on both sides underwent a fundamental adjustment. Data relating to patient charges differ noticeably from that in (and before) 1925 in that many record "free or payment according to means," with many associations relying on the nurse to make that judgment or "means-test" (very few of the 1931 entries record weekly subscriptions, although that situation changed significantly by the end of the decade). Hitherto, the district nurse had often acted as educator and social reformer among the poor, but the increasing inclusion of middle-class patients often called for greater tact and social skills on the part of the nurse.

Table 2.1 suggests a very high percentage of the cases attended in connection with local authorities were cases with respiratory diseases and childhood infections. This was reaffirmed in 1934 when for the first time the figures for the previous year were published in full by the QNI. They included statistics for maternity nursing and maternal mortality and on the nursing of patients with notifiable diseases such as tuberculosis, puerperal pyrexia and other postnatal (and antenatal) complications, measles, chicken pox, and whooping cough.[76] These had been collected by the QNI from their nurses through a nationwide survey, and the editorial's forceful encouragement to nurses to study the statistics in detail reflects the importance attached to promoting a professional and scientific approach among their membership. Particular attention is drawn to public health concerns such as "undernourishment and unsatisfactory housing conditions," which the editor considered might be underlying causes of otherwise preventable deaths and should therefore be of primary concern to district nurses.

District nurses and HVs were also engaged in many vaccination campaigns. In addition to the network of nurses routinely working in the

Table 2.1 Cases Attended by District Nurses in Connection With Local Authorities in England and Wales (1932)

Disease	No. of Cases Nursed	No. of Visits Made
Pneumonia	13,470	13,997
Tuberculosis (all cases)	4,764	167,463
Puerperal pyrexia and fever	465	9,067
Influenza (uncomplicated)	4,812	43,542
Measles	2,668	26,015
Measles with pneumonia	639	11,732
Ophthalmia neonatorum	776	17,415
Chicken pox	349	1,943
Whooping cough	695	6,806
Infantile diarrhoea	446	3,531
Pemphigus neonatorum	145	2,003
Other diseases (children under five)	12,925	152,419
Other cases paid by local authority	845	10,955

Note. Data from "Report on the Nursing of Patients in Connection with Local Authorities," QNM XXVI:2 (1933): 77.

prevention and treatment of tuberculosis, a specifically designated district nursing post was created in the 1930s to tackle what was now a growing problem. The high incidence of tuberculosis was a matter of great concern in the Highlands and Islands of Scotland and in an effort to combat its spread the QNIS in conjunction with the National Association for the Prevention of Tuberculosis, the Royal Victoria Hospital Tuberculosis Trust, and the British Red Cross Society, appointed a Queen's trained district nurse commissioner for tuberculosis in Scotland. Nurse Weir, the first nurse commissioner, began her appointment in September 1934 by accompanying the Medical Commissioner of the National Association for the Prevention of Tuberculosis, Dr. Harley Williams, on a tour of Shetland, Orkney, and Caithness, meeting public health officials, medical men, and nursing committees. By October, Nurse Weir had visited twenty-seven schools and numerous notified cases at the request of the Medical Officer for Health as well as having given several lectures and attended public meetings. Her itinerary for November included visits to twenty-two schools in Western and Southern areas, nine evening lectures and home visitations, taking her up to the end of November, after which she moved her work to Orkney and on to Caithness in January 1935. Thereafter she continued to operate in Shetland, Orkney, and Lewis, dealing only with tuberculosis cases and related prevention work.[77]

In August 1934 the Advisory Committee on the work of the Nurse Commissioners for Tuberculosis in Scotland discussed a plan to support a substantive post based in Inverness-shire with responsibility to cover tuberculosis work in Lewis. The proposed nurse was to be attached to the county association under the direction of the county superintendent, although she would be specialising in tuberculosis work. It was decided to forward this suggestion to the Inverness County Nursing Association for consideration and approval. Despite initially declining the suggestion, the following year a second nurse was appointed to cover Inverness-shire.

Nursing commissioners nursed tuberculosis cases in the home but their main task was to educate the public in prevention by giving lectures in local community halls and visiting schools:

> The education part of the work consists in visiting schools and talking to the young children on general hygiene and how to live healthy lives. I also show films of children of many lands carrying out the laws of health, etc. The older children are taught how infection is spread and how to prevent it. Films, which are provided by the National Association for the Prevention of Tuberculosis, are shown. Lectures on the prevention of tuberculosis are given to Women's Rural Institutes, Church Guilds, Debating Societies, Scouts, Guides, etc.; in fact, to any bodies who appear interested.[78]

This role for the district nurse was unique to the specific areas where tuberculosis was prevalent and continued to be so until the late 1940s. The existence of such a role indicates that not only the physical but the epidemiological landscape affected district nursing employment and practice.

The economic depression of the 1930s also affected the health of the district nurse. The report of the Queen's Institute's own Welfare fund, the 1930 Fund, notes "It is evident that the strain of the times has told heavily upon those who come within its scope. Breakdown in health tends to occur at an earlier age; provision for the future, adequate a few years ago, is no longer; Nursing Associations find it more difficult to raise money to help their nurses; amidst widespread unemployment those handicapped by age or weakness have less chance than ever."[79]

Following abolition of the London Metropolitan Asylums Board and the 25 boards of guardians by the Local Government Act (1929), responsibility for public health administration was transferred to, and divided between, the London City Council, the Metropolitan Boroughs Councils, and the City Corporation.[80] Dr. Hogarth, who carried out a survey of London DNAs, noted in the general conclusions to her report the additional roles of a district nurse compared with a private nurse, notably educational and preventative health care. It was more demanding where "the actual necessities of life are hard to procure."[81] For these reasons she felt it became "more a vocation than a profession."

TERMS OF EMPLOYMENT AND CONDITIONS OF SERVICE DURING THE INTERWAR PERIOD

Set against this ideal of vocation, however, was the short-lived tenure of many district nurses. An article in the *QNM* a few years earlier explained the proposed introduction of a Long Service Fund.[82] The main points of its rationale were listed as:

1. The comparatively late age at which Queen's Nurses join the Institute; the average age of the entrants for the years 1913 to 1924 being 32.48.
2. The comparatively early age at which the pension would have to begin, as owing to the character of the work many nurses have to give up about the age of 55.
3. The large number of nurses who only remain a few years in the service. The average length of service of the Queen's Nurse is five years.
4. About half the nurses left within five years.

The trend noted in the last two points, of district nurses in many areas wishing to remain in post for a very short time, remained largely unchanged at least until the outbreak of World War II. A "long service fund" therefore provided some incentive to remain in district nursing, and there is evidence that in some districts the associations provided other small incentives such as coal and lighting, domestic help, a salary slightly above the standard rate, free transportation passes, or a pleasantly furnished cottage.

Bearing in mind the increasing numbers of DNAs being established after World War I, a preoccupation with the provision of adequate nurses' accommodation was expressed through the *QNM*. Although felt particularly in urban areas, it was also increasingly difficult to find suitable rooms for district nurses in the large number of rural associations springing up. For example, the Clydach-on-Tawe DNA in South Wales described itself as an association entirely managed by local workmen, the funds being raised chiefly by a levy on wages. A letter from the honorary secretary of that association stated:

Through the generosity of three donors, the District Nursing Association here has received the splendid gift of a very nice house at a cost of £1,250. It is a very nice villa, very central, and with all modern conveniences, including electric light. Through the generosity of others the bill for furnishing will also be paid without any cost to the Association.

I have put a man and his wife in as caretakers, giving them free rent, coal, light, and 10/- a week for looking after the nurses, so now I think they will be very comfortable.[83]

A rise in salaries demanded by the QNI for its nurses, but not necessarily applicable to employment of non-Queen's Nurses, was held to be responsible for some disaffiliations such as Criccieth in Wales, which had been affiliated since 1905, notable because it was the home of the Prime Minister, Lloyd George. Nevertheless, Mrs. Lloyd George was actively supportive of district nursing and spoke at the opening ceremony of a fête and bazaar in Sketty, South Wales, congratulating Swansea on "having begun to think seriously of the nurse's welfare."[84] Despite this, it is clear that district nursing—and particularly Queen's Nursing, which involved the more expensive employment of a Queen's Nurse and affiliation costs—were casualties first of the coal miners' strike in 1921, and subsequently the 1926 general strike and ensuing economic recession. The latter hit certain industrial areas of Britain particularly hard with the effects of economic depression on health and welfare provision persisting well into the 1930s. For example, lack of funds "owing to the coal miners' strike"[85] resulted in suspension of the Treherbert DNA in the Rhondda from its affiliation to the QNI and consequently their nurse was relocated to Swansea.

An analysis of a list of seventy-three recorded resignations for the year 1933 published in the *QNM* provided the breakdown of reasons for nurses leaving shown in Table 2.2.[86] Further training as a midwife was an expected reason for leaving, although quite often this appears to have been only a temporary resignation. Occasionally the DNA would have paid for this further training.[87] However, numbers leaving to return to hospital work, for other work, and for a move into private nursing were relatively high, suggesting some discontent among the workforce. Those leaving for marriage confirmed the belief noted earlier that resignation for marriage was an unwritten rule.[88]

For all Queen's Nurses, off-duty consisted of a minimum of one half-day per week with occasional weekends and one month's annual holiday.[89] Welfare provision consisted of "full salary and allowances for six weeks, less the benefit received under NHI, with half salary and allowances for a further six weeks." The possibility of a more generous allowance was made through benefits in recognition of long service plus some grants available from the QNI or from the Tate Fund and convalescent care at the Home of Rest for Queen's Nurses at Bryn-y-Menai. By the end of the 1930s this was established as a standard provision for Queen's Nurses by the local committee's subscription to the Long Service Fund of the Institute or the Federated Superannuation Scheme.[90] Following enrollment, a Queen's Nurse would be "recommended for work with an affiliated Association which is not in a position to give district training itself"—the nurse had to sign an agreement "to work for at least one year as a Queen's Nurse wherever her services may be required," although any personal preferences in location and post were

Table 2.2 Resignations From District Nursing

Reason for Resignation	Number
For marriage	17
For midwifery training	9
To return to hospital work	9
For other work	8
Retirement	7
Due to health reasons	6
Private nursing	5
For home duties	4
To work abroad	3
To work in an unaffiliated district	2
School nursing	2
For work as health visitor	1

Note. Data from "Institute News: Resignations",
QNM XXVII, no. 1 (1934): 54.

often taken into consideration. On completion of her first year of service she was then free to apply for alternative posts. Likewise, nurses might be given free midwifery training following district training, but the agreement also stipulated that they must agree to practise as a midwife for at least a year afterwards. HV training for Queen's Nurses was reduced from six months to four months and some scholarships were made available to support this.

A series of recruitment leaflets[91] published by the QNI from 1931 onward and aimed at student nurses nearing completion of training emphasised the similarities to hospital nursing before concentrating on the more autonomous aspects of the work that made it distinctive:

> She [the district nurse] has no appliances with which to work beyond which she carries in her bag, and no one in authority at hand to whom she can turn for help and advice. She has to work on her own initiative; to act in critical situations and frequently to carry out medical instructions under the most difficult conditions—work which calls for skill, courage, promptitude, and resource, but which is peculiarly satisfying, as all nurses will understand. There is surgical nursing, including preparation for, and attendance at, operations both major and minor; there is medical nursing; there is midwifery for those willing to practise.[92]

These recruitment pamphlets outlined the unique public health and educative role before detailing the training and minimum salary: "The *clear* salary for a Queen's Nurse must not be less than £63 for the first year (£5 more if required to hold the CMB certificate) rising by £3 annually up to £75." In addition there was a standard annual uniform allowance to each nurse of £8, together with an allowance for her board, lodging and laundry. The equivalent inclusive recommended salary ranged between £125 and £137 dependent on seniority "with furnished rooms (or cottage), fire, light and attendance." In the second of these three leaflets, a handwritten amendment was made to the prepublication draft (presumably for addition by editor or publisher): "It is understood that a Queen's Nurse will resign her post on marriage." However, this clause was not included in the published revised version five years later, in 1938. Instead there was a new addition advising that "where districts are wide a car is usually provided," suggesting some modernization in outlook regarding conditions of service between 1933 and 1938. By 1939 the starting inclusive annual salary for a Queen's Nurse was between £180 and £200 so that salaries can also be seen to have doubled those offered in 1916 (see Table 2.3).

Table 2.3 Changes in Queen's District Nurses' Pay and Allowances from 1916 to 1937

Year	Minimum Clear Salary	Allowances
1916	£35 per anuum rising annually to £37	Weekly board and laundry: 15s
	£40 per annum (CMB) (candidates at £30 per annum)	Annual uniform: £5
1918	£40	Weekly board and laundry: 15s
		Annual uniform: £6
1919	£50 (candidates at £40 per annum)	Unchanged
1920	£63 per annum rising to £75 and £68 per annum rising to £80 (CMB) (candidates at £55 per annum)	Weekly board and laundry: 25s
		Annual uniform: £10
1937	£70 per annum rising annually to £100	Weekly board and laundry: 21s
	£80 per annum rising to £110 (CMB) with additional £5 for HV certificate where required (candidates at £55 per annum)	Uniform: £8
		Cost of two rooms or rent of cottage, plus fire, light, attendance, household laundry, and incidental expenses to be defrayed by the Committee

Note. Data from QNI *Summary of Evidence Submitted to the Interdepartmental Committee on Nursing Services* (1938): 2.

CONCLUSION

This chapter has demonstrated the difficulties faced by a professional group in promoting and advancing their interests in an economically depressed era, particularly when confronted by the professional rivalry of doctors (some of whom were also struggling at times to make a living), and the rising fortunes of the HVs employed by local government rather than being reliant on fund-raising and subscription. Added to this, district nurses were handicapped in establishing their professional role and status by a confusing, three-tiered hierarchical system. This consisted of the fully trained Queen's Nurse; followed by the lesser trained registered nurse who learned her district techniques on the job rather than through prescribed training; and finally the village nurse-midwives, cottage nurses, and handiwomen, who represented a broad band of trained, semitrained, and untrained carers. Communication among these three groups was recognised as being far from ideal. Likewise, contact between the nurses and their superintendents was often limited to twice-yearly inspections based more on maintaining standards and discipline than encouraging any form of constructive interaction. As a result of this and the blocking by GPs of recommendations for a team approach to community health care made in the *Dawson Report*, there is little evidence of any widespread cooperation between community health professionals.[93]

In the community, this applied to the relationships with professional colleagues, with the lay employers, and with the general public in failing to create a better understanding of the particular roles and skills of district nurses. Limited face-to-face contact of district nurses with both GPs and HVs perpetuated distrust and misunderstandings, and prevented the exchange of ideas on which a more mutually respectful relationship might otherwise have been founded. Similarly the need for better hospital liaison was felt to have contributed to difficulties in recruiting trained nurses, and created a "them-and-us" mindset, which hampered attempts to employ nursing resources more economically. Nevertheless, real gains were made through institutional improvements such as the move toward streamlining of salaries, conditions of service, the professionalisation of QNI superintendents, the establishment of a number of Queen's training centres across England and Wales, and a widespread introduction of subscription membership to DNAs through a determined campaign to promote the Provident system. This last point was largely responsible for extending provision of district nursing care to the wider community rather than restricting it to the sick poor as originally intended.

The chapter's title question, "What Became of the Lady?" was intended to highlight the subtle changes and power transfers that took place in district nursing's management over this period. The move away from an untrained, voluntary Lady Superintendent to a trained supervisor of nurses employed by the QNI marked a move from lay philanthropic control to a figure of professional authority. At the same time, the ladies of the committee of local

DNAs retained the earlier philanthropic image, and as lay men and women were nevertheless able to exercise considerable control regarding the employment, payment, and living and working arrangements of "their" nurses. The social divisions between these ladies and the nurses they employed meant that the power held by them greatly diminished the true professional autonomy of the district nurse in a way never experienced by the GP or HV, especially where there was no cushion provided by QNI affiliation.

3 War to Welfare State, 1939–1948

Writing in 1942, a Chief Superintendent of the Queen's Institute described district nursing as a " 'front line' occupation and an essential war service."[1] In addition to providing a chronological overview of the development of district nursing through this period, this chapter evaluates the extent to which this front line image was an accurate picture and how the district nurse's role changed during World War II (1939–1945) and in the immediate post-war period. Bearing in mind the ideological reconstructions that inevitably surround accounts of wartime experiences, we provide a context for some of those written at the time. Together with others related through oral history, these provide an impression of how events were seen at the time, how and why nurses' roles and responsibilities were extended, and how daily workloads increased in different parts of Britain. Through this it will also be possible to assess the part played by district nursing in restructuring health care leading up to the NHS Act (1948). The effect this reorganisation had on relationships between the district nurses and other members of the emerging community health care team is part of this consideration.

RAIDS AND ROUTINES: THE INITIAL
DISRUPTION OF THE EARLY WAR YEARS

Shortly before the outbreak of war, in March 1939, a note of considerable optimism was sounding from *QNM* editorials as a result of the recommendations of a government interdepartmental committee's report. The opening paragraph of this report stated that "nursing is a service for the nation because it serves a national need, therefore the time has come when the public health authorities and the State should realise that it is a service of outstanding importance."[2] At this stage, shortage of recruits to the nursing profession as a whole was a cause for concern, and the recommendations of an interim report enquiring into the conditions of nursing were eagerly awaited. Proposals for a forty-eight hour week and improved off-duty and holiday arrangements, better living conditions, and an improved scale of salaries were all anticipated from the report. At that time the QNI's

President and Chairman, the Earl of Athlone, was the chairman of this inter-departmental committee. Unfortunately no final report was ever issued, as by September 1940 the Earl of Athlone had been appointed Governor General of Canada. The QNI was well aware of its considerable loss of political influence, but it was by that stage far more focused on the immediate needs of helping its nurses cope with the difficulties presented by air raids, evacuation, and the exceptional conditions of wartime.[3]

One of the departing actions by the Earl of Athlone in his QNI presidential role was to send a letter to all Queen's Nurses discouraging them from volunteering for military service, stating "You will best serve your country by remaining at your post" and outlining the emergency measures to be introduced in case of war.[4] Unlike during World War I, when district nurses were actively encouraged to volunteer for active service, during World War II they were actively discouraged. As evacuation meant the closing of most school and welfare clinics, many DNAs felt they could no longer afford to keep a nurse because of loss of income from local authorities, so "many nurses resigned and went to other areas or began to do a different kind of work. Some were lent to air-raid shelters and first-aid posts under the control of the local authorities"[5] and others left district nursing altogether, returning to hospital work or joining the Armed and Civilian Defence Services. By 1942 this had resulted in an acute shortage of district nurses, particularly in central London. It was not until 1943 that a Control of Engagement Order was introduced, preventing nurses from leaving their posts.

Figure 3.1[6] shows a slight fall in numbers of Queen's Nurses and village nurse-midwives in the period from 1939 to 1945, but a more marked drop in those labelled "other district nurses." It seems likely, therefore, that it was these women who were lost to other areas of war work, but uncertainty over this underlines their obscurity. These nurses were often trainee district nurses or nurses working for non-affiliated DNAs. As a result of their move into war work, a number of affiliation agreements were signed with the QNI in 1940 and 1941 in an attempt to solve the problems of recruitment experienced by independent associations. Their lack of commitment to the wider ideals of the QNI was to rebound on the QNI in postwar negotiations over the NHS, discussed later in this chapter.

The *QNM* through the first three years of the war provides a vivid picture of district nurses living and working under a range of very difficult conditions. From the outset they were provided with steel helmets, respirators, and a distinctive white strap worn across one shoulder and over the back with a metal disk in the centre of the back, so that they could be seen cycling at night during blackouts. In the early months, some Queen's Nurses also disregarded the call to stay at their posts and volunteered for the Queen Alexandra's Imperial Military Nursing Service. One wrote a remarkable description of her experience in France during the severe winter of 1939, including the difficulties of an outbreak of rubella on an overcrowded ward,

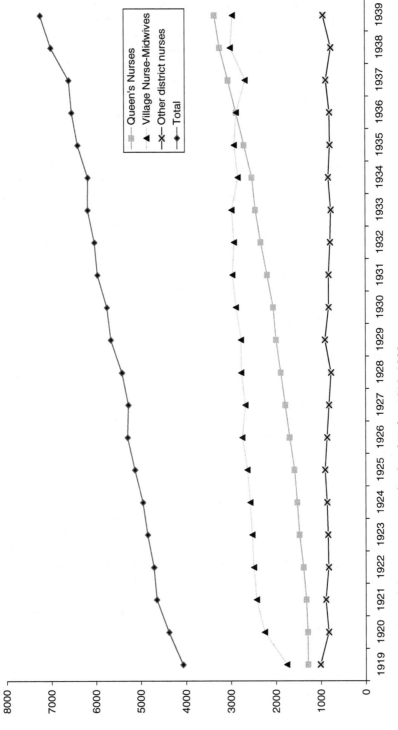

Figure 3.1 Numbers of district nurses, England and Wales, 1919–1939.
Note. Statistics from SA/QNI Box IBB-37 and Box 2 B38-45 Published Annual Reports 1910–1947.

and ultimately the evacuation under fire at Dunkirk and the (unnamed) port at which her makeshift hospital was based.[7] Another left her district in Preston to join the Queen Alexandra's Imperial Nursing Reserve and was made an Associate of the Royal Red Cross for attending patients during a heavy German air raid while serving in Italy. On the other hand there were a number of foreign visiting members of staff in several of the larger district nursing training centres who needed to be repatriated, and for some this proved impossible, forcing them to remain in the United Kingdom for much of the war.[8]

Despite the dangers, many district nurses remained at their posts in the cities and some also found themselves working under enemy fire, particularly in the heavy air raids of 1940 and 1941. In East London alone, a third of all living accommodations were demolished in the Blitz and approximately ninety percent of the remainder suffered some damage from bomb blasts with resultant additional dangers and practical difficulties to district nurses working in affected areas.[9] In addition to the personal stresses of living through the air raids, there were often difficulties in locating their patients, together with the practical problems arising from interrupted water, gas, and electricity supplies, working through blackout conditions, and frequently having to cope with punctured bicycle tires as a result of broken glass on the roads. An example of this sort of dilemma was provided through an account of a visit to give a Jewish diabetic patient his insulin injection: "Houses were down, rubble everywhere. . . . Nobody had seen Mr. Geist. In the rubble I saw his Insulin tin, complete with all his equipment and I collected it." Assuming he had been killed in the raid, this nurse was surprised and delighted to find him a few days later and be able to resume his treatment at a nearby Rest Centre.[10] Insulin was particularly expensive and the results of untreated diabetes, including gangrene and glaucoma, became increasingly common as patients focused on spending their rations on what was perceived to be nourishing food rather than paying attention to a more healthy diabetic diet.

The nurses were expected to include new areas of work such as emergency casualty treatment at Air Raid Precautions (ARP) first-aid posts, and provision of a variety of care and attention to people at air raid shelters, reception centres, and rest homes. Much of this seems to have been undertaken remarkably calmly, demonstrating an apparent detachment that characterised several oral testimonies, but was probably part of the necessary survival response to such a challenging experience. This is demonstrated by the following description given when a nurse was asked about her wartime district nursing training experience. She described watching bombs dropping from a hill overlooking Woolwich, adding:

We used to sleep in the basement at one time, but we decided, well if we were going to be killed we might as well do it in comfort so to speak in bed![11]

This kind of dark humour appears to have been an essential attribute to nursing in these conditions. One nurse described carrying out a postoperative dressing in Millwall, East London when a bomb dropped nearby and the nurse threw herself across the patient to protect her:

> The patient being eighteen stone, the ceiling on top of them. Suddenly the patient tried to sit up—"Hey, it's a good thing I didn't try to cover you, isn't it?"—both nurse and patient laughing at the resultant scene of devastation![12]

In contrast, a nurse writing for the *QNM* in 1940 described rather more soberly a particularly bad week of blitz bombing she had experienced in East London when her nurses' home became a shelter for those made homeless, prior to evacuation elsewhere. Despite being under bombardment themselves:

> By candle light we decide that we are all right and thank him [the ARP warden] the house is still standing, though not the front door; windows out, curtains and blinds all over the road, houses down either side but no casualties. We bring in the homeless and shocked ones, and attend to them, and as soon as it is light set off for the schools and church halls to help tend and feed the homeless.[13]

Nurse Thomas, a district nurse transferred from Llanelli, was one of several nurses awarded the George Medal for her brave action in a London air raid in which she "crawled through a small hole to administer injections of morphia to a man and woman trapped in debris."[14] Later in 1941 a nurse in Plymouth described the damage done to many areas of that city rendering them uninhabitable, and a similar experience of having to turn out during an air raid because:

> The call of a woman in childbirth must be answered . . . managing to bring her baby into the world while the woman was lying in a narrow passage in the pitch dark, and high explosive and incendiary bombs were falling and nearby buildings crashing to the ground in a heap of ruins [. . .] Miss McCarthy arrived at one patient's house during a raid to find three incendiary bombs blazing in it. Before attending to the sick person she extinguished the bombs with the help of an elderly man, and then went on with "business as usual."[15]

Comparable stories all presenting similar images of nurses carrying on despite dangers and difficulties were reported from other towns and cities such as Coventry, where they lost their nurses' home but continued to practise, living together in an air raid shelter, as well as from Liverpool, Hull, Southampton, and Bristol (see Figure 3.2).[16]

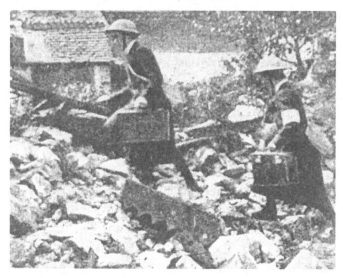

Figure 3.2 Plymouth Queen's Nurses Cantrill and McCarthy picking their way over the debris from a bomb raid to the house of a patient. From "Plymouth Nurses Carry on," *QNM* XXX:9 (September 1941):47. Reproduced by kind permission of the Queen's Nursing Institute.

As a result of the bombing, patients, potential patients, and many of the association's voluntary collectors left the cities. Unfortunately, this often included a number of the wealthier contributors who willingly paid high fees or gave generous donations to their local DNAs.[17] As a result, associations suffered financial hardship compounded by losses incurred from withdrawal of some local authority provision such as the closure of school clinics. At the same time, district nursing was not included in the Emergency Medical Service (EMS) despite the fact that early discharges from the hospital forced by the hospitalisation of numerous war casualties greatly increased the district nurses' workload. Set up in 1938, the EMS, which was also known as the Emergency Hospital Scheme, did not take domiciliary care into consideration as, unrealistically, the Civil Nursing Reserve was intended to cover all eventualities. Similarly, the nurses were expected to provide nursing cover at rest centres, which were makeshift areas for those bombed out of their homes but not requiring hospitalisation. This required a wide range of care, from general attention to hygiene, feeding babies and small children, and dressings of minor injuries, to care of those psychologically traumatised.[18] In general there was no compensation payable to nurses for this type of work. GPs, on the other hand, were able to claim compensation for treatment of civilian casualties not covered by national health insurance. The London County Council did in fact pay compensation when a nurse was taken away from her district to work at a rest centre, and the Ministry of Health provided payment at 9d per visit for transferred workers (those men and women compulsorily sent to places of work away from home and therefore housed in local lodgings).[19]

Not all the action was restricted to the cities. One village nurse in Sussex was reportedly killed when her cottage was bombed.[20] Another, dug out of her Kent cottage after a bombing raid, immediately went to the aid of a patient injured in the same raid.[21] A greatly increased workload was also a major problem for the nurses working in the rural areas, as they were expected to include duties such as inspecting child evacuees at reception centres and caring for those found not to be in good health on arrival or needing to be temporarily isolated due to infectious diseases such as scabies and respiratory infections. The subsequent increase in local populations was rarely reflected in any increase in the nursing workforce, with the exception of the early period, when there was an attempt to transfer some district nurses from city to rural districts to help overworked colleagues cope with the first batch of evacuees.[22] They therefore had to incorporate new patients into their caseload. Although later there were attempts to move nurses according to areas of greatest need, the emphasis was on midwifery rather than domiciliary nursing support.[23] In addition, the numbers of women providing informal care to the elderly and chronic sick substantially decreased,[24] as did numbers of GPs. This effectively combined to place a far greater burden on the district nurses both in workload and in responsibility.

As with World War I, numbers of GPs were severely depleted with the older practitioners having to manage understaffed practices,[25] but this problem was increased substantially by additional duties such as ARP and hospital casualty work.[26] Therefore the rise in midwifery noted earlier, plus the civilian casualties and a fluctuating population with all the medical, psychological, and social complications that went with caring for the civilian evacuees and the homeless, provided a considerable increase to the workload of GPs and district nurse-midwives alike. Remarkably, the figures provided by the QNI record a fall in maternal mortality from 1.64 per 1,000 births in 1939 to 1.00 per 1,000 in 1944,[27] although there was a slight rise in the infant mortality figures over the same period. Less well documented, but equally taxing for the district nurses, was the high death rate between 1939 and 1942 for those over sixty-five, and also a rise in deaths from tuberculosis.[28] Both of these placed considerable strain on the district nurses' workload.

Irven stressed the particular public health role of the district nurse as educator (of the whole family as opposed to the restricted access available to social workers or HVs), seeing this as particularly vital to the war effort where healthy workers were badly needed.[29] She also addressed the urban–rural divide, noting that there was "less continuity of health education in urban than in rural areas" because the "rural district nurse is often nurse/midwife/HV and school nurse, thereby seeing the family throughout the formative years as well as in later life, through her care of the elderly family members."[30] Compared to the urban situation where health, social, and nursing services were more disjointed, the rural district nurse had the opportunity to make more of an impact on the health and welfare of any one family and the community as a whole.

The records of the QNI quantify some of the war work in lists claiming payments for treatment of air raid casualties by Queen's Nurses.[31] These do not refer only to care at the time of the air raid but to subsequent nursing care following initial trauma. It was the source of a long-running dispute between the QNI and the Ministry of Health starting early in 1940 when a letter was sent to the ministry requesting clarification of payments for district nurses attending air raid casualties in line with arrangements for doctors. The reply states rather ominously, "Some of the cases may admittedly require nursing attention, but it does not seem likely that they would be numerous enough to exceed the capacity of the normal nursing agencies of the district."[32] In other words, the same rules were to apply as to ordinary need for nursing care, therefore the nurse or nursing association would have to look to the patient for payment. As if to underline this, the Ministry of Health claim forms for treatment given to air raid casualties, issued the following month, were specifically designed for use by doctors with no provision for nursing care other than in the hospital situation. A letter received from the ministry later that year in response to a second enquiry from the QNI reinforced this stance.[33]

In May the following year when the intensive bombing was revealing the existing and potential increases in demand for nursing care of air raid casualties, a letter from the QNI General Superintendent, Miss Wilmshurst, to the Minister of Health gave the total number of nursing cases following air raid injury for England and Wales as 1,206 cases and 10,365 visits.[34] The figure for 1941 was later updated, numbering 1,268 cases, to whom 21,120 visits were paid. Clearly many of these were not single-visit cases, and some required long-term care. The largest numbers were in the counties of Lancashire and Cheshire, with the lowest in rural counties.[35] In June Wilmshurst wrote again to the Minister of Health pointing out the problems of casualties returning home with serious injuries requiring long-term nursing care that would present a "very heavy liability to the Nursing Associations in the same way that the ex-service men were after the last war and will be after this one."[36] In this letter—perhaps hoping to appeal to the compassionate instincts of the minister to strengthen her case—she also described the heroic action of a district nurse candidate attending a midwifery case during an air raid: "With the flats she was in on fire she remained with her patient when a land mine had to be fired and protected her patient from the blast and as much as possible from shock."[37] She explained that although £411.9.6d had been recovered in fees, where the liability for nursing care of these patients fell on associations running a contributory system, these schemes had not been formed with the anticipated demand from war injuries in mind, again asking that the minister urgently respond to this situation with compensatory payment to the associations.[38] The eventual reply stated that the minister felt that "the position is not such that would justify him in seeking the consent of the Treasury to any formal scheme for making payments to district nursing associations beyond the limits of the Statute, particularly as the associations are in many cases subsidised in other ways from public funds."[39] Wilmshurst responded, requesting this decision be reconsidered, pointing out that the government had promised that victims of air raids would not incur any expense in connection with treatment, but despite private meetings and deputations, this situation remained unchanged.

A copy of a letter received by Lady Richmond (nee Elena Rathbone), Honorary Secretary of the QNI Council, refers to this impasse, shedding a little light on the background, stating:

> There was no chance of altering the decision to pay grants through the Local Authorities. The principal reason, I gathered, was that a number of small, unaffiliated associations had definitely said they were unwilling to receive payment through the Institute. She [Miss Horsbrugh at the Ministry of Health] said that district nursing was not on a par with voluntary hospitals, on account of these small associations employing a few nurses, affiliated to nobody; . . . She is very anxious to see that the Queen's Institute receives every reasonable safeguard against interference by Local Authorities.[40]

Mrs. Beatrice Wright M.P. received a more detailed explanation of the ministry's view of the case in a letter from Henry Willink repeating that as minister he was limited to paying only for the hospital treatment of war injury cases. Pointing out that in some cases hospitals contributed to the cost of nursing for discharged patients, the Minister went on to suggest that with casualties lower than in the first year of the war, the level of service provided by DNAs did not merit funding from the Treasury.[41]

In response to an enquiry from QNI headquarters for details of nursing of air raid casualties for the year ended December 1944 (see Table 3.1), it was nevertheless clear that there was still a continued demand being placed on district nurses for immediate care and aftercare of casualties. Details available for Sussex, Essex, and Kent demonstrate this continued demand and the anomaly between numbers of air raid cases and resultant need for nursing care, signified by numbers of nursing visits.

This is less a story of government and voluntary sector cooperation as it is one of exploitation. Hiding behind the duress of war, government placed the burden of community care on district nurses in a way it did not expect of the medical profession and hospital service. It seems surprising that the district nurses accepted this situation with such little argument until we take into consideration the fact that this was a male-dominated Conservative government operating in a traditional way that made far greater allowances for a predominantly male medical profession. It highlights the extremely

Table 3.1 South Eastern Region of England Air Raid Casualties Requiring District Nursing (Year Ended December 1944)

Place	Report	No. of Cases	No. of Visits
Kent	Beckenham nurse helped with the hospital convoys and Penge nurses attended a few patients for shock at the rest centre and slept there with the people as their houses had been bombed.	11	50 (total): 29 to one elderly patient in Bromley, 8 to three patients in Hawkhurst, 9 to three patients in Shoveham, plus 4 first aid attendances
West Sussex		25	95 nursing visits
East Sussex	Most initially first aid calls, many required subsequent nursing visits. Further two cases not included as nurse attended them with a doctor: one was removed to hospital and the other being already dead.	25	285 visits
Wimbledon, London	All elderly patients suffering from shock and bruising after air raids and fly bombing; one had to be removed to hospital and there were a further four cases of "Shelter legs" needing treatment.	3	26 visits
Dagenham, Essex		3	20 visits
East Kent		67	390 visits
Essex		19	201 visits

vulnerable position of the district nurse as a woman working in the largely unseen domestic environment of community nursing.

The debate over compensatory payment betrayed tensions in district nursing relationships at an organisational level. Some independent nursing associations expressed misgivings over the fact that the QNI would be accorded the right to handle the proposed compensatory payments should they be made. This disunity later affected negotiations over the role of the QNI within the new NHS.

In a similar way to other members of the home defence system such as ARP wardens, the fire brigade, and ambulance services, district nursing was a front-line occupation, although this has subsequently been less well recognised or publicised. Nevertheless, it would be wrong to present this situation as being consistent nationwide or even regionally. In Bacup, Lancashire, for example, there was minimal disruption and, despite its proximity to Manchester, only one air raid was recorded and there is no record of evacuees being received. In addition to differences in demands between urban and rural situations, and at different times during the war, there were also considerable variations from one place to another. Some districts were seemingly untouched, whereas others felt the full impact of war and the immediate results of bombing campaigns from death and injury to homelessness and the longer term resultant devastation. In addition there were secondary effects from this such as early hospital discharges to make room for fresh casualties being admitted to an understaffed hospital service. In addition to the many stress-related illnesses not normally such a large part of the district nurse's workload, and having to cope with the combination of large-scale movements of patients and inadequate community staffing levels, this made the wartime workload far heavier than that of peacetime.

Despite this, it is striking that very few local nursing associations had references to the war in their monthly meetings. Business appears to have continued to revolve around everyday issues of collecting fees and maintaining the nurses' home, with only occasional reference to rationing or transport difficulties to remind the reader that the period was in any way exceptional. The business-as-usual ethos seems to be pervasive, excluding descriptions of conditions that would have been part of the common experience at the time; it is only later, in postwar discussions (including oral testimony), that these details are addressed in any depth. In one oral testimony, a nurse recounted her daily wartime work in terms that would have been routine both before and after the war before adding almost as an afterthought:

> It was all barbed wire along the sea front, not a lot of traffic, of course. We were on bikes. One or two walked. . . . I remember coming along on my auto-scooter, I think we called it, and seeing the bombs coming over, the planes dropping the bombs, coming over the electric works at Portslade, you know those big chimneys—the power station, I saw them coming over the power station, and I saw the bombs coming out of the planes . . . I got off my bike and got under a tree, as though that would save me from a bomb. . . . Anyway, that was a major incident, and then of course we had the incidents all around, bombs dropping in Brighton and various places—we were very busy![42]

REORGANISATION AND RECONSTRUCTION

The minutes of a meeting of the Interdepartmental Committee on Social Insurance and Allied Services, War Cabinet, chaired by William Beveridge, noted that at that time there were approximately 7,200 district nurses working in the United Kingdom, of whom approximately 1,000 were employed by independent (non-QNI) associations.[43] The contributory scheme was described to him as being carried out by voluntary collectors in rural areas with nearly every district having its "penny a week" plan, and in Leicester 95,000 contributors out of 260,000 (representing 27.3 percent of the population) were registered as belonging to the system, mostly through direct deduction from the payroll or through groups. The DNA representatives urged the minister to nationalise the system, thereby making it compulsory and ensuring a standard rate of contribution and removing the problem of excluded employees whose employers refused to participate, or where there were differences between place of employment and place of residence.

Miss Pilkington, Honorary Secretary to St. Helen's DNA, explained that having only 25,000 contributors out of a population of 107,000 was partly because 3,000 to 4,000 "worked in factories outside the town where there were no facilities for pay-roll deductions."[44] It was also noted that in rural areas the cost was higher (2d per week). Discussing the relationship between recruitment and pay, Mrs. Kevill-Davies (Honorary Secretary of the QNI) expressed the frustrations felt at the grassroots level: "I think in a large way it is financial, we are all waiting to know what the salaries are going to be, if they are going to be increased. The nurses want to know what their standing is going to be." Miss Wilmshurst explained the cause was partly the differential that existed between pay scales for district and hospital nurses in the past, stating "It was more so on the old scale but not the rather heterogeneous salaries that are being paid out now. There is a great deal of competition all over the country."[45] She also emphasised the importance of specialised training, saying there were thought to be approximately 1,000 registered nurses working as district nurses, not all trained Queen's Nurses nor village nurse-midwives, but mostly "older" nurses.

The comments about recruitment and pay had been articulated more strongly the previous year by a nurse writing anonymously, highlighting the inherent insecurity not only of the wartime situation in which she found herself, but also of more deep-rooted financial uncertainties:

> I am hoping for a plan of reconstruction. I hope no nurse, choosing District work, will have the burden of worry I have had. Very few nurses in training know how District Nursing is financed, and it would be a shock to many working on Districts if they knew the financial outlook of many associations. Hand-to-mouth existence in many [. . .] The Health Visitors and School Nurses are financed by the rates, yet they only serve a section of the ratepayers; the District Nurse serves all.[46]

This anticipated the Rushcliffe Committee's recommendations for nurses' salaries that were published in 1943. Although representing a considerable improvement for the nurses, these might have increased the difficult financial situation being faced by many DNAs at that time, although they were initially to be subsidised to cover some of the salary increase.[47] A rise in the nurses' salaries added to the difficulties caused by wartime demographic flux, which hindered promotion of the Provident system, collections of subscriptions and donations, and the National Gardens Scheme, all of which constituted important sources of income locally and nationally. From the QNI's viewpoint, the recommendations of the report from the Rushcliffe Committee were important because the pay differential recognised the extra value of a registered nurse or nurse-midwife with district training (almost synonymous with Queen's training[48]) as well as the inferred acknowledgment that State Registration should be a standard requirement for district nursing. Nevertheless it can be seen from Table 3.2 that there were also financial advantages to be gained by the independent, non-Queen's Nurses who could work from private premises.

From as early as 1942, district nurses had joined GPs, social workers, local government officers, and central government, in planning for the public health needs of the anticipated postwar period.[49] The QNI was involved in negotiations between official bodies, such as county councils, and the Ministries of Health and of Labour, in providing evidence to the Rushcliffe Committee (on nurses' pay) and the Beveridge Committee (on the future role of district nursing in an NHS).

Fox described the unsatisfactory negotiations between the Ministry of Health and representations from the QNI, the Ranyard Nursing Association, the London Central Council, and the RCN, concentrating on the period from 1944 onward, stating that "meetings went on from 1944 to 1947 without the consultations finding common ground," and that "in the end, compromise was forced upon it [the QNI]."[50] Furthermore, she

Table 3.2 Rushcliffe Recommended Salaries (District Nursing)

District Nurse Category	*Resident*	*Nonresident*
District candidates in training	£95	Not applicable
Registered nurse and midwife with district training	£140–£200	£260–£340
Registered nurse and midwife without district training	£130–£190	£240–£310
Registered nurse with district training	£120–£180	£230–£300
Registered nurse	£110–£170	£220–£290
Village nurse-midwife	£110–£170	£210–£270

Note. From Lord Rushcliffe (Chair) MOH Cmd 6487 *Second Report of Nurses' Salaries Committee: Salaries and Emoluments of Male Nurses, Public Health Nurses, District Nurses and State Registered Nurses in Nurseries* (1943). This scale was updated in November 1946 together with a London additional allowance.

criticised the QNI for claiming to represent district nursing as a whole, and for failing to take account of independent associations or consulting its own membership.

Certainly the QNI saw itself as the obvious (and probably only) choice to run a national district nursing service, with the possibility of contracting this out to the Ministry of Health, while retaining its voluntaristic identity. There is evidence to suggest this was not popular with the independent nursing associations that remained unaffiliated to the QNI and even with a few associations that were affiliated.[51] However, these were not numerous[52] and their hostility was based on a long-held and strong resentment of the monopolistic and hierarchical system run by the QNI that threatened to control and dictate, or even exclude them completely. In retrospect, it seems misguided and arrogant for the QNI to have claimed to be representative of district nursing as a whole without consulting these independent district associations. Yet bearing in mind that many village nurse-midwives came under the regulation and control of the QNI, on a percentage basis it could clearly be said to represent a large sector of the workforce.[53] To have represented all its membership, let alone the entire workforce, would have been an impossibility even in peacetime. In fact, the QNI also represented a large number of village nurse-midwives employed by affiliated associations, and was the only existing professional organisation prepared and able to represent district nurses. Taking the figures for Lancashire in 1939 as an example, there were 155 (QNI) affiliated associations employing a total of 576 nurses, of whom 507 were Queen's Nurses, compared with 12 unaffiliated societies employing just 13 nurses and two private associations.[54] Similar figures exist for the other fifty-one (out of a total of sixty-two) counties in England and Wales (see Table 3.3), which were affiliated with the QNI. At the time that negotiations began in 1942, therefore, its claim to represent district nurses would seem a more reasonable one than Fox suggested.

Despite the difficulties imposed by war restrictions, the QNI did attempt to consult their membership as far as was practicable: The Queen's

Table 3.3 Wartime Queen's Nurses Percentages of Total District Nurses Working in England and Wales

Date	Number of Queen's Nurses	Total of District Nurses	% Queen's Nurses of Total
1939	3,337	7,204	46%
1942	3,123	6,298	50%
1945	3,315	6,726	49%
1947	3,428	7,439	46%

Note. Figures taken from SA/QNI Box 1 B8-37, Box 2 B38-45 Published Annual Reports 1910–1947.

Superintendents had their own society that met on an annual conference basis. In addition, the Queen's Nurses' League was formed in 1941 from the ordinary membership of the QNI to provide a local forum for discussion and a mouthpiece for (Queen's) district nurses, "the great aim being for the profession as a whole to be of one mind and one speaking body to the Government when the time comes [for postwar reconstruction], *as come it will.*"[55] This reflected a growing concern that the RCN did not represent district nurses as a single specialist group, there being no District Nurse Section within the College at that time.[56] At that time district nursing fell under the broad banner of the RCN's Public Health Section together with HVs, school nurses, and public health nurses, and district midwives were represented separately by the Royal College of Midwives.

In fact, the RCN did not share the opinion voiced by the QNI, that dependency on voluntary schemes was the best way forward in raising the professional status of nurses. Without wishing to defend the QNI's blinkered vision on this particular point within these negotiations, the Labour Government's emphasis on nationalisation and regionalisation included the abolition of contributory health insurance schemes on which most DNAs were dependent for their finance.[57] Likewise, the transfer of power to local health authorities presented the QNI with some impossible choices, perhaps the most difficult of which was to relinquish its powers of inspection when regular monitoring was seen by them to be fundamental in the maintenance of standards of practise and employment—without this the QNI felt a district nurse could not practice as a Queen's Nurse. A compromise was eventually negotiated, which resulted in the QNI conceding to allow counties and boroughs the less expensive and restrictive "membership" rather than full affiliation with the QNI with all the rules and regulations this implied. Nevertheless, foreseeing fragmentation of the district nursing service, in 1947 a cautionary note was expressed regarding local health authority responsibilities for training and supervision of nurses. It was feared that, without imposing the safeguards of regular supervisory inspections, standards would fall and the QNI's professional ideals would be forsaken.[58] A one-time grant of £4,000 was paid to the QNI by the Ministry of Health in 1949 toward the costs of training district nurses, but the balance of training costs had to be found by the QNI and no further assistance could be promised.[59]

AFTER THE WAR: RECRUITMENT AND THE PUBLIC AND PROFESSIONAL IMAGE

In 1947 the QNI commented that, "The improved conditions under which such nurses now work and the greatly increased salaries payable to them under the Rushcliffe Committee scale should do much to encourage recruitment to this most important branch of the Nation's health service."[60] At the end of the war, London experienced a considerable and rapid return of its evacuated population: For example, in 1945 in East London just sixteen district nurses paid 77,600 visits to 2,445 patients, and almost 2,000 of these were cases from whom no financial contributions were due to the Society from any public authority.[61] Nationally, staffing shortages inspired a number of recruitment appeals, which were combined with appeals for public financial support for the QNI at national and local branch levels, both during and immediately after the war.[62] For recruitment purposes, the appeal leaflets contain descriptions of wartime devotion to duty shown by district nurses, coupled with the presentation of an instantly recognisable image of a respected and dependable figure within the community making an essential contribution to the nation's health. The opportunity to develop high standards while "meeting emergencies" and "reducing chaos to order" are the qualities that are most heavily stressed. The uncertainty of the approaching NHS resulted in a fall in contributions to DNAs, creating a crisis in 1947 as the associations still had to fulfil their financial commitments. Where patients did not belong to a contributory scheme, nurses would often have to decide what fee the patient should pay. Guidance on this was that:

> If the family is necessitous and is in receipt of public assistance, or is an old age pensioner without other means, nursing will be given free of charge. For other persons the nurse will judge what payment is appropriate. The actual cost varies from 2s. 6d. to 3s. 6d. per visit, and those who can afford it are asked to pay this amount. If this appears difficult, then a proportion of this or a weekly charge is made.[63]

This was an aspect of their work many nurses disliked intensely, finding it "embarrassing and distasteful asking the patients about their income and expenditure"[64] and having to issue receipts for payment and entering the information in their case books, "the amount varying from as little as threepence to as much as two-and-six per week or per visit."[65] In the towns this money was handed to the superintendent, who kept the accounts of patient payments, thereby retaining a certain degree of patient confidentiality. However, in the rural situation this information was less well protected, as one nurse described:

> You collected as much money as you could and indeed you encouraged the patients to pay a penny a week and they had a card which was marked and then once a month you took any money that you collected to this good woman who called herself "the Secretary."[66]

In contrast, another nurse-midwife who worked in Hertfordshire before the NHS Act, when asked if she had to collect money from the patients, seemed more comfortable with the situation saying:

Oh, yes, yes we collected money—they paid me but I couldn't keep it for myself of course. I think for midwifery it was 25/-, and I think it went to the secretary. Well, we kept them in bed for ten days and we went to see them each day. . . . And you always used to carry a bag as an emergency, because people were very poor then you see, so you needed a bag of things in case of an emergency. But then of course if you are on a district for a time you get to know the people, don't you? I used to visit them in their own homes and go through the things they'd want, you see?[67]

District nurses were—and still are—at the front line in witnessing hardship and poverty as members of the primary health care team with perhaps the most prolonged contact with the sick in their own homes, and this comment concerning an emergency "bag of things" reflects many others from our interviewees. The nurses were expected to recognise neediness and would either apply to the nursing association's comforts guild or linen guild or would hold their own supply of baby clothes, bed linen, and sometimes even nursing equipment such as commodes and wheelchairs. Our interviewees stressed that considerable tact and diplomacy were needed, especially in the pre-NHS era, to avoid causing offence either in offering this kind of material support or in offering advice. This was particularly so during the war period where, for example home sanitary conditions were often far from ideal and food rationing presented additional problems where diet was a significant factor in recovery or healing.

CONCLUSIONS

At the end of the war, the Earl of Athlone wrote a letter to all Queen's Nurses thanking them for their hard work and stating, "I commend you all for your steadfast service, so quietly and cheerfully carried out, and for your courage, so often unsung. I know that District Nurses can be relied upon to continue to serve during the stress and strains of post-war life which throws increasing demands on us all."[68] This echoed an earlier sentiment first expressed in the first editorial following the outbreak of war, at which time many hundreds of patients were being discharged from hospitals to be nursed in the community and, "in the reception areas the nurses will be looked to by mothers and the foster mothers in the billets for advice and help [. . .] This work may seem less spectacular than that of nursing the wounded, whether from the Services or civilian population and may not be so realised by the general public."[69] Apart from a few surviving illustrations of the more spectacular and undeniably courageous actions of district nurses, there is little record of the continuously heavy caseloads and understaffing, nor of the increased responsibilities resulting from depleted numbers of medical colleagues, experienced on a daily basis by many district nurses throughout the country during wartime.

The lack of formal recognition of district nursing lies in its location in the "unseen" female domestic sphere. Interestingly, those interviewees who described their war experiences away from district nursing—either in the armed services or in hospitals—displayed a similarly understated attitude to their own personal contribution, so that it is possible this was symptomatic of an outlook that accepted the hardships and dangers as a wider communal experience. War might also have been a positive experience, a means of empowerment with nursing being offered as a career to some women for whom this might not have been considered an option before.

The battle for the district nurses' role in reorganisation and reconstruction of the health service that began as early as 1942 appears to sit uneasily with a wartime ethos based on making the best of a bad situation, but was in fact consistent with the widely held rationale that the war was being fought for a better future for the nation as a whole. The failure of the QNI to win its case with the Ministry can be seen as the rejection of the old order, which it typified in many ways. Their insistence on retaining a voluntaristic support system was an anachronism that, combined with lack of support from the RCN and some apparent animosity from a section of district nursing, explained the political stance that was taken toward the QNI.

4   Changing Places, 1948–1979

The thirty-year period from 1949 to 1979 marked a time of rapid and wide-ranging social, demographic, economic, and cultural change in Britain, all of which considerably affected urban and rural communities, not least in their attitudes towards and expectations from community health care provision. In the previous chapter we discussed the introduction of the NHS and the obstacles that prevented the representatives of district nursing from participating in its formulation. We consider in this chapter the transfer of responsibility for the district nursing service from the QNI and voluntarily organisations into the hands of local government. The effects of consequent changes in the training, supervision, and employment of district nurses will be viewed alongside other changes that directly affected their role, working arrangements, and consequently their professional outlook and image. A key aspect to this was the move towards a practice-based, community-care team and the drive for a nationally, professionally recognised, specialised district-nurse training. Drawing on oral histories, these changes as well as the later implications of NHS reorganisation in 1972, are explained in more practical terms to show how the nurse and patient (and informal carers) were affected and what impact this had on their intra-relationships as well as professional inter-relationships.

POSTWAR ATTITUDES TO DISTRICT NURSING: CHANGING PUBLIC AND PROFESSIONAL IMAGES

Lewis wrote that the range of occupations open to women in the postwar period increased substantially, but she pointed to a "persistence of sexual segregation of the work-force, whereby women find themselves doing different tasks from men either in the same occupational category (female teachers, male headmasters), or in different jobs (female nurses, male coalminers)."[1] This separation of roles effectively reinforced the idea that work in the female, domestic sphere was of lower status. Furthermore, although the marriage bars that had earlier forced women's resignation from most professions on marriage (including district nursing), had been removed during

World War II and were not widely reinstituted, even as late as the 1980s a majority of men and women considered that a married woman's primary responsibility was to her family.[2] This was born out by our interviewees, most of whom left nursing to marry and raise children, taking career breaks typically of ten to fifteen years, and returning as part-time employees. On their return they often accepted posts where they did not have their own districts but provided relief for full-time single women. There were a few exceptions to the lifting of the ban, such as marriage during training (including postregistration training) in some hospitals, and within the Ranyard Nursing Association. A nurse could no longer practise as a Ranyard Nurse if she was married, although several were employed on a part-time basis as relief nurses.

There was also a perception among the public at this time that district nursing did not constitute proper nursing. Implicitly, district nursing was viewed as an extension of home nursing, a support to the family carers, thereby making the nurse seem in some way inferior to, or less skilled than her hospital counterpart. Two examples taken from the oral histories demonstrate this: Both nurses worked on the district in the 1950s and 1960s. The first is from a nurse who worked in central London, and the second worked in Lancashire:

> The people who had District Nursing care worshipped the District Nurse—I mean she was absolutely wonderful. At the same time they felt she was less educated than the Hospital Nurse. I remember patients saying to me "When are you going to qualify as a nurse?" and that sort of thing. [. . .] People don't perceive hands-on nursing as being skilled nursing.[3]

> I have been asked, in a home, "Have you ever worked in a hospital?" And I said, "Yes. District nurses have all had to do their training in hospital. And when you're in the community, you're actually being nursed by qualified nurses, whereas in the hospital, although they're supervised, you may be being nursed by a student nurse."[4]

The continued existence of village nurse-midwives contributed to this misperception in the public mind where community-based nursing was viewed as the provision of basic care that did not require the same skills as those of the acute sector. Roberts described "discernible changes in attitudes to welfare provision"[5] taking place in the interwar period that included a widespread belief within the working classes that they would be better cared for in hospitals. The view that district nurses were less proficient than their hospital counterparts might well stem from this.

As part of a move toward greater integration between hospital and primary health services and the development of the health care team, the organisation of district nursing was revised in the 1960s. Following on the heels of the NHS was the proposed creation of health centres throughout the country that would include district nurses as part of the team. However, by the 1960s high capital costs meant that these were still few and far between, so GP attachment schemes were encouraged as an alternative. Under these schemes district nurses remained employees of the local health authorities but drew their caseload not from a geographically bound district, but from a given GP's patient list. The schemes also allowed district nurses to work in the GP's surgery. However, they remained distinct from *practice nurses*, who also worked with a given GP's patients but who were employed directly by that GP and did not make home visits. This system of GP attachments took over from the geographical system and has continued to prevail in most areas throughout Britain. Although it is still the case that district nurses serve remote areas, most are no longer bound to a district but to a GP or health centre and the relevant patient list. This has been the formal organisation of district nursing services since the 1960s but in practice, district nurses in remote areas remain relatively isolated and as a result have and can still experience a different level of nursing responsibility. The term *community care* first appeared in health policy documents in the 1950s[6] and Berridge pointed to the subtle changes in emphasis that it implied, notably a rise in dependence on professionals to advise on health issues. By the 1980s and 1990s community health care encompassed a range of care providers operating in an environment where rights, responsibilities, and expectations of community services had changed considerably from the early days of the NHS.

OUTCOME OF TRANSFER OF RESPONSIBILITY OF DISTRICT NURSING TO THE LOCAL HEALTH AUTHORITIES

In many cases the transfer of full responsibility for provision of home nursing was not actually made on July 5, 1948 (otherwise known as the Appointed Day, when the NHS Act officially came into effect). The greatest change to affect the district nurses was that responsibility for much of the funding, including their salaries, could be immediately transferred away from the nursing associations, effectively making the Provident schemes redundant. At this time there were 2,716 county and local DNAs affiliated with the QNI nationwide, employing a total of 8,294 district nurses, of whom 4,760 were Queen's Nurses.[7] Negotiations took place among the Ministry of Health, the County Councils' Association, the Association of Municipal Corporations, and the QNI in 1948. The outcome of these negotiations enabled local authorities, as county and county borough councils, to opt either for direct employment of district nurses or to continue using the voluntary organisations.[8] The voluntary organisations in Liverpool, for example, handed over the district service to the city's Public Health Department as late as 1959, and the London Council for District Nursing was not dissolved until March 1966, although after the Local Government Act (1963) most nursing associations had been absorbed by the new London Boroughs.[9] By September 1948 in Scotland "in one third of the Counties, the work had been delegated to the district nursing associations, and in the remaining two thirds, the local authorities (LAs) had taken over the service."[10] So, with the coming of the NHS, in a third of the local authorities there, district nurses were still recruited by the associations but employed by the local authority and accountable to the MOH.

Given that nurses had had little to do with financial matters or the cost of their service, their practice hardly changed under local authority control. The most notable practical change to their routine was that records kept by the nurses were no longer sent to the association committee for inspection but to the MOH, who would comment on the home nursing service in the MOH annual report. This shift away from the traditional authority of the association committees represented a possible threat to the quality of district nursing. It also weakened the bond between the associations and the QNI as the affiliating institution and standardising body for good practice. Expressing its continued interest in maintaining high standards of nursing in the home, the QNI encouraged county council nursing officers to forward a brief report of the nurses' work to the QNI, but under local authority control this could not be obligatory.

Furthermore, the QNI had long presided over home nursing by encouraging associations to affiliate with the QNI and to recruit only Queen's Nurses and it operated a system of inspections of district nurses' work by Queen's-appointed superintendents. The QNI was anxious to ensure the continuance of the Queen's superintendent and feared a drop in standards if the task of inspection were to be undertaken by the supervisors of midwives and HVs already employed by the local authorities but who had no district training. They suggested that where Queen's Nurses were employed by an authority not allowing inspections by a Queen's superintendent, these nurses should automatically lose their status as Queen's Nurses. After some months of discussion, a national agreement was reached whereby either county council nursing officers, who would oversee district work on behalf of the local authority, could take their Queen's district training and be placed on the Queen's Roll as soon as possible, or the QNI would be allowed to send in an inspector triennially.[11]

St. Helen's in Lancashire was one of the last voluntarily run associations to be handed over in the 1970s[12] and therefore retained a considerable degree of control over the service until then. A nurse working in St. Helen's in 1963 described a situation very similar to the conditions of work 30 years earlier, apart from the concession that she was able to work as a married woman and live outside the nurse's home once training was completed, suggesting that those associations that remained under the old system retained many of the authoritarian constraints of the past:

Some of the nurses did live in. But when you were on duty, you were expected to have lunch at the Home. I think it was because then the Superintendent knew where you were, and you had to be in for a certain time . . . but you always got a good meal! So she was making sure you were well-fed as well. . . . we had to be in for one, and you had a break till half past two, and then went out again, but you went in pairs in the afternoon, because the morning was the bulk of the work. And then you were on call until eight o'clock at night.[13]

Issues surrounding the transfer of control from voluntary associations affiliated with the QNI to local authority were discussed continuously within the QNI throughout 1948 and into the 1950s, focusing mainly on the transfer of association assets, payment for training, and the salary and superannuation of district nurses. In November 1948, the QNI distributed a circular to all affiliated associations encouraging them to transfer their funds to the QNI at the time of their dissolution. Even the smaller associations had accumulated certain assets such as property or a car. By 1948, precedents were set as assets were handed over to the local authorities. In Shetland, for example:

The County clerk reported to the Public Health Committee on the decisions indicated on a form of return sent to the associations. Fetlar had just purchased an auto-cycle which was handed over free and told the Council that they [the local Fetlar nursing association] had been granted permission to erect a garage and coal store. In Northmavine the nurse's car and garage at North Roe will be given free while Delting took the same action on their nurse's car on the stipulation that it will only be used by the nurse in that district.[14]

Some associations had been able to provide a car for their nurse from very early on, whereas others either did not have the funds or did not consider it necessary. One nurse who worked in Maybole district, Ayrshire, in the 1940s told how a local gentleman wanted to buy the nurse a car but then discovered that the committee had enough money to provide one, but was not prepared to do so. The committee later purchased a car and the gentleman in question donated a garage.[15] Under the voluntary scheme the financial burdens on the smaller associations had been considerable. Not only had they been responsible for collecting subscriptions and donations, the nurse's salary, accommodation, transport, and all administrative costs, but also the materials used by the nurse such as gauze, bandages, preparations, and all other consumables which the patients could not provide. Under the NHS these would be provided through the GP's prescription, by the pharmacist, at a cost to the state. With the burden of cost removed, financial discrepancies between associations from one area to another decreased and therefore the more extreme discrepancies in provision no longer existed.

As agents of the local authority, local associations under the NHS could apply to have their nurses admitted to the government superannuation scheme "but no allowance would be made for past service" and they would have to make payment for this on a noncontributory scale. Under a moral obligation to provide for its nurses, the burden for this would fall on the QNI Pension Fund, so the need to replenish the fund was crucial. However, association constitutions did not always allow for the direct transfer of funds and many, as in the case of the Comrie and Crieff DNA, used their cash assets by reforming as benevolent societies for their community.[16] Some associations responded immediately to the new system by insuring their nurse's car for one month only and freezing their funds from that date "until such time as their disposal was thought desirable."[17] For all, the important issue was to ensure a nursing service continued.

In fact many local authorities continued to subcontract responsibility for training and inspection of district nurses to the Queen's Institute or the Ranyard Nursing Association, and a number of voluntary-run nursing associations continued to raise funds by subscription to provide "patient comforts."[18] However, in other areas the local authorities placed responsibility for recruiting and managing district nurses on the department of the MOH, and in-service training was provided at a local level on a rather haphazard basis. In turn, he or she often devolved this task to the senior HV in that department, adding to growing interprofessional tensions, as discussed later. We would therefore argue that apart from standardisation of salaries by most local authorities, the immediate outcome of nationalisation was less national standardisation rather than more, as might have been expected.

As we have seen in previous chapters, recruitment drives have always been an issue in district nursing and this period proved to be no exception. An article promoting recruitment published in 1951 stated that in 1948 there were affiliated with the QNI in England and Wales, Scotland and Ireland, 2,716 county and district associations employing nearly 9,000 district nurses and midwives, of whom 4,760 were Queen's Nurses. The same article also noted that "the only national body providing training in district nursing is the Queen's Institute which trains over 600 nurses annually."[19] However, financing this training remained sufficiently haphazard that an appeal had to be launched in 1949 for annual subscriptions to the QNI to cover costs of training, research work, and its international work together with the long-service and welfare funds for retired Queen's Nurses.[20] In 1951 a similar appeal outlining the work of the QNI in more detail explained the need for well-structured training and effective regulation through regular inspections by the QNI Visitors or County Superintendents.[21] The appeal then added a disturbing comment that "the reports are considered at the Central Office of the QNI, appropriate entries are made on the nurses' record cards and suitable recommendations are sent to the employing authority. In addition, the nature of the reports makes it possible for the Central Office to have a knowledge of the standard and nature of work undertaken in each area and also of the suitability of the nurses for such work, thus mutually benefiting employers and unemployed." It is difficult not to view this from a contemporary perspective with the rights of the employee in mind, but even at that time this must have seemed heavily authoritarian and weighted in favour of the employers.

At this time the village nurse-midwife was being steadily replaced by (hospital trained) state registered nurses some with midwifery training, but many of whom had no district training and later, by assistant nurses and state enrolled nurses. District nurses were often interviewed and appointed by an MOH with little knowledge of the content of nursing training, but with the expectation that the nurses could learn district practice and technique on the job, as did the GP at this time.[22] The haphazard nature of this situation is illustrated by a district nurse who worked in Middlesex:

> This friend persuaded me to go and see the Doctor, the Medical Officer of Health, about the post and off I went and she welcomed me with open arms and said just try it for a fortnight to relieve the nurse. I said, "Well I haven't done any training, I don't know what to do at all—I've no idea what to do with dressings, dirty dressings"—I mean in a hospital everything is laid on for you. Well she said, "You can have a week or a few days with the nurse that's going on holiday and you'll soon get used to it. It will be quite all right." [. . .] So that's what I did. I did a few days and learned the rudiments of District Nursing with this particular nurse. At the end of the fortnight—I had quite enjoyed the work.[23]

This casual attitude contrasts dramatically with the QNI's earlier emphasis on professional training and regulation, and later demands for a postregistration qualification that would reinstate professional status and respectability.

TO TRAIN OR NOT TO TRAIN: THE DILEMMA

From the viewpoint of diminished professional status, the attitude typified by this quote places district nursing at a disadvantage compared with other members of the emerging community healthcare team. This was also reflected in a lack of recognition by the wider nursing profession. For example, at a district nursing conference held during World War II, regret was expressed that no district nursing experience was included in general nurse training, which inevitably was having a significant impact on recruitment: "Most delegates had experienced a lack of interest in district nursing in their hospitals, and some had taken it up against the wishes of their Matrons."[24] Another nurse commented, "Many nurses on completing their hospital training . . . are wishful to take up another branch of the profession, but fear to do so as they know so little about nursing outside of hospital."[25] Indeed, Dora Williams OBE remembered that the RCN branch in Plymouth to which she was appointed chairman, was run "by what appeared ageing hospital matrons who took it in turns to be Chairman, Secretary and Treasurer for no one dared to propose lesser fry."[26] Her appointment as a practising district nurse marked "the first time a nurse not living in hospital had held office." The situation was the same in the higher office of RCN College Council to which she was elected in the 1960s.

As both White and Baly recounted, the issue of training featured in debates surrounding home nursing provision under the NHS and ultimately in the struggle toward professionalisation for district nurses that continued into the 1960s.[27] After the institution of the NHS there was disagreement on the matter of responsibility for district nurse training within the new structures being mooted. Following the Wood Report of 1947 (set up to examine the recruitment and requirements of nurses) the Nurses Act 1949 amended the constitution of the General Nursing Council (GNC) and rendered it unfit for this responsibility, as it did not include postregistration training among its new institutional functions. In this context, the QNI, as providers of postregistration training, continued to lobby for a position within the new organisation, finally gaining its voice in the appointment of the General Superintendent of the QNI, Miss E. J. Merry, as one of two nurse members of the Central Health Services Council. The issue of training was addressed again in 1953 after some of the local authorities questioned the value of district training when they could save the cost of further training by using general nurses. A prolonged debate over the length and quality of training ensued, with the QNI trying to protect its high standards and the need for a training course of at least six months. The working party, influenced by the growing cost of the NHS and the economic benefits of a shorter training period, found in favour of a four-month training course as the requirement for local authorities.

In an attempt to remedy this, in 1955 a Ministry of Health Report recommended introducing a compulsory, postregistration training for district nurses.[28] It recorded that in England and Wales, for the year ended December 1952, there were a total of 8,884 district nurses practicing, of whom 4,123 were Queen's trained. A small number of the remainder (130) were Ranyard-trained nurses, leaving 4,631 with only minimal district training. However, the report's working party was seriously split on accepting the length (four months) and content of the proposed training and three of the sixteen members of the working party would not agree that this was sufficient. It is not surprising to find these members were Miss Merry, General Superintendent of the QNI; Dr. Struthers, Chairman of the QNI Training Subcommittee; and Miss Treleaven, Senior Superintendent of the Ranyard DNA. All three had strong opinions based on their personal experience of district nursing as well as reflecting the interests of their institutional backgrounds. They expressed their disagreement with the majority's conclusions both through dissenting and by publishing a minority report that argued strongly against shortening the training, pointing to the need for supervision and guidance for practical work as well as theoretical training. The report outlined the difficulties and poor standards of living that still existed in some rural areas for which special training was needed before a nurse could effectively apply skills learned in the hospital environment.[29]

A leader article in *The Lancet* in 1955 compared training for general practice medicine and for district nursing, stating that a doctor entering general practice requires at least a year to learn his job "to look after patients without the resources of the hospital behind him" together with acquiring the administrative and bureaucratic knowledge necessary to do the job and "to gain not only the full confidence of his patients, but sufficient confidence in himself."[30] In comparison, the writer felt the district nurse required at least as much extra training because she had to "learn these things too, at a more fundamental level; for it is one thing to call and give directions about the care of a patient, and another to carry them out in any and every kind of home, whether clean or squalid, well equipped or bare of the simplest amenities." It was strongly in support of the minority report and noted that The College of General Practitioners, whose members worked closely with district nurses, favoured extending training to a year in line with that of GPs. The article noted that by 1953 "some 4000 district nurses in England and Wales—about half, that is of the SRNs in the home nursing service—had had no special district training."[31] The majority working party report itself observed that "the district nurse is no longer working in isolation: she is a member of the public-health team, and is in constant touch with colleagues working in parallel professions."[32]

The idealism that underpinned the desire for national training and qualification reflected a growing belief in specialisation and professionalisation that was pervading society as a whole. More specifically, the emphasis on specialisms could be seen permeating the fields of medicine and nursing extensively, highlighting the importance of the training system and new academic model. One of the responses to this was the setting up and development of courses in community health run by the Queen's Institute through the William Rathbone Staff College established in 1960 in what was formerly the central home of the Liverpool Queen Victoria DNA.[33] These were initially intended for district nurses as refresher courses and a three-month course in administration, but later became more multidisciplinary, to include hospital nurses, HVs, and social workers.[34] The inclusion of the latter, which was instigated in the early 1970s, illustrates a broader acceptance of the team approach toward community health care from the nursing establishment. In 1963 the QNI also appointed Miss Lisbeth Hockey as Nursing Research Officer. Hockey conducted several groundbreaking studies gathering information on the changing role of district nursing and GPs' understandings of this role, and on how hospital discharge arrangements could be improved to make more efficient use of district nurses.[35] These and other reports underline the extent of the lack of interprofessional communication and understanding at this time.[36]

No longer feeling able to argue its case, in 1968 the QNI passed all responsibilities for training and examining district nurses to local authorities. Training centres had already been established in many areas and a National Certificate in District Nursing was awarded after successful completion of courses, with the Department of Health having responsibility for overseeing training arrangements. However, concern was expressed ten years later that this was still not statutory, nor was the National Certificate a prerequisite for service.[37] The QNI's correspondence with the Briggs Committee highlighted the importance of quality teaching and support in recruiting the more highly qualified entrants.[38] It also stressed the importance of adequate assessment of students, recommending a national, rather than a regional register for external assessment. In addition, concern was expressed that there should be strong representation of community nurses on GNC education boards and committees. The Briggs Report[39] did stress the need for specialised training for community postregistration courses of comparable standard to other hospital-based courses and the RCN underlined the importance of this, reporting an eighty percent increase in total numbers of persons nursed by the home nursing service in 1971–1972, including a significant rise in the younger age group and the acutely ill. However, the failure to change the 1968 arrangements by providing district nurses with their own statutory body when HVs and midwives had their own independent training councils perpetuated the professional inequality between district nurses and their colleagues in community health care. It was not until 1979 that legislation sanctioned the establishment of a District Nursing Joint Committee under the newly formed United Kingdom Central Council for Nursing, Midwifery and Health Visiting (UKCC).

CHANGING INTERPROFESSIONAL RELATIONSHIPS

Throughout this period, HVs were frequently seen as representing a major threat to the professional status and autonomy of district nurses. At the first Queen's League Conference held in 1942 several points had been raised demonstrating a growing concern together with portents of escalating intraprofessional tensions. The first of these was an appeal concerning their respective pay structures, proposing that the salaries of Queen's Nurses should not be less than that of HVs to "attract the young, the keen and the best who are in search of a profession."[40] Second, concerning training, the question was raised whether it would be possible to include the HVs' training for Queen's Nurses as it would create greater unity with the public health services and establish the QNI as a more complete training body. In reply, the General Superintendent of the QNI recorded that just such a scheme for combined training was currently with the Ministry of Health awaiting governmental approval.[41] At this time both midwives and HVs had their own examining bodies and to be qualified and certified in these areas did not require the SRN as a prior qualification, whereas in district nursing this was a prerequisite. Although the QNI aspired to become the national examining body for district nursing, the fact that by 1948 no such body existed represented a major professional disadvantage.

During the period following the NHS Act, and before the Nurses, Midwives and Health Visitors Act (1979), the relationship between district nurses and midwives and HVs became undeniably uncomfortable. All claimed membership of a community team in which an external harmonious professional image was projected to the public although the private face was often one of resentments and discord. This situation was rooted in the nineteenth-century origins in which duties were not clearly demarcated and therefore overlapped, particularly in public health's highly prized role of health missioner and the postnatal care of mothers and babies. The resultant misunderstandings and rivalries increased following 1929 when local authorities took responsibility for the employment of HVs, providing them with far greater security than their district nursing colleagues, and enabling them to work closely with MOHs. Baly argued that the older midwives and district nurses resented the new, younger, college-trained HVs, and the better educated nurses also resented them because HVs were perceived as rivals. District nurses from the latter group were aspiring to extend their range of community health expertise into the potentially more lucrative fields of public health nursing. HVs represented a major obstacle to that progression.[42]

In addition, HVs were themselves feeling professionally insecure and undervalued due to the perceived threat of replacement by social workers from the late 1940s until the early 1960s.[43] Miss Sankey, herself an HV and district nurse, expressed what many interviewees also confirmed as their perception of the problem; that is, she believed the HVs "felt they were a superior race and the DN was a poor relation. I remember how surprised a HV was when I told her I too was a HV!"[44] She found many HVs to be "officious," giving themselves "airs and graces," and related how, when working as a trainee Health Visitor, "it came as a shock when a door was slammed in my face," yet when visiting the same house dressed as a nurse the following day, she was made welcome.[45]

A nurse in South Wales gave a similar account, describing her relationship with HVs:

> Not a very good relationship in the very beginning because they thought they [HVs] were the highly qualified people and knew exactly what was going on and this that and the other, and yet the District Nurse could prove to them that they were quite as knowledgeable too. Because a few instances occurred in the community, especially on a Saturday when Health Visitors didn't work, I could never understand why problems then ended on a Friday at five o'clock—with Health Visiting—because District Nurses took over on a weekend! [. . .] It did improve when I got

the job [of Nursing Officer] because I would not tolerate the fact that we were lesser than them, you know in any way at all and I think that our nurses proved it because a lot were doing diplomas, and degrees at the time.[46]

The situation was exacerbated by the fact that in some areas district nurses were now supervised by HVs, fuelling this atmosphere of resentment. In 1957 an anomalous salary award giving five percent to district nurses but fifteen percent to HVs, increased this friction still further.[47] A letter from P. J. Morland, Director of QNI (c. 1972) expressed concern regarding the new grading of community nursing posts, particularly noting the District Nursing Sister was to be rated as Grade II when the HV was to be a higher paid and higher status Grade I. This was seen as "a disincentive to recruitment and retention at a time when the need from the role of district nurse has never been greater."[48]

However, an HV who worked in St. Helen's pointed to an additional factor, left over from the previous decade, that was clearly region-specific but that must have added to this feeling of acrimony and resentment to greater or lesser degrees according to the local authority under which the system operated:

When I was riding round in a car, as a Health Visitor, our district nurses were still on bikes, because they were working for a charitable organisation. . . . Pilkington's provided the building that they worked from, and a certain amount of money . . . I remember, in 1974, when it was . . . the whole sort of affair—district nurses, Health Visitors, district midwives—went under the auspices of the Health Service, rather than the County Borough Council and charity and whatever. And I remember one of the bosses telling us that the district nurses were so short of facilities, you know . . . beds . . . walking aids, things like that.[49]

Many felt the GP attachment system introduced in the early 1970s changed the relationship through more regular encounters and therefore improved communication:

We never bothered with Health Visitors—the district nurse and the Health Visitor was like you know chalk and cheese . . . well when the new amalgamation came round we got, we were in the clinic with them you know, and I got very friendly with the Health Visitors then and then we used to—we had much more communication with them. We hadn't—in the beginning there was no communication with the Health Visitors.[50]

Similarly, several of the GPs expressed an antipathy toward HVs. For example, a doctor from Rotherham said he thought the HVs "were a bit of a useless crowd, on the whole," whereas the nurses "were very good; I never had any fault to find with them."[51] Similarly, a doctor from Ulverston described the district nurses he worked with as "very useful—taking stitches out at home that would save you a job" and "dressing chronic leg ulcers and bathing people,"[52] but admitted not understanding what the HVs were meant to do and consequently, not getting on too well with them. To what extent this was a matter of poor communication and unfamiliarity is not certain, but it would seem likely that this played a significant part, as things changed according to some interviewees when the team began to work from offices under the same roof. Even though the NHS Act largely removed the competitive element, communication problems certainly still existed between GPs and district nurses in the 1960s. One example was described by a district nurse:

> I remember one night, it being very very foggy, and I was on duty, and at ten to eight, we got a call to go and give an injection. And Matron said, "Well, it's too foggy for you to drive, you'll have to walk." And I had my little black bag, and I walked all the way to . . . about four miles from here. And I walked it there, and walked it back, to give a morphia injection. Well, it had to be done. Someone had to go. Someone needed it! (Prompt: Could the doctor have done it?) I suppose so, but some doctors wouldn't, would they? Some doctors just wouldn't give the injections, that was a nursing duty. It depended on the doctor. (Prompt: How did you get on with the doctors, generally?) Fine. Being a geographical area, of course, we weren't doctor-attached, so you went to . . . to different doctors . . . Still very much, I suppose, if you look back, you were the handmaiden, because what they said went. You didn't query things the same as sometimes you could now.[53]

Although this quote applies the term "handmaiden" to district nurses, this implied relationship of subservience was one established in the hospital wards. Oral testimony presents a strong argument to suggest that the situation was altered in the community context.[54] The relationship between nurses and the GPs they worked alongside in the community was more akin to Stein's doctor–nurse game theory where the nurse should "be bold, have initiative, and be responsible for making significant recommendations, while at the same time she must appear passive. This must be done in such a manner so as to make her recommendations appear to be initiated by the physician."[55] On the other hand, many district nurses felt no need to enter into such a game. Where they were confident in particular skills, they neither took the subservient role nor reverted to the manipulative ways of the doctor–nurse game:

> I could say such and such a person's got tonsillitis . . . all I would do is say to the doctor, such and such a person, I'm sure he's got tonsillitis.

He'll need you to see him and give him antibiotics or something, and that was done.[56]

Nurses opting for careers in the district saw that priorities in the community were different from those in hospitals. Reasons commonly given for moving into district nursing included a desire "to be my own boss" and the opportunity to deal with patients as people, with lives and families outside the hospital setting. A holistic approach to health care was part of the language of district nursing and part of its attraction. Although recognising the doctor's status as the medical authority, district nurses freed themselves from it by clearly delineating nursing from medical practice. They invariably defined their relationship with doctors as good, not by virtue of being social or professional equals, but by being able to reconcile the nursing care and medical cure of the patient in a relatively unproblematic way. They viewed district work as nursing in a partnership with medicine, where the distinction between caring and curing, and nursing and medicine was not so much a matter for negotiation but a defining factor in professional relationships.[57]

Communication among members of the emerging community care team appears to have been the main stumbling-block in its effective teamwork and cooperation. Merry described contact between doctor and district nurse as taking place largely by telephone or written message, or via the doctor's letter handed to the patient's relative, but added that in a country district the nurse-midwife would be more likely to meet HV and GP face-to-face and know each other well.[58] This rural–urban difference was reiterated by a GP who described the inadequacies of contact, "by a series of notes or telephone calls and hastily scribbled thanks" but felt the "lucky general practitioners and district nurses in this respect are those in isolated country areas who are brought by circumstances more closely together, and, for geographical reasons, care for the same population of patients," adding, "What hospital physician would contemplate the care of patients without periodic discussion with the ward sister?"[59] Prior to GP practice-based organisation of district nurses, a typical method of communication between doctor and nurse or between central office and nurse during the daytime would be messages left at the post office or chemist, as described by a district nurse working in Nottingham:

Another way was, each nurse, in each area or district, or part of . . . a portion of it, that's her "patch" as we call it, and the males as well, we used to have a chemist's shop, local chemist, I had one attached here . . . two mile away, and I used to go twice a day, morning and afternoon, mid-morning and mid-afternoon, "Any messages?" you know?[60]

Although most interviewees agreed that if they wanted to see the doctor it could be arranged on an informal basis during surgery times or at the patient's house, having an office within the GP's practice clearly made a big difference to work organisation.

THE TEAM APPROACH AND THE MEDICALISATION OF NURSING

The concept of a primary multidisciplinary health care team was suggested in 1920 by the Dawson Report as part of its recommendations for health centres.[61] An article written by Dr. Fisher, a GP working in Lewisham and Bromley, noted the problems in interprofessional communications at that time, stating that there was "no common meeting place and communication was usually limited to the telephone."[62] The HV, district nurse, midwife, almoners, and other community-care workers were curiously described collectively by this GP as the "social workers."

A more enlightened view was expressed by a country doctor who wrote about the (community and rural-based) district nurses working with him a decade later:

> The district nurses are to us in the villages exactly what the house staff are to the consultants in a hospital. They know the set-up, the social background, the oecology [sic], of the people in the village very much better than we do, and it is from them that we general practitioners obtain a great deal of information that we do not get from the patients themselves. It is very often the things that the patients themselves want to gloss over and keep away from the practitioner that are the things which matter, and it is those things, such as the anxieties and difficulties in the homes of the people, that the district nurses can and do tell us. Therefore in the country villages, where the district nurse is living among the doctor's patients, she is the absolute key-point. In the country we are rung up by the district nurses and we ring them up ourselves, and we also meet them. There are six district nurses in my neighbourhood and I meet every one of them at least once a week, either because she is in the patient's house when I call there or because she comes to see me about a case, or I go to see her about a case when I am in the village.[63]

Although this GP seemed to have had more interaction with the district nurses than many, his perception of their role continued to be as subordinate assistant. This view is consistent with that expressed by the GPs interviewed by ourselves and by Bevan, many of whom described the district nurse as "very helpful."[64] Most also provided a very vague description of what the nurse did, such as "dressing varicose ulcers and this, that and the other,"[65] or "Well, nursing . . . seeing what people needed in their own home, reporting back . . . Mainly a matter of tradition and good sense."[66] Not all saw the move to GP attachment and primary care team as a positive move. A doctor who worked in Sunderland preferred the earlier system, saying he felt communication was simpler, being more direct and to the point: "In the 1950s you would find a little note behind the mantelpiece [. . .] from the nurse."[67] Similarly, a GP from Worcester explained there was "none of this ringing some office or whatever. No you just rang them up and talked to them, and said 'Mrs. Jones is out, could you pop in and have a look at her?' And she popped in and if she was worried she rang you. And if she wasn't she got on with the job."[68]

Baly attributed the general recognition of the need for a much closer, community health team approach, to a response to changes in the pattern of illness and the demands for different types of care. She believed these to have been urged for more than sixty years by would-be reformers of the system, unsuccessfully, and asserted that resistance came largely from the "family doctor who feared loss of independence and interference with the doctor–patient relationship."[69] Accepting this viewpoint, the removal of a significant portion of the competitive aspect afforded to GPs by the NHS Act, opened up possibilities for a closer professional relationship between the GP and the district nurse. This was enhanced by increased demands from technicalisation within medicine, creating a need for increased teamwork and a widening of the nursing role to encompass some jobs previously reserved for doctors. Walby et al. referred to this as "the glorious ideal of the ethical professional" in which "each profession sees to the achievement of its own standards of work."[70]

The establishment of the Royal College of General Practitioners in 1952 and subsequently a successful negotiation for a new pay structure for GPs in 1956 might be seen as indications of changes in medical education and of the organisation of GPs' practices that effectively provided the family doctor with a raised professional status.[71] This contrasted with the professional doldrums in which district nursing was placed during the same period. In *Good General Practice: A Report of a Survey*, a study of general practice medicine published in 1954, Dr. Stephen Taylor gave considerable attention to district nursing.[72] In particular, he drew attention to the "outstandingly good" relationship between district nurses and GPs "with very few exceptions," adding that this was not merely fortuitous. The general impression of the report is very supportive of district nursing. However, he wrote that "she [the district nurse] and her superintendent are used to taking their marching orders from the doctors in clinical charge of the patients." This remark is evidently not intended to insult but merely reflects the wide difference in professional standing between the two at this point, with the GP confident in his professional ownership of the patient. Taylor stressed that many nurses were being underutilised, particularly in towns where "GPs fail to realise what the nurse can achieve" or "fail to organise contact with the nurse," quoting one area where of the forty-eight GPs, only twenty were regular users of the local district nursing service.[73]

Most members of the medical profession therefore welcomed the Gillie Report in 1963, which revived the idea that community nurses should become attached to specific groups of doctors and their practice populations.[74] This used similar language in explaining that the GP "should use the domiciliary team of workers (Health Visitors, district nurses etc.) as the consultant uses his ancillary staff in hospital," describing them as "tools to do his job properly," itemised alongside equipment and premises.[75] A GP writing at the time emphasised:

> If general practitioner and district nurse are to work usefully together, loyalty to each other is essential. The GP's decisions may be right, or wrong; but he (or she) will expect support from the district nurse or midwife in carrying out the treatment or management ordered, in all her dealings with the patient or household. [. . .] She will do nothing but harm if she instils a suspicion in the patient's mind that the doctor has misjudged the seriousness of his condition and that hospitalisation would be safer.[76]

The tone of each of these examples strongly underlines the relationship that was envisaged by GPs in reducing the autonomy of the district nurse to a more subservient role. An article by a county nursing officer considering setting up nursing teams attached to GPs noted a few cautious words, in particular that it must be emphasised that "nursing staff are there to work as colleagues and not in any inferior capacity."[77]

By 1969 after a sprinkling of experimental attachments, the move to GP attachment of district nurses widened. Combined with an increase in larger, purpose-built practice premises and health centres, this new system was viewed as successful in developing the concept of the community health team into a workable reality where family care was comprehensive and those providing it were professionally supported.[78] Interviewees emphasised the effects of change from geographical allocation of patients to attachment to GP practices as the key factor in this change of relationship. A nurse remembered working in North Kensington in the 1970s:

> We all met as a large group of district nurses . . . [but] I can almost on a hand tell you the number of contacts I actually had directly with a G.P. or who was a Health Visitor, or social worker, so the contacts with other health care professionals was very very limited [. . .] [however after moving to a GP attachment in Chester] I had more contact with other health care professionals in the team and valued very much being part of that team.[79]

An HV who was working in St. Helen's, Lancashire, in the 1960s and 1970s felt there was a good working relationship at that time between herself and other members of the community team but felt the problem was more with communication between hospital and community. Asked to comment on this she explained:

> Well, there was no communication at all at that time. That was where the big gap was. Not the District Nurses, or the District Midwives. It was . . . you very rarely went into hospital, prior to 1974 . . . the child went into hospital, the child came home. You saw it before it went, and you saw it when it came home, but you had nothing whatsoever to do with it while it was in.[80]

Firmly based within the community, the district nurse's role continued to expand throughout the 1970s and into the 1980s. According to a chief nursing officer of the time, it was the district nurse who led the primary health care nursing team. Supported by RGNs, [S]ENs, and auxiliaries, she took professional responsibility for the assessment of patient need and the subsequent delivery of appropriate care by the nursing team. In delegating tasks, such as bathing the patient, to the lesser qualified nurses, she was also responsible for monitoring the work to ensure that it was carried out to a high professional standard. In the community context, health encompassed general welfare and it was the responsibility of the district nurse to see that all appropriate social and financial needs of the patient and his or her family were being addressed.[81] These roles of assessment and empowerment, coordination, and supervision (leadership, delegation, teaching, monitoring, and regular reassessment) were all new to the pre-NHS job description of the grassroots district nurse. In addition, the role was being extended to include more specialised areas of work such as focusing on the elderly, the mentally ill, screening and preventative work, counselling, or working more closely with social services, for example, in providing high-dependency care for acute, chronically ill, or terminally ill patients and their families. Health promotion and health education continued to be seen as focal areas of district nursing, although this was (and still remains) often implicit rather than explicit practice compared with the evangelistic attitude toward health education of the early decades of the century. The separation of HV and midwife from district nurse and clearer delineation of the roles of each was therefore achieved in all but the most remote areas by the mid-1970s. An interesting parallel can be drawn with the declining role of GPs in hospitals following the NHS Act and this boundary-drawing creating specialist fields within community nursing.[82] In effect, both generalists—the GP and the district nurse—had their professional wings clipped by the rise of specialism in the larger medical and nursing arenas.

Bliss and While argued that the arrangement agreed at the beginning of the century between the BMA and the Queen's Institute that ensured that nurses undertook to work under the directions of the GP, together with the involvement of the medical profession in the training of district nurses, led to the understanding that "some GPs or indeed district nurses still view the

GP as the leader of care."[83] We would suggest that although this was almost certainly the case and is indicated by the GP oral histories referred to earlier, it was probably no more so than in the hospital environment, and quite possibly less so. Nevertheless, the nurses working during this period often described the later development of the community care team (from 1972 when GP attachment was introduced) as a mixed blessing that represented a move away from professional autonomy and toward shared responsibility and increased communication. On the one hand it gave them increased personal privacy, the support of a team, and more regular working hours, but on the other it brought about a change in identity that impacted on their relationship with the community and included a degree of compromise in their professional autonomy.

ROLE OF WELFARE STATE: CHANGES IN PATIENTS' NEEDS AND IN NURSES' RELATIONSHIPS WITH PATIENTS AND COMMITTEES

A change that was accepted most willingly and with immediate effect from the appointed day in 1948 was the transfer from patient payment to government payment for nurses' services. "Never again would they be required to look over their shoulders at the strivings of a hard-pressed voluntary committee to raise money for their services. Never again would they feel an obligation to assist at bazaars and local fetes, buy tickets for concerts, or function as uniformed exhibits in support of charitable appeals." Nurses had also been asked to assess and collect fees from individual patients.[84] Numerous nurses interviewed described this last task as particularly unpleasant:

> And in those days you also had to charge your patients for your visits, which obviously I didn't, but we had to you know officially, pre NHS, officially you had to charge them half a crown per visit. Some patients had an insurance system which was called a Provident Scheme and they had the little yellow card on the mantelpiece so you could see it and our hearts just, you know, were very, very pleased to see the little yellow card because it meant that you didn't have to ask them for half a crown. But just imagine an old lady given an enema and she could hardly afford to buy her meals and she had to give you half a crown—you had to account for the number of visits. You had to do your accounting—number of visits money or insurance system—they had to equate and I remember more than once putting our own money in because you know if you didn't you were accused of not having done the visit. It happened relatively often, I mean those of us who were really committed and people couldn't afford to pay we just put our own half crowns in.[85]

Testimonies indicate that the exchange of money between nurse and patient was not a standard feature of the work but varied from region to region, with many nurses reporting that they never handled money at all. The following anecdote from a nurse working in an Edinburgh district in 1947 suggests the lack of direction young nurses were given in the matter of charging fees:

> I remember an evening in this rather opulent district of Edinburgh . . . one of my new patients was this person who was a professor of mining engineering. And I was quite out of my depth as to what to do, the first visit was the one where you had to mention the fee. He was not a member, if the household wasn't a member of a district nursing association you had to pay out a fee, so I weighed matters up in my little mind, and I thought, oh well, if he pays ten shillings a week, that's reasonable I thought, in view of what a membership fee for a year would cost . . . And when I came back, I mentioned what the fee I had applied to this man. But when the nurse of the district came, she was horrified that this person, who could afford to pay much more, was only charged ten shillings. So I was kindly taken aside and told, well this is, you've made a faux pas here, this really should have been far more because nurse so and so has now to put this up to thirty shillings a week. And I had priced her at ten shillings, so I had cheapened the service.[86]

Others recall taking fees, retaining the sums in their own homes, and depositing them with the nursing association on a weekly or monthly basis. However, the collection of fees from patients was not a strict regime to which the nurses always adhered:

> Patients were charged fees if they were able to pay . . . Unless you were a member, each area in Glasgow, in Edinburgh . . . they all had their local district nursing associations. And probably for perhaps half a crown a year you could become a member, and that entitled you to the services of a Queen's nurse free. If you weren't a member, then, and it was apparent that you could afford to pay, then you were charged a fee. But in the district I was allocated to, they were neither members, nor could they afford to pay. . . . So they weren't charged.[87]

Another nurse described the transition to nonpayment with the NHS as being quite confusing for the patients, some of whom equated nonpayment with charity:

> She said "The envelope is in the hall on the hall stand," and I picked up the envelope and I went back to her, and in the envelope was half a crown, and I went back to the lady and I said "I'm sorry but I don't know."—"Oh that's my, . . . that's the money"—and I said "No, no," I said, "Oh no it's all free now.' No way, no way, she wasn't going to

have me if I didn't and I went back to the doctor. [. . .] He said "If you can't use half a crown then," he said, "forget it, but she must have it [her treatment] done."[88]

The reorganisation of health services inherent in the NHS Act brought a widespread fear of change, particularly in rural areas. When the idea of regrouping district nurses was put forward there was fear that familiarity with the local nurse would be lost to the implicit economies of personnel and administration.[89] This loss of public recognition as *the* district nurse is also a common theme noted by many when remembering the 1972 reorganisation. At this time, it was exacerbated by the almost universal move to car transport, which for many occurred around this time and meant that friendly meetings on the street were less likely. In effect this increased the separation of the nurse from her local neighbourhood and was felt by some to be efficiency at the expense of community knowledge and personal identity:

> We then went GP-attached, so you weren't actually in one area, you were all over the place . . . which had its advantages and disadvantages. I don't think you quite got to know the area, the patients in the area, the same, because you were actually specifically nursing a patient at that residence, not the whole street any more.[90]

Rising numbers of public pressure groups bringing a new awareness of patients' rights was one aspect of the changing role and relationship between nurse and community in the late 1960s and 1970s that produced some of the most strongly felt comments from the district nurses interviewed. After the NHS Act, this changed relationship was felt to represent a wider social adjustment and the suggestion was made on several occasions that relatives were then less willing (or able) to cooperate with the nurse or take such an active part in patients' nursing. In addition there was felt to be less expression of appreciation or allowances made for flexibility of timing for visits. To what extent this is a case of remembering a golden age that never really existed is unclear. However, it was surprising to see this substantiated by one of the GPs who worked in Bolton, Lancashire, who remembered that in later years his district nurses "had a very rough time, sometimes" as the "irritable old people would expect them to arrive on the dot of nine o'clock [. . .] Oh, I've had to go on several occasions, and warn them off."[91] In an address to a group of district nurses in Cardiff, a local GP described this changing public attitude: "There is far too much demand from the public today, who grow helpless and less self-sufficient. More and more they make demands particularly in the industrial areas, on doctor and nurse. 'I have a headache, doctor, is it safe for me to take an aspirin? A Sunday paper says it gives me ulcers.' "[92]

Roberts's study showed that despite popular perceptions to the contrary, there is little evidence to suggest a weakening of neighbourhood kinship attitudes in poor urban areas during this period, nor that support given to elderly family members by the extended family reduced significantly before 1970.[93] A nurse in Lancashire remembered this vividly:

> Oh yes. Because I can remember . . . you'd get a patient in a street, and you'd go in, and there was no question of who would bring their dinner in. One of the neighbours would. (Prompt: There was always some-body?) Oh yes. Or they'd come and make the bed, and they'd come and look after them, and they would . . . the only trouble was, if they knew you were a nurse, in that place . . . "Now, while you're here, nurse . . ." And you'd have the whole street in![94]

However, certain time-consuming tasks, such as bed-bathing, disappeared from the district nurse's list of duties in some areas by the late 1970s to be done either by nursing assistants or (more recently) by social service "car-ers," and other menial domestic tasks were done by the home help service, although where these tasks overlapped, conflicts of interest could result. Indeed, Abbott claimed that district nurses, in protecting their own status and professional expertise, were sometimes using a form of occupational closure toward home help in much the same way as GPs had previously done towards district nurses by "defining an area of expertise over which they claim a monopoly."[95] She recognised that there were grey areas in the division of labour, particularly following the introduction of home help and home care assistants. Her research suggests that although "clients preferred nurses to perform personal care tasks," they "expressed greater satisfaction with the home help service" largely because "district nurses were seen to keep a professional distance and partly because of the working practices of the nurses."[96] Nevertheless, many of the (trained) district nurse's tasks involved much briefer visits to carry out specific procedures such as injec-tions or dressings, again resulting in a changed relationship and perceived role within the community as one of several health workers. This was both regretted and to some extent also resented:

> I think the Care Assistants have a certain training, but they can't always spot things the same as you would yourself. And to me, bathing was part of it. You got a relationship with the patient, sometimes some of them wanted too much of a relationship, should we say! But . . . you noticed things. You could see whether they . . . if they'd had a stroke, whether the grip was there, or whatever, or if they were covering up incontinency and things like that.[97]

This helps to explain an element of contradiction between the comments relating to changes in relationships with patients that had begun by the late 1970s and increased with the awareness of patients' rights in the 1980s and the earlier quotes claiming lack of recognition of the district nurse's professional status. According to the later comments, the patients seemed to show less respect for the nurse's authority as a detached professional, despite recognising her as a trained professional. It seems likely that the answer to this enigma lies more in a change in the patient's self-perception as a client and with increasing access to information about his or her own care, rights, and treatment, and that this change in attitude was not restricted to district nursing but applied to health care generally. In addition, by the end of the 1970s the public image of the district nurse had changed from a mixture of dedicated vocational, but familiar member of the community, to a less accessible member of a team who had abandoned some of the more "female" roles or those traditionally associated with nursing.

The postwar period, in addition to undergoing considerable social change, was also marked by rapid innovation within medicine and surgery. Elizabeth Roberts identified the rapid decline in infant mortality rates in England and Wales between 1900 and 1969 as signifying an overall improvement in health, which accelerated in the post-World War II period, and noted particularly the benefits of the NHS that had not previously been enjoyed by many women and children.[98] She also commented that jobs previously done by older women in the community such as laying out the dead and caring for mothers and babies, were substituted in this period by professionals: "There was a strong feeling that professional services were better than those provided by well-meaning amateurs [. . .] Increasingly, the advice of doctors and Health Visitors was preferred to that of older women in the family or neighbourhood." She went on to ascribe this to an increasing emphasis placed by government and the media on the value of expertise and professionalism. In the earlier, interwar period, this had not been the case despite the fact that "an increasing number of mothers had visited these [infant welfare] clinics."[99] Roberts suggested this was responsible for a decline in self-reliance and self-confidence, toward greater dependence by the public on professionals.

CONCLUSIONS

1948 to 1979 was an era of numerous rapid changes affecting many aspects of district nursing and its professional standing. From within, the gradual loss of controlling influence on the part of the QNI made the first two decades of this period a low point for district nurse training and regulation, with a recognized curriculum based on just three months of training only being introduced after a considerable battle. The weak position of district nursing as it fell under local authority control exposed differentials in salary scale, grading, and status between district nurses and HVs that contributed toward the creation of intraprofessional rivalries standing in the way of true teamwork. On the other hand, the move away from the voluntaristic system and lay-controlled employment and into the NHS represents a move toward professional equality with other nurses as pay and conditions of service gradually became standardized throughout England and Wales. Throughout the 1960s and 1970s, changes in the nurse's role resulted from several factors, including the introduction of improved transport and communications and the creation of the GP attachment system. In addition the move toward more technical or sanitized tasks and equipment was accompanied by the need for nursing of more acutely ill patients in the community, due to rapid advancements in medicine and surgery throughout this period combined with changes in policy toward length of inpatient stays. This all combined to create a professional image more closely associated with medicine and the hospital, but it simultaneously removed the district nurse from her traditional one-to-one relationship with the community and thus diminished her professional autonomy.

In the postwar period there were extensive adjustments made by district nurses in responding to the challenges presented by evolving professional and public relationships; the changes resulting from a wide range of technological innovations; and enormous adjustments to their professional administration, organisation, and training. By 1979 the primary care team had become a physical reality rather than an elusive concept, facilitating interprofessional interaction and communication. A shifting relationship with the community these nurses served also reflected wider social changes, including a more critical public awareness of health issues. The difference between the ideals of the NHS and the realities of delivering a comprehensive "cradle-to-grave" health service was often all too obvious in the profession of district nursing by the end of this period.

Part II

Themes and Issues

The District Nurse and
the Changing World of
Primary Health Care

5 Town Nurse, Country Nurse: District Nursing Landscape

INTRODUCTION

This chapter explores the relative impact of regional demography and local community on the working experience of district nurses. We introduce the urban–rural split that was and remains particularly evident in British district nursing. Although in theory district nursing practice adhered to strict standards, the conditions of work varied widely between nursing situations, most notably between those of the city and rural areas, with remote or island districts providing the most extreme examples. The picture used on the front cover of a 1964 recruitment leaflet (see Figure 5.1) depicts two quite different lifestyles: on the left, the modern, industrial urban setting with its factory chimneys and back-to-back houses, and on the right, an idyllic rural image reminiscent of a previous century. The district nurse transcends both.

Nurses in rural or remote districts (and in some small towns) were often organised differently, in that they were invariably employed as double- or triple-duty nurses: As well as district nurses, they also acted as HVs, midwives, or both. Strictly speaking, triple-duty nurses should have held the relevant qualification for each role but dispensation to work without the HV's certificate was given at the discretion of the QNI with the qualification to be gained at a later date. The responsibility of triple-duty nurses to their community was more keenly felt and wide ranging than that of the single-duty nurse. Triple duty also provided a continuity of care within the community that was disrupted in the cities by the involvement of separate midwives and HVs. Those who worked as triple-duty nurses recall the long hours of work necessary when they were the only nurse, midwife, or HV serving a community. Despite this multiplicity of roles, district nurses were clear about the distinction between the nursing duties of the district nurse, those of the midwife, and the education and preventive duties of the HV, remaining aware of the possibility of overlap. "A health visitor can't encroach on the district nurse's territory . . . but the district nurse can encroach on the health visitor's area."[1]

In contrast, city districts were served by a range of separate visitors: HVs, midwives, welfare workers, hospital almoners, and so on, all of whom might

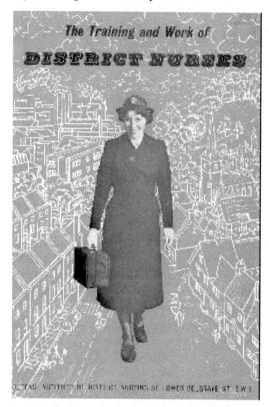

Figure 5.1 1960s recruitment leaflet, front cover. From Queen's Institute of District Nursing, *The Training and Work of District Nurses* (London: QNI, 1964). Image reproduced by kind permission of the Queen's Nursing Institute.

have had occasion to visit in the homes of the district nurse's patients. Hence city districts were generally single districts with the nurse responsible only for home nursing matters. Small towns varied in their home health care provision, with some local authorities providing separate midwives or HVs and others doubling up the duties of the district nurse to provide a double- or triple-duty nurse. The triple-duty post was the most isolating in professional terms. By its nature, it provided no other colleagues such as midwife or HV with whom the nurse could discuss professional issues.

Although stories of district nurses throughout Britain refer to the nursing of the same illnesses and conditions (leg ulcers, childhood fevers, diabetes, arthritis, injuries, stroke, midwifery, etc.), the nursing experience is not expressed by one consistent narrative. Similarities in experience help to define the nature of district nursing but this is enriched by looking at the differences that emerged from a variety of sources including regional studies of DNAs, oral testimony, biography, and registers and inspectors' reports of the QNI.[2] In this chapter we look at several case studies of district nursing in Lancashire, Dorset, and particularly in regions of Scotland and South Wales. In addition to providing fascinating snapshots of the localities and the particular requirements imposed by them on the community health providers, this exposes more general aspects of evolving patient needs and problems. These regional studies serve to contrast the different work experiences of nurses in rural dual- and triple-duty practices with those working in urban practices where duties were restricted to general nursing only.

Before focusing on specific district nursing situations we offer a sample of the level of district nursing provision within England and Wales. Although comparable figures are not available for Scotland, it is probable that the range was similar, with the more urbanised counties faring better than the largely rural ones. The original aim of the 1935 QNI survey from which the data for Table 5.1 were extracted was to demonstrate the need for more district nurses, simultaneously showing the extensive development of the service nationwide. London and Lancashire are shown as extremely well provided for in terms of availability of nursing staff, whereas Monmouth and Glamorgan were underserved at that time. So, too, was rural Dorset, but in Glamorgan the average population served by each nurse was almost four times that of Dorset. However, this ignored the variations in nursing workload that resulted from differences in local topography as well as patients' social circumstances.

CITY AND TOWN DISTRICTS

The details of a select number of Welsh associations are presented here to demonstrate some of the differences between urban and rural districts, the ways in which these districts were managed, and the conditions under which nurses worked.

South Wales is diverse in character, ranging from the cosmopolitan cities of Cardiff, Newport, and Swansea to the mining valleys such as Neath, Rhondda, Mountain Ash, and Ebbw Vale, providing a contrast in nursing experience. The more rural nature of coastal districts such as Gower and South West Wales and the mountainous region of Brecon offer a further alternative.

The expense of employing a Queen's Nurse was not an uncommon concern for DNAs in all areas, but this was usually offset by the support offered by the QNI in finding holiday or illness relief nurses. They also helped to supply regular replacements when nurses stayed in a post for only short periods, as was common during the interwar period. Hence, the traditional image of the district nurse as indigenous to her community did not always hold true. On the contrary, records suggest that in cities such as Cardiff and Swansea, the cosmopolitan population of the city was reflected in the diversity of cultural backgrounds of the district nursing staff, many of whom came from elsewhere in the United Kingdom or Ireland. In contrast to the

Table 5.1 District Nursing Provision: Selected Counties (England and Wales)

County	Population (1931 Census)	Population Included Within Area of County DNA	Population Remaining "Unnursed"	Number of Nurses Employed	Average Nurse: Population Ratio	Extra Nurses Needed (Estimated)
Lancashire	5,039,000	5,013,308 (99%)	26,147 (1%)	503	1:9,987	184
Dorset	239,000	209,870 (87%)	29,482 (3%)	80	1:2,623	14
London	4,389,000	4,388,645 (100%)	—	335	1:13,100	211
Glamorgan	1,225,000	1,039,301 (84%)	186,416 (16%)	118	1:8,808	67
Monmouth	435,000	326,499 (75%)	108,459 (25%)	49	1:6,663	26
Caernarfon	121,000	120,209 (99%)	620 (1%)	54	1:2,226	1
Total (England & Wales)	39,864,000	38,206,8679 (95%)	1,657,317 (5%)	7,170	1:5,329	1,625

Note. Constructed from data in Queen's Institute of District Nursing, *Survey of District Nursing in England and Wales* (1935).

single nurse in a small community, nurses in city areas operated in a more collective environment, made possible by the large size of the urban populations there. Sociocultural demands on a district nurse working in the city were quite different from those in rural areas, but wherever they were, district nurses were central to their communities. Whether rural or urban, districts could present equally difficult challenges arising from deprivation, the effects of hard physical work often combined with heavy responsibilities, and consequent ill health. A GP who was working in (urban) Merthyr Tydfil in the 1930s described "bad living and working conditions, there were many deaths from diphtheria and scarlet fever," adding that there was high unemployment and poverty.[3]

Cities each had their own characteristics that impacted differently on the experiences of the nurses. Cardiff, for example, like Liverpool and London, had for a long time been a richly diverse and culturally mixed city; by 1900 it was second only to London in the percentage of its population that was foreign-born (see Figure 5.2). In 1919 Cardiff was the first city in the United Kingdom to experience race riots, and in the 1950s and 1960s it experienced a second wave of immigration from the West Indies and Asia.[4] The need to understand the problems of rapid urbanisation and a multicultural mixture of people was part of city life and so made its own contribution to the requirements of the nurse.

QNI district nurse training, which took place in city areas, gave nurses experience in a comprehensive range of public health aspects including maternity and child welfare, the school medical services, and the prevention and treatment of infectious diseases such as tuberculosis. It was noted that "They afterwards follow up and nurse patients from these clinics in their own homes."[5] In cities such as Cardiff the high levels of respiratory diseases

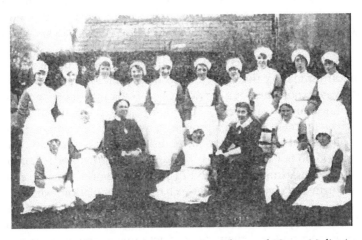

Figure 5.2 Superintendent and assistant superintendent and (Queen's) district nurses at the nurses' home in Cardiff (1926). From "Cardiff," *QNM* XXII:6 (1926): 135. Reproduced by kind permission of the Queen's Nursing Institute.

including tuberculosis and silicosis they encountered added a particular specialist dimension to this training. An interviewee who had been a district nursing officer in the 1960s and 1970s explained how caring for patients in a more deprived district of a city who lacked amenities such as indoor bathrooms, running hot water, and basic items of household equipment, combined to make the nurse's work far more onerous and time-consuming than attending the same number of patients living in better conditions in more affluent districts of the same city:

> You look now, take now, down in Langland Bay, the numbers—this is just hypothetical. The nurses were finishing by one o'clock. In Townhill, in the middle of Swansea, they were still working at eight o'clock at night. They had the same caseload, but there were differences in terms of . . . well, ecological differences, environmental differences, ageing, poverty, all come into it. The more poverty there was, the more time it was taking. In the town, they couldn't park, for example. By the time they find somewhere to park, there's half an hour gone in walking to the patient . . . so we just had to see what we could do about making the workload more evenly dispersed. . . . Take, for example, if you went into a home where they had bathrooms, indoor toilets, they had trays, they had dishes, . . . you know, they *had* things! You know, the nurses could just go in, everything would be laid up ready. . . . But you go into some of those other homes where they had nothing . . . They had nowhere even for you to lay up. They didn't have a bowl for you to wash your hands. I've seen me plug in an enamel bowl, or a plastic bowl, with a piece of bandage, to put water in it, to wash a patient. [. . .] And again, if you go to the rich people's homes, they have the beds, they're standard size. But they've got bed linen they can change. They've got sheets that you can use as draw sheets if you wanted to, or what have you. But, I mean, you go into other places, and mattresses are heavy and sodden and wet.[6]

Table 5.1 does take into account the different demands of rural and urban nursing in estimating the desired ratio of population to nurses. London's density was responsible for a far greater ratio than the more sparsely populated rural counties of Dorset, Monmouth, and Caernarfon. The county ratios given for these regions, although showing regional variance, probably mask considerable differences in nurse distribution between city, town, and country, and do not indicate areas of population growth or reduction. Taking Wales as an example, the QNI inspectors' reports show several towns such as Porth and Cymner with little change in population, whereas others, such as Neath and Swansea, reflect large population growth between 1900 and 1931. As for all cities experiencing such growth, this would have had a major impact on the demand for district nursing and associations had to work hard to keep staffing levels up to meet this demand, to raise the money to pay their nurses, and to maintain the nurses' homes provided for them.

Adequate levels of pay were crucial in retaining staff. Nurses often resigned posts to take up midwifery training, as this dual qualification improved their chances of promotion and higher salaries. Nurses from South Wales often went over the English border to Bristol, Gloucester, or Cheltenham for this, although by the late 1920s this was increasingly done during an extended leave of absence. By the 1920s the nurse's annual salary in Cardiff averaged between £63 and £68, falling below the QNI's recommended national average of £68 to £75. There were exceptions to this pattern such as the unusually high annual salary of Nurse Fynn working in Cardiff in 1924, recorded as £80 plus 2/6d weekly for coal for 7 months of the year and 5/- weekly for attendance plus 23/- weekly for board and laundry. She remained for 11 years, leaving only because of ill health. From 1927 the QNI salary scale was usually adopted as part of the terms of engagement nationally but individual districts remained at variance with this move toward standardisation. The salary in 1929 of Nurse Emily Kennard was detailed as "£72 rising to £75 p.a. plus board and laundry allowance of 23/- weekly and fire and light allowance of 17/6d (winter)- 15/- (summer)."[7] These emoluments presented attractive inducements to new recruits, as did passes on railways, which had been issued to district nurses working in Cardiff since 1909. From 1934 half-fare was charged on trams and buses to district nurses, midwives in uniform, and candidates or pupils in Cardiff. In addition by this time, the association was participating in the federated superannuation scheme to which the QNI encouraged all associations to subscribe.

Table 5.2 shows the disparity between the numbers of nurses serving the population and the level of GP support afforded them, particularly in urban districts.

This distribution of workload was further complicated by the type of caseload (chronic medical cases and care of the elderly being more time consuming than acute surgical aftercare, short visits to diabetics, or hospital aftercare), duality of role (as midwife and perhaps HV or school nurse), and mode of transport. A report of the inaugural meeting of Glamorgan County Nursing

Table 5.2 Relationship Among Nurses, GPs, and Population Served

Type of Borough	Population	Number of District Nurses	Number of GPs	Ratio of Nurses to Population	Ratio of Nurses to Doctors
Mixed industrial county borough	295,000	30	180	1:10,000	1:6
Mixed borough	185,000	7	66	1:26,000	1:9
Rural district	9,000	3	4	1:3,000	1:1

Note. S. J. L. Taylor and Nuffield Provincial Hospitals Trust for Research and Policy Studies in Health Services, *Good General Practice: A Report of a Survey* (1954):369–371.

Association[8] emphasises the public health role of the district nurse with Dr. Colston Williams, the MOH for Glamorgan, speaking of "the need for more district nurses in such a large industrial area as Glamorgan." Penarth, for example, is listed as employing one Queen's Nurse covering an area of two square miles and a population of 17,719 by 1931. The nurse, Mary Warriner, was appointed in 1901 and although not undertaking midwifery as part of her nursing duties, remained in the post for 29 years, an unusually long period at this time. Similarly, the smaller mining town of Treorchy DNA employed two nurses (one for midwifery), who covered an area of just two square miles, charging no fees, and were provided with a "comfortable little home."[9] Their above-average rate of pay (£100–£105 per annum) and good conditions suggest there might also have been a wealthy benefactor or possibly the Miners' Federation, supporting this otherwise fairly poor association.[10]

A different scenario is presented by Bridgend DNA, which also employed one Queen's Nurse who lived in her own cottage and similarly covered an area of two square miles serving a population recorded as 10,000 in 1926. The entry in the QNI records at this time notes the association was supported by Provident club subscriptions of 1d per week and voluntary collections. Patients who were not weekly subscribers, paid according to their means from 3d to 1/- per visit but the association appears to have suffered an insecure history as it disaffiliated at some point after 1909, reaffiliating in 1926, only to disaffiliate again in June 1929. This second period of disaffiliation might well have been in response to the pressures of the severe economic depression and is consistent with experiences reported elsewhere.

Perhaps one of the most commonly recounted differences between rural and urban districts throughout Britain was that of travelling and transport. Whereas rural nurses undeniably encountered more extremes of terrain and the effects of bad weather, the city district nurse had her own regular travel difficulties, going mostly on public transport or on foot often over widespread or hilly areas, and up and down stairs. In rural districts local support was not infrequently given by the donation of a motorised vehicle. In the towns and cities this was less common, although not unknown:

> General care can be very heavy especially if you are wheeling a push-bike up Penylan Hill or somewhere, you know, which I did, I had all this area to do . . . I used to go all up Pencoed all down by the lake and part of Llanishen—and we'd be wheeling those bikes all loaded down, and I was doing that for ages and . . . there was a doctor, Doctor Bense, and he used to be on the Council. And one afternoon going up to this patient at the top of this hill and I got to the top and we got to the gate at the same time and I was puffing a bit and I said to him, "Well you're very lucky I can see to this patient! . . . It's taken it out of me going up this hill." I said, "I'm puffed." And he looked at me and he said, "Oh I'll see what I can do," and I didn't think any more about it at all. I didn't realise he was a councillor at the time. I just thought he was the

doctor and about a couple of days after the matron rang me up and I could almost sense her sniffing at the other end of the phone and she said, "Your friend's on the phone ... Doctor Bense, he wants to see you." She said, "I've got to take you in to City Road to" somewhere and wherever it was I had a little scooter anyway—I did have it and it made such a difference![11]

It was not until the late 1960s that urban nurses were given a car allowance as commonplace. In a Scottish town where several nurses shared a nurses' home, the local council used to send a taxi to the nurses' home to take the gas and air equipment to midwifery cases, whereas the nurse on-call for confinements had to make her own way on foot or by public transport. Only between the hours of 11 p.m. and 7 a.m. was the nurse allowed the luxury of taking a taxi to a case.[12] Whatever the means of transport used and whether in town or country district, the district nurse of the past was more visible to the public. This was partly due to the fact that, before the nurse's car became ubiquitous, the nurse walked in her area and became commonly known and recognisable. The keeping of a tidy uniform worn properly was a factor in this recognition. It was a physical identification with the district nursing service, notably the QNI, and a sign to the public that reinforced the image of the nurse as knowledgeable, authoritative, and professional, an image remembered with fondness by district nurses:

> Our shoes were polished, our hats were brushed, our coats were brushed, we wore white gloves and everything was so proper. And we had to wear our coats and caps, even although we had a car. In the summertime you felt like taking them off, well we did. We were allowed to take our coats off, but you had to have a cardigan, a navy blue cardigan, and your peaked cap. We had peaked caps with "QNIS." And we had epaulettes on our coat "QNIS."[13]

RURAL AND SEMIRURAL AREAS

In contrast to the average of two square miles covered by the urban district nurse, nurses working in rural areas covered a larger geographical area, but would often be provided with a furnished house and transport. Duties often included midwifery as well as general nursing. An example was the Welsh district of Gower with a population of 2,000 rising to 5,172 by 1931. The two nurses (one a Queen's Nurse) covered an area of six square miles, their remit again including midwifery in addition to general nursing, plus "inspection of boarded-out children." They were provided with either a bicycle or pony and trap as necessary, the QNI salary scale had been adopted, and by 1934 the report records this as "£175 p.a. plus furnished house provided." Surprisingly, considering the beauty of this gently rural area, the good pay and conditions and the company offered by the shared practice, the records show mostly short stays in post (one or two years or even less) and there is evidence in the comments of some friction with the employing body with notes recorded by the Inspector stating, "did not give satisfaction," and "left at a moment's notice though satisfactory." This suggests an uneasy relationship with the DNA managerial committee that was perhaps over-zealous in its duties.[14] The following testimony gives an idea of the character of such a district:

> Well, it's very rural, very agricultural, plenty of nice narrow roads . . . wonderful narrow roads. Welsh-speaking community, largely, 99 per cent, although there were other people that had moved in, country . . . holiday cottages and things. A few largish villages Llansawel, Llany-bydder was a bit bigger. Then we went to Cwmann, which was on the outskirts of Lampeter, which was more urbanised. But apart from that village, apart from Cwmann, the rest of it was very rural, and you had probably about . . . I'm trying to think. It would be about eight miles to Llanybydder, then it would be about another six, seven miles over to Cwmann, then another 10, 12 miles via places called Powderbrenin, Pumsaint, Caeo, and back round to Talley, and then back to Llansawel again. You had about, oh, I don't know, it must have been about 20/30 mile round journey [. . .] Oh, of course, you had to walk miles . . . leave your car here, because you couldn't take it any further. You had to walk down all these fields, gathering mushrooms on the way! Of course, opening gates, shutting gates. Opening gates, shutting gates![15]

A level of cultural conformity by nurses was often preferred in the more rural districts. This was particularly true in areas of distinct cultural character throughout the country. As in Scots Gaelic-speaking areas, in Welsh-speaking districts an ability to speak the language was a prerequisite for nurses, and in some parts this persisted into the 1970s at least. One nurse from Ammanford in South West Wales commented that "it was much simpler if you did speak Welsh . . . even the GPs were Welsh-speaking."[16] In Carmarthen the affiliation record notes the district requires "one Welsh-speaking Queen's nurse for general nursing only." Likewise in the Edinburgh training home, only Gaelic speakers were appointed to many of the Scottish islands. Where a nonnative speaker was appointed, this served to limit the district in which she could work:

> She was Welsh-speaking. Well, the lower part of the Valley, were very Welsh-speaking, so they wanted the Welsh-speaking nurse. Well, as you go up the Valley, there were more incomers, because there was work here, as you can imagine, from Merthyr and all round there. Well, they were like myself, not Welsh-speaking, and I was allocated the top part of the Valley.[17]

In contrast, a nurse who worked in the more urban and industrial coal mining towns of Aberdare and Hiruain in the 1960s commented that the need to be Welsh-speaking was a fast disappearing characteristic of the old regime in her area.[18]

Although not crucial, familiarity with the local environment, families, and particular cultural rituals concerning birth, illness, and death was a distinct advantage in smaller rural areas but less so in the large towns and cities. Local characteristics impinged on the experience of the nurse.

> So there was a huge difference between London, which had always been very very multi-racial, and, you know . . . certainly in Lambeth I'd grown up with a lot of racial integration there, and so I'd seen mixed families right from the start, and all the problems that that created. But in Dorset, they were really just Dorset people. And in, certainly in Bournemouth, relatively affluent. I mean, it still is a relatively affluent area. We have pockets of deprivation, certainly in terms of youngsters, young families growing up. But I suppose our main majority of elderly population are indigenous, and fairly well to do.[19]

Until the end of the 1930s a nurse would cover her district either on foot, by bicycle, or perhaps a pony and trap, often conducting midwifery in rural areas, and restricting her practice to general nursing in the more urban districts. Although in theory she worked under the direction of the GP, in practise her contact with him appears to have been minimal throughout this period. In the rural situation this seems to have been quite an isolated professional existence, whereas the nurse living with others in the nurses' home would have been able to share the day's experiences and professional concerns with her colleagues and superintendents. Here a district nurse working in rural Wales typifies the hazardous conditions met by many rural nurses in midwinter attending to patients in deep snow. Although she had a telephone, contact from the patient's relative was made via the postmistress nearest to the farm, who warned that neither doctor nor ambulance could get through because of the road conditions. The nurse got a lift as near to the farm as possible in a lorry from the local garage owner, then walked the remainder of the way across several fields waist-deep in snow. She found the patient suffering from hypothermia but managed to revive her using ginger-beer bottles filled with hot water placed around the patient. The report notes the particular difficulty of the "big oak bed on which the patient lay being very heavy and difficult to prop up at the foot."[20] This cameo demonstrates not only the remoteness of this work, but the need for resourceful adaptability and good local knowledge as a valued member of the community. In addition, the mountainous terrain made nursing quite physically demanding before the motorcar became a standard mode of transport for the district nurse:

I was thin as anything because I used to walk miles . . . In the winter I walked up the Tram Road as a short cut and found myself up to my waist in snow—silly me!—I had to go back on to the main road which was a very mountainous road and got to the top walking in a blizzard.[21]

Is it possible to suggest there is something unique about any particular region? Obviously daily routine in general nursing tasks is universal—this was implicit within the (national) training and practice laid down by the QNI which (in theory) was intended to equip a district nurse for practice anywhere in the United Kingdom. Urban district nursing was essentially different from rural nursing wherever it was practiced: It took place in a much more heavily populated community, did not include midwifery, often entailed nurses living together in a home, and the likelihood of knowing all the GPs was greatly reduced compared with the rural experience. A nurse who worked in St. Helen's described her training, which was divided between St. Helen's and Liverpool with some time spent in rural Oxen-holme, which could be applied equally easily to rural practice in Dorset or parts of South Wales:

And we went there for a week. I remember it well, with a Miss King. And they taught us, they took us round. And, of course, they were Health Visitor trained as well, so they used to take us round. But they didn't have as many patients, that's what struck me. They didn't have as many patients as we did, because it was a more rural area. (Prompt: They'd be covering a larger mileage, presumably?) Mmm, mmm. Much bigger. We went to the farms, and they would do, like, general nursing care, and the Health Visiting . . . weighing babies and . . . (Prompt: Were they doing midwifery as well?) Yes, yes. There were all three. They were . . . triple duty, I can remember her weighing the babies and that, when I was there. Yeah, very pleasant.[22]

However, there are differences in the cultural backgrounds of the communities in which these nurses worked, which also come through in the oral histories but apart from the obvious aspect of language or dialect, are particularly elusive. These were often attributed to a particularly strong sense of community or to parochial attitudes toward outsiders, although the intimate relationship established through the practice of district nursing seemed to lessen this. In addition, the nursing in some areas of South Wales included industrial injuries from mining accidents and respiratory diseases attributable to the coal-mining, tin-plating, and steel industries. Some of these could also be found in the Lancashire mines—the same nurse described receiving the injured from a mining accident at St. Helen's at the beginning of her general training—and there were also many industrial injuries from the glass-works and textiles factories in Lancashire. This would have been totally outside the everyday experience of a nurse working in Dorset or other southern regions of England, where rural nursing meant working in an agricultural community.

The Welsh example has already shown that rural district nursing work presented quite different demands from those required of a nurse working in a large town, and that it would therefore attract a nurse for totally contrasting reasons. One of the interviewees described the occupational hazards of visiting a patient in the rural district of Charminster when she was a county superintendent:

> We opened the gate and these four geese came charging out—you know how geese are—frightened me! I was frightened to death. I stood behind the nurse and said "Are they—are we safe to go in there?"—and she just marched on and said "Just walk on behind me, they won't take any notice of you—they are used to me." And then you went in to the house, it was all dark inside, there were about six cats running around and this little old lady.[23]

Ironically, the patient being visited had once been a "handiwoman" [untrained nurse] herself, demonstrating how recent (in historical terms) the transfer was from that informal system of local village nurses to this more formal one of professionally trained and organised district nursing. In Dorset, a largely rural and farming county, triple-duty nursing, as opposed to the dual-duty of nursing and midwifery described in the Welsh rural examples, was common practice in many areas until the 1970s. Grants were received from the local government board for midwifery and for health visiting carried out by suitably qualified district nurses, where they were available and by superintendents where they were not. According to the Dorset County Nursing Association records (1916) the district nurse might therefore undertake health visiting that included "mothers, babies, T.B., mental deficiency and school cases."

For a small town, Blandford in Dorset supported a relatively large population of around 3,000. The Blandford DNA employed a triple-duty Queen's Nurse carrying out "chronic medical and surgical work, midwifery and maternity care, school nursing, Infant and Maternity Welfare Centre, Health Visiting and Tuberculosis work."[24] Her salary was £130 in 1919, but despite this high salary, nurses stayed only an average of two years until 1926 when Nurse Hurrell stayed five years, finally resigning for "home duties." By this time the annual salary had increased to a strikingly high £140 plus the attraction of a furnished house.

The wide-ranging job description of triple-duty district nursing demanded considerable versatility from the nurse as well as careful planning of her working day to prevent cross-infection from patient to patient. Maternity visits were always done early in the nurse's day with infectious cases coming last. Postsurgical cases were always visited and their wounds dressed before attending to cases such as infected leg ulcers. Clinics were generally held in the afternoons but the nurse would still have to carry out any outstanding nursing duties in the evenings, making her day exceptionally long.

Rural–urban differences also affected the way the nursing associations organized their finances. Miss Peterkin, the General Superintendent of the QNI, described in a paper presented at a nursing conference in 1931 how each local DNA was responsible for "finding the money to support the number of nurses required for the work in the area for which it undertakes to provide nursing" and explained "there are, of course, nursing associations not in affiliation with the [Queen's] Institute, but they work more or less on the same lines, though not united together in any way."[25] She outlined the usual methods of fundraising, clearly differentiating rural from urban areas. According to this paper, the rural areas widely implemented the Provident system of asking a penny-a-week minimum subscription from each household, often supplemented by fundraising events and philanthropic donations plus fees and grants for midwifery and maternity nursing and for "work done for Public Health Authorities and other Bodies having power to pay for nursing." However, the more urban associations, although increasingly turning to the Provident system, relied more heavily on arrangements with public health authorities,[26] together with charging fees for services given according to means. This was supplemented by collecting on a house-to-house basis, through charitable subscriptions, or any other means thought appropriate to the area.

In 1934, Miss Crothers, the County Superintendent for Worcestershire, was seconded from her nursing duties for a year to act as organizer of Provident schemes including the appointment of paid secretaries to supervise the Provident funds. She also differentiated between urban practice that usually required general nursing only, and rural practice, which was more often general nursing and midwifery and might include public health nursing as some combination of health visiting and school nursing. Nurses in the urban setting usually lived together in a nurses' home, whereas the minimum accommodation provision for a rural nurse was "two furnished rooms including fire, light and attendance" plus a minimum of 21s. a week as board and laundry allowance. In Dorset there were seventy-one affiliated associations employing seventy-five nurses, suggesting a high number of single-nurse practices, whereas in the rural counties of Cornwall, Shropshire, and Cumberland some areas were reported as remaining completely "unnursed."[27]

We look finally in this section at district nursing provision in rural Lancashire. [Hawkshead and District is now part of Cumbria but was included in Lancashire until the boundaries were changed in the 1970s.] This has been included because the experiences of nurses in this remote, rural setting were quite different from those described so far. Like the rural nurses in South Wales and Dorset they covered a particularly large area recorded in 1924 as 6x2 miles and increased to 25 square miles in 1934. It was described as a "country district, rather hilly" adding "cyclist necessary" but from as early as September 1925 a Morris Cowley, two-seater car was provided. A committee that ran a Provident system of subscriptions and donations managed the DNA, which employed just one Queen's Nurse who covered both general nursing and midwifery. The first, Nurse Filkin, stayed from 1919 to 1924 and was paid £75 annually, plus 21/- board and laundry weekly, and £8 uniform allowance, having "two furnished rooms with fire, light and attendance provided," and later a furnished cottage was provided. She was succeeded by Nurse Edwards who stayed fourteen years from 1924 to 1938, broken only by three months out in 1930 for a hospital postgraduate course (although unfortunately there are no details of where this was undertaken or what it entailed). The role of HV is not mentioned, although it is probable that this work was undertaken if somewhat informally.

REMOTE DISTRICTS: THE HIGHLANDS AND ISLANDS OF SCOTLAND

We have alluded to the fact that conditions of work were affected by local geography, local weather patterns, local transport services, and local health service provision. This is particularly true of the Highlands and Islands of Scotland where historically, conditions deterred the development of comprehensive health services. In the mid-nineteenth century the highlands and islands were relatively well supplied with nurses but this situation deteriorated at the turn of the century. The shortcomings of the National Insurance Act of 1911 spurred an increase in nursing provision in the Highlands and Islands, but health care services remained generally inadequate. A new initiative to improve medical and nursing provision became necessary. The setting up of the Highlands and Islands (Medical Services) Board in 1913 tackled this problem. More trained nurses and doctors were supported in the region with salaries and subsidies to allow much needed housing for them as well as financial incentives to improve communication and mobility; doctors were expected to furnish themselves with motor cars. Telephones were installed for their use. By the 1940s, largely due to the impact of the Highlands and Islands (Medical Services) Board coupled with the proliferation of nursing associations affiliated with the QNIS and employing highly trained nurses, access to health care services improved in remote areas, particularly in the provision of nurses. In 1900 there were thirty-two Queen's Nurses engaged in the Highlands and Islands.[28] By 1937 this figure had increased to more than 200 and the 1940s saw a substantial number of nurses from Gaelic-speaking Highland and Island areas in training for district work.[29] Such was the success of the health scheme for the Highlands and Islands that it was cited as a model for the national health service for Scotland under discussion in the 1930s.

Whereas the cities of Scotland presented the same range of conditions found throughout Britain, many more of its districts were rural or remote (including the numerous non-doctored islands). Curnow provided a working definition of *remoteness* in the context of health services, noting that "geographical isolation is of course important but it is not the only consideration."[30] He contrasted an offshore island in calm waters having a good weather factor with the same island set in the North Sea. In this scenario remoteness is not defined by distance but rather accessibility and "transfer time to a clinical facility providing sufficient medical services." Given the weather and terrain of much of northern Scotland, which makes travelling difficult and time-consuming, even many of its mainland districts qualify as remote. District nurses in these areas might have had to travel miles over difficult terrain to reach a patient, or deliver babies in isolated situations with no recourse to distant medical services. Hence, work in the district varied, with those working in a small border town such as Hawick developing different relationships than those nurses working in large cities like Edinburgh or remote rural districts such as Caithness, with the small islands presenting a different experience yet again. With the exception of tuberculosis, where numbers of epidemic proportions prevailed in specific highland and island areas—even compared to the notorious scale in Scotland's cities—the kinds of nursing cases encountered did not vary dramatically throughout the country. What was noticeably affected by geography was the experience of being a district nurse in social and professional terms. In the remote rural or island districts the district nurse was commonly the only person trained in matters of health other than the doctor. She would frequently have been the first on call to an emergency; in the absence of a doctor she might have had to make a diagnosis, assess the need for a doctor, and perhaps organise transportation to a mainland hospital.

In contrast, the city nurse was never too far from a GP's surgery or hospital and had the benefit of an accessible public transport system. Although not accountable to the GP, the city nurse's caseload was largely determined by the local GP's referral patterns and she was less likely to be called on directly by patients. Rural and remote district nurses frequently fulfilled triple duties that extended their role, whereas the city district nurse was usually confined to general nursing. To some extent these differences were reflected in the social relationships the nurse had within the community. In city districts the nurse could live outside her district and maintain an independent private life away from the gaze of her patients, whereas the island or rural nurse was compelled by geography and culture to live as part of her district community. The all-encompassing nature of triple-duty nursing brought nurses into a more intimate relationship with their patients and they were accorded the same respect as other figures of authority, such as the minister, the policeman, and the teacher. The single-duty nurse worked in conjunction with other colleagues in the health professions such as midwives and HVs, thereby dissipating personal responsibility for, and involvement with the patient. Rural nurses often had little or no collegiate support except for the infrequent visits from the nursing superintendent. Single-duty rural nurses might share cases with an HV or midwife but few reported a close professional relationship with them until the inception of the working healthcare team in the 1970s. Combined-duty nurses did not even have this; for them, the local GP was their closest colleague but, although most described working with their GPs as a partnership, this was not always an easy relationship to manage and has been analysed in terms of playing the doctor–nurse game or by establishing a negotiated order. It is our contention that both these frameworks, although they did operate effectively, did not recognise the level of autonomy that district nurses displayed in their daily work. As is still the case today, district nurses in isolated areas could be called on to make diagnoses and this was not uncommon for the triple-duty nurse where the doctor was not nearby. One triple-duty nurse in an isolated district was regularly called on to make diagnostic decisions that could be crucial in determining the treatment given:

> In one case a lad had a condition—torsion of the testicle—now this is not seen very often and I'd never seen one before . . . and when I phoned the doctor he diagnosed something else and when I hesitated he asked what I thought . . . so he said to give some Pethedine for relief of pain and phone back in an hour . . . within the hour I phoned back to say I thought he needed to go to hospital—he was in the operating theatre within about two hours of the original phone call and they were able to deal with it.[31]

Sometimes arrangements were made with the doctor whereby the nurse held prescriptions and sickness certificates presigned by the doctor that the nurse then issued at her own discretion. Whereas this was a practice illegal but not unheard of in remote districts, on non-doctored islands it was a necessary arrangement to allow quicker access to appropriate medication or benefits.

In common with the rural Welsh districts, travel in rural Scotland was an ubiquitous problem. Difficult terrain was rendered almost impossible in bad weather:

> In winter when the weather was bad, you just had to manage . . . not a big lot of snow . . . you could always get out . . . sometimes the gales would stop us . . . gales would bring down the telephone wires and there would be damage.[32]

Scottish winters were not sympathetic and in country areas the lie of the land could be lost under deep snow. The attitude recalled in nurses' testimonies demonstrates a nursing ethos where commitment and determination to make it to the patient was the guiding principle. Reminiscent of a devout dedication to duty there is a sense of quiet subservience to the responsibilities of nursing, whatever circumstances prevailed.

Although rural areas could encompass many miles and a sparsely spread community of patients, those on the islands bore an added burden of isolation. With no doctor on many of the islands, emergency cases had to be transported to the mainland quickly for hospital treatment. Emergency referrals to hospitals had to be authorised by the doctor. However, one Shetland nurse proved an exception to this rule. She recalled attending the confinement of the local schoolteacher's wife who had suffered bleeding during her pregnancy. Having eventually delivered the baby, the nurse called the doctor who was on a nearby island at the time:

> The doctor sent me word that he would come in the next day. So he came in with a fishing boat . . . it was 12 miles between Skerries and Whalsay and it took the boat an hour and a half to go and back again that was three hours . . . I had written him a letter telling him that Mrs W. had had her baby, but he didn't know and he said, "What! Well I was wanting to get to her," because she had an APH [ante-partum haemorrhage] during her pregnancy. So he took his bag up to the manse which was also the school house . . . by then she was dried up . . . and when he came the next morning I told him I couldn't take the risk another time, I would just send her to Lerwick. He said, "No it'll not happen again" . . . and he wasn't half way back to Whalsay when I got this frantic call and the Earl [the local transport ship] was coming up that day and she was lying at Baltasound . . . and I arranged for them to pick her up and I went with her . . . and I sent a message to the doctor to meet the Earl when it came to Whalsay . . . and when he came he'd been on the phone to the surgeon . . . but from that day onwards I got permission that if I needed to send a patient to hospital I could send her.[33]

Early in the twentieth century emergencies entailed calling up the local boat-man and hoping the seas would allow a safe crossing, but the 1930s saw the welcome introduction of air ambulance service to some areas. Small planes were made available to transport the sick to central hospitals but the service covered only a few routes at first and had to be paid for by the patient. Local funds were often started for this purpose and added to with the proceeds of ceilidhs, concerts, and dances. The service gradually expanded to cover all remote districts and later became free to the patient under the NHS.[34] On islands with no doctor the nurse was expected to assess the need for emergency treatment and contact the doctor to arrange the airlift. Given the high cost of the service, the district nurse sometimes found herself having to argue that the case was a true emergency, and therefore worthy of the costly airlift, and more often than not was then required to accompany the patient on the flight. The nurses then had to make their own way back and so an emergency of this kind could take them out of their district for some time:

Occasionally the doctor would go ... one pregnant patient haemorrhaged at 31 weeks in the middle of the night ... it really was touch-and-go ... the airstrip wasn't equipped for night flying ... it took three of us to deal with it ... intravenous drip was needed ... the pilot eventually was persuaded to do it, but cloud cover was low and it was difficult.[35]

In the 1960s a central hospital-based air ambulance service was operated carrying nurses from the city out to the islands. Nurses at Glasgow's Southern General Hospital who had enrolled for the air ambulance service were given on-call rotas during which time they could be called at any time to staff an emergency flight. This system relieved island nurses from the need to leave their post (and their home) for days to accompany emergency cases and the air ambulance began to feature in the working lives of general nurses in the city:

Another attraction of the Southern General was the air ambulance ... When you got, there was a casualty or a sick person or a woman in labour having to come in from Barra, Islay, you know, the outlying places, Kirkwall, used to go to Kirkwall. That was a challenge for us all. You had to do an observer flight first of all. And then you did ten, you had to go on ten flights following that to gain your silver wings. So ... that made it exciting. You didn't, you know, you'd be sitting down at your lunch, the call would come through. "Right, you, you're down on call for the air ambulance, off you go." Maybe it was Barra, maybe it was Kirkwall. Barra, you know, we landed on the beach, there was no airstrip. That was, the tide had to be out. And I remember going to Islay to bring in ... one of my friend's ... her father was unwell and I was the one that went to bring him in. We got paid a guinea for each flight.[36]

INDUSTRIAL AREAS

In addition to the rural–urban split there are significant aspects to the district nursing experience and working conditions that applied to nursing in industrial areas in particular. The similarities between Lancashire and South Wales are noteworthy examples, as both comprise large areas with mixed heavy industry (including coal mining), and busy ports with large hinterlands of rural countryside. Many of the industrial areas of Britain presented a far more desperate socioeconomic picture than we have expressed for the urban and rural areas thus far. Arguably they were subject to the harshest effects of recession with few, if any, alternative occupations to provide a livelihood for the workers. For such communities the district nurse played a pivotal professional role in liaising among employer, employee, GP, and hospital, and where there was one, with the specialist industrial nurse, so much so that in 1940 the RCN proposed to the government that a comprehensive nationwide industrial health service be established with the Queen's Nurse or district nurse at its core.[37]

This chapter would therefore not be complete without reference to the prolonged depression of parts of this region, and the effects this must have had on the health of its inhabitants and the consequent heavy workload on community health workers. A nurse who worked in Oldham, Lancashire in the late 1920s and early 1930s described the prevalence of diseases related to poverty, particularly malnutrition, rickets, and high maternal and infant mortality rates, and to the hardship of work in the cotton mills, including high levels of respiratory diseases and cancers of the mouth from handling and spinning the raw materials.[38] She vividly described attending an emergency confinement in a dirty and very poorly lit home with no electricity or running water, and with the mother lying on two orange boxes in an otherwise bare room and having nothing in which to wrap the baby (this had to be borrowed from a neighbour). She commented on the widespread ignorance of effective contraceptive methods, which she felt exacerbated many of these hardships.

Similarly, Blackburn, which in the 1930s was considered "typical for the whole cotton area," was described as "grim . . . everywhere is a forest of tall brick chimneys, against a sky that seems always drab, everywhere cobbled streets, with the unrelieved black of the mill girls' overalls and the clatter of wooden clogs."[39] Unemployment among women was considered to be a major problem in these areas, and signs of stress and malnutrition were also most evident in the women.[40] Nurses interviewed in a BBC documentary set in Lancashire[41] commented that the ill health of women often contributed an additional burden to their heavy workload as district nurses and midwives, as GPs' fees before the NHS were prohibitively expensive for those excluded from national health insurance. They commented on the problems of infestation with lice, fleas, and house mites, and in providing a layette for new babies, before describing the problems in procuring abortions and getting family planning advice, commenting that home remedies such as epsom salts were commonly used. The community they served clearly depended heavily on the nurse and midwife. Several Liverpool district nurses described similar experiences. One interviewee spoke of her experience while training as an HV in Liverpool in the 1950s:

> [The Wash houses] were in . . . you see, most of the houses in Liverpool that we went to had no facilities for . . . for washing, and hanging the washing out. They just had yards, didn't they, you know, and . . . and a brown sink in the back kitchen, and a cold water tap. But the Wash Houses, they had in various areas round Liverpool, and for the women, it was a day out, really. They used to put all their dirty washing in a pram, and push it up to the nearest Wash House, take their own soap

powder with them, and . . . I think . . . I can't remember how many sinks there were, they took us on a visit there, probably about . . . there might have been as many as 14 or 15 sinks, and they had the hot water and everything, and they took their own powder. And I remember, Tide had just come in at that time, and they wouldn't let them use it, because they thought it was wrong for the sinks. But they were there most of the day, you see, and they all knew one another, and it was a . . . a social outing!! Because, you see, people didn't have washing machines then. They were just beginning to come out at that time. And I remember the Tide, because when I came on the District, as a Health Visitor, an awful lot of women had dermatitis on their hands then, and they all said it was due to the washing powder, the new ones that were just coming out.[42]

She also commented that two of the major problems she encountered when first working in Liverpool and St. Helen's in the 1950s were infestation of the heads with lice and impetigo in children.

Decisions impacting directly on the health and welfare of industrial communities were often in the control of the local industry owners. For example, in Ammanford, Carmarthenshire, an area of collieries and tin plate works, we find, "the committee decided to leave the district without a nurse for a time as the people did not seem to appreciate one enough" and disaffiliated from the QNI for several years, reaffiliating in 1924 only to disaffiliate again in 1931 "on account of low funds." This meant that the services of a district nurse were withdrawn from the entire community during these periods of disaffiliation, leaving them to fall back on the care of untrained local women. Apart from the care provided through the NHI (which applied only to those workers paying NHI contributions) it was to the district nurse that most people would have turned in the first instance of illness or injury in industrially deprived areas. In industrial regions the district nurse was a crucial link between the workplace and the home and for many people was often the only recourse to the kind of holistic care that district nursing epitomised. Without the employers' financial support toward the DNAs, the social and material effects of periods of economic slump were exacerbated by the absence of a trained nurse.

Conversely, relations between industry and district nursing were often harmonious. Barry provides one such example of a benignly paternalistic relationship. An urban district of South Wales comprising busy docks and railway works, Barry employed five Queen's Nurses to cover an area of approximately six square miles. They were well provided for, with a purpose-built home and employed on the QNI salary scale. Despite this apparently good support, their average stay throughout the interwar period was just two years, often resigning for marriage or occasionally due to ill health, but also several taking leave for midwifery training. Although there might have been support from local philanthropist Lord Bute, Barry's nursing association also had close links with Barry Railway Company. A ward for nursing the sick poor was bequeathed in 1927 by the wife of a director of Barry Railway Company,[43] with patients on the ward being looked after by the association's district nurses before and after their rounds. Beds were also available to other patients able to pay their maintenance at a cost to the Insurance Committee of 10/- per day.[44]

This example underlines the complex dynamic between the local industrial elite and local communities, which underpinned the provision of district nursing and health care. In November 1927 the association was being run by the Lady Superintendent, with her staff of two Queen's Nurses and two temporary nurses. At that point it was the intention to employ another Queen's Nurse and there is a reference to the 1,067 visits made in the preceding month and to "the growing practice of the local doctors in asking for nurses to attend and assist with operations performed by specialists." The resolution is recorded in the minutes "to write to the doctors bringing the claims of the association to notice, and the nurse to leave circular letters with the patients and to endeavour to receive a reply when she ceases to attend." A temporary nurse was paid £60 per annum and at this time the Welsh Nursing Board tried to persuade the association to accept the cost of employing two Queen's Nurses to replace the temporary ones. This would have meant losing one of the temporary nurses (Nurse Evans), as she was asked to train as a Queen's Nurse but declined. It was therefore resolved to only accept one Queen's Nurse and to retain Nurse Evans, an interesting choice of the experienced local nurse over the professionally trained unknown. There is no reason given for Nurse Evans's decision, but it seems likely that she felt no wish to travel to Cardiff to undergo further training. This was an attitude expressed by most non-Queen's interviewees, who considered practical experience to be the key to good nursing and felt this could not be taught in a classroom.

Charity of the kind described in Barry did not always come from the immediate locality. Following the 1926 General Strike, the Society of Friends (the Quakers) set up an organisation of poverty relief in the extremely deprived communities of the Rhondda Valleys, establishing self-help groups that rapidly grew to become a substantial centre based at Trealaw called Maes-yr-Haf (see Figure 5.3), combining health and welfare provision with education and retraining. From this a number of Unemployment Clubs, Sewing Groups, workshops, and allotments were created. They also supported the formation of the Mid-Rhondda Nursing Association in 1931, which employed two Queen's Nurses who were continuing to work there in 1933, making more than 4,000 visits in their first year. The Rhondda was chosen to represent an area of severe economic deprivation in a study of unemployment and the voluntary social service movement between 1929 and 1936 conducted by the Pilgrim Trust.[45] This showed the Rhondda to be one of the most economically depressed areas, yet one demonstrating considerable social solidarity and supporting an unusually high number of societies such as these, as well as political and religious institutions and social clubs.[46] Unfortunately

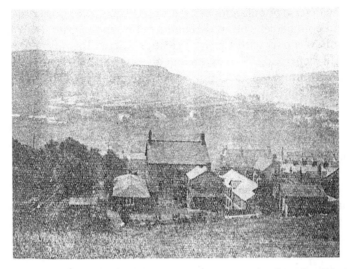

Figure 5.3 Maes-yr-Haf, opened Spring 1927. From "In the Rhondda Valley," *QNM* XXVI:1(1933): 12–17. Reproduced by kind permission of the Queen's Nursing Institute.

unemployment and resultant economic depression had resulted in large-scale emigration of younger men to other parts of Britain, leaving behind the elderly and a high number of physically disabled ex-miners suffering from chronic diseases, particularly nystagmus, silicosis, and dermatitis.[47]

Elizabeth Roberts noted the diversity of Lancashire's economic base from the heavy industries of Barrow and Liverpool to the textile towns of Preston, Bolton, and the broader spread of Lancaster's mixed economy. Lancashire's district nursing service was extremely proud of its contribution toward the founding of district nursing by trained nurses, and it might have been this sense of tradition that made them more ready to pioneer new developments in this field. Among these were the William Rathbone Staff College in Liverpool, which ran refresher courses for district nurses, courses in community health administration and ward management, and for "overseas nurses."[48] Lancashire was also the first county to train students in their own districts while attending lecture centres at either Manchester or Liverpool. A report referring to this innovative experiment noted, "There are a few district nurse/midwife/health visitors in the north, about sixty district nurse/midwives in the other rural areas, and general district nurses in the more urban and industrial areas." Table 5.1 shows Lancashire to have had a much larger population than the whole of South Wales in 1931, and only one percent of that was considered to be "un-nursed" at that time, although it was then felt that 184 more nurses were needed to cope adequately with the heavy workload.

In Liverpool itself, as in Cardiff, there was a QNI training centre and nurses' home that was very proud of its long tradition and served a similarly culturally diverse population, as Liverpool was a major port and centre for trade and commerce. The study conducted by the Pilgrim Trust described Liverpool as "a port with a past of great prosperity but now suffering from prolonged depression"[49] that included heavy and long-term unemployment. Queen's nursing probationers were drawn from across the north of England and North Wales, and could be placed for one year after training wherever they were most needed. Nevertheless, concern was expressed in 1934 that "The population of Liverpool is about 866,013. Of that number only about 1,000 contribute to the support of the District Nursing Association, whose nurses last year attended 7,288 cases, and paid 177,393 visits."[50]

As an industrial region Lancashire provides us with evidence of particularly direct and open participation by philanthropists and employers in providing nursing care for their employees. An example of this is Summerseat, affiliated with the QNI in 1914. Its nurse covered a small area (one square mile) succinctly described in the QNI inspector's affiliation report as "industrial, cotton mills," and a population that was fluctuating between 1,000 and 3,000.[51] The association was managed initially by "Messrs. Hoyle Bros. with a small committee," and from 1919 this became just two trustees: Horace Hall Esq. and Mrs. Sydney Whitehead, with the "Nurse paid by Mill owners for the benefit of their employees." The Queen's Nurse performed "general, monthly and midwifery cases" and by 1923 undertook infant welfare work, receiving "usual salary and allowances" while renting a furnished cottage. Initially this work also included health visiting but that appears to have been discontinued by 1918. The first nurse left within the first year, for military reasons and her replacement, Nurse Palmer who stayed until 1923, was paid a generous annual salary of £115 inclusive rising to £150, being replaced by Nurse Simpson who was paid £155 yearly rising in annual increments to £164, and the record notes that even her gas bill was paid by the DNA.

A second example is the town of Littleborough, which covered an industrial area just northeast of Rochdale, of approximately three square miles and a growing population.[52] In this case the DNA was managed by a general and executive committee, and unlike Summerseat, this supported two nurses through house-to-house collections and paying patients. In 1917 the records note midwifery was undertaken "owing to shortage of doctors."[53] However, this work was discontinued in 1921 after which it was felt just one nurse was needed for general work only until 1932, suggesting that midwifery had accounted for a large part of the workload. When there were two nurses, a furnished cottage and bicycles were provided, but this changed to rooms in 1921 and at some later point a car was provided. Unusually, terms are included for the early period noting that "The nursing of better class patients is undertaken and reasonable fees charged." These charges varied according to how much of the nurse's time they occupied, averaging between seven to ten shillings per week for a daily visit (approximately

30p–50p in modern currency), or five and sixpence to ten and sixpence for assistance at an operation done in the home, to ten and sixpence to fifteen and sixpence per month for regular attendance (i.e., three or more visits per week) of chronic cases, whereas a single visit would be charged at between 1/- and 2/6.[54]

In 1919 the records note that annual grants were received (£10.10s from the Cooperative Society, £6 from Gatside's charity, and £21 from Board of Guardians), together with income from midwifery undertaken. This example serves to demonstrate the very business-like way in which many of these DNAs were run, particularly following the move toward more inclusive nursing care provision for the whole community. The care provided by the nurses was the same whatever the social background of the patient, but it is clear from this and similar examples elsewhere[55] that a means-related system existed.

Nurses came to and left the district in pairs until 1921, consistently staying about three years. From 1921 an unusually high starting salary was provided of £150 per annum plus furnished rooms with the addition of "fire, light and attendance." These two examples bear similarities to the mining towns of South Wales, but time in post was longer and the salaries and living conditions offered to the nurses were considerably better. It might be that higher female wage rates being paid to textile workers in Lancashire dictated these higher salaries for trained nurses.

There are numerous similar examples of privately financed or works-funded DNAs such as Ashton in Makerfield, largely funded by The Lady Gerrard but with £100 support from the Colliery owners; and Irlam and Cadishead, an industrial and agricultural district located between Manchester and Warrington, the nursing association of which was managed by a committee and was supported:

> by all large works. The employees have consented to a levy of ½d per week which brought in a total of £300 annually, together with grants from Barton and Irlam and Cadishead Boards of Guardians.[56]

However perhaps the ultimate example was the DNA at St. Helen's, which was supported by the Pilkington family, a large, family-owned glass-making company. This included the provision of a purpose-built nurses' home opened in 1927 and enlarged considerably in 1935,[57] as well as a tradition of committee membership by a member of the family and private donations. The DNA was established in 1884 and was originally run by six ladies including Mrs. R. A. and Mrs. W. W. Pilkington. By 1935 they employed a staff of twenty-five district nurses supported through a contributory scheme. This was felt to be so successful that Mrs. Pilkington gave evidence to explain and defend the voluntary system in 1942 to Sir William Beveridge.[58] A district nurse who trained at St. Helen's in the 1950s described the hierarchical administration of this top-down organisation:

Oh yes. Each . . . what happened, when we first started on the District, our District in St. Helens, was run by a private Committee. It was St. Helen's District Nursing Association. Lady Pilkington was the Chairman . . . Chairwoman. And Mrs. Greaves was on the Committee, and Mr. Laylum, and so on. And it was run by this private Committee. It wasn't attached [controlled by the local authorities] . . . you know. I think we were like a little service on our own. And we had a Matron, an Assistant Matron, and a Chief Nurse.[59]

To those at the top of this organisation, the move to nationalisation following the 1948 NHS Act represented a step backward, and handing over "their" nursing association to local government was only done with considerable reluctance and trepidation when there was no other option. This was in many ways a little empire ruled by the privileged social elite of St. Helen's.

CONCLUSION

The particular combination of varied topography together with unique cultural backgrounds presents a distinctive scenario for each region—and arguably, for each district. In addition, socioeconomic contexts had a considerable impact, whether this was unemployment throughout Lancashire in the interwar period,[60] the miners' strikes and subsequent depression in the South Wales valleys, or the Blitz in cities such as Liverpool. In each case the resultant effects would have been felt acutely by the district nurses through increased workload, the types of disease or injuries resulting from poverty or war, or even occasionally by making their employment unsustainable. As a result, although nursing associations were theoretically set up and run on formulaic lines so that Queen's district nurses were all trained to the same standards and with the same basic techniques, there had to be adaptations to meet the special needs of each particular community. Terms and conditions of employment varied until a national standard was imposed through the NHS in 1948. Even then, variations in emoluments offered by individual associations might have been used to entice nurses and persuade them to stay in post.

The nostalgic image of a district nurse who lived in, and felt part of her community was of only limited reality. These case studies have revealed far greater mobility between district placements among nurses than this image would suggest. Although some of these can be explained by the QNI's policy of compulsory one-year postings immediately following qualification as a Queen's Nurse, it would seem likely that these first placements were often used to staff positions that were otherwise difficult to fill. The idea of the district nurse staying for most of her life in one post, certainly before 1948, seems to be a popular stereotype with little foundation in reality, although there were certainly a few who did. This can be compared with a similar pattern discovered among GPs, again refuting the popular image of the family doctor staying in one practice throughout his professional lifetime. In fact, they too usually moved several times during their careers, and like the nurses, sometimes returned to hospital work or went abroad to practise after a period of time, particularly during the interwar period.[61]

The work and experiences of district nurses have been shown here to be subject to geographic, socioeconomic, and cultural influences.[62] First was the local and regional culture that must include the more individual elements that might have made one town or village distinct from another, together with the individual characters of the nurses and of the association's committee. These influences are difficult to evaluate and appear to some extent masked by the more obvious urban or rural factor. This dictated, for example, whether a nurse was also the midwife and the HV covering a large, and often lonely, district on her own, with or without access to a resident doctor or the support of another nurse, or whether she was one of a community of nurses in a town or city, living together and practicing general nursing only, under the much tighter supervision of a home superintendent. However, we would argue that the topmost layer in this model was the overriding one. The work the nurse did, and her place in society, was substantially similar and familiar to her, wherever she practised.

6 Technology, Treatment, and TLC

This chapter evaluates the role of practice-related technologies in the changing work pattern of district nurses. The introduction of disposable materials and equipment, the Central Sterile Supply Departments (CSSD), materials technologies, pharmaceuticals, and further developments in communications and transport each made a contribution. The intention here is not to suggest a fully deterministic theory in which technology directly governed the development of district nursing. Rather we aim to demonstrate the powerful influence technological change had on what nurses did and how they did it, even at what is popularly considered to be the least specialized end of the profession.

In the postwar period, the rapid development of pharmaceutical treatments meant that fever nursing was no longer such a key aspect of the district nurse's skill, whereas before the arrival of sulphonomides and penicillin, an acute case of pneumonia had been thought of as a challenge requiring intensive nursing and several home visits per day through the critical phase. However this was countered by a steady rise in surgical cases. Although most surgery was performed in hospitals by 1948, there were still some operations carried out in the home, and assisting the doctor with these was still included in the district nurse's training. "Kitchen table" surgery included "circumcision, tonsillectomy, incision of abscess and minor gynaecological conditions, such as curettage."[1] In addition there was a gradual rise in the number of increasingly complicated postsurgical cases that required nursing care in the home after being discharged from the hospital and that demanded a different nursing expertise. Introduction of revolutionary new drugs (e.g., Mersalyl and insulin) used in the treatment of chronic diseases such as cardiac and renal failure and diabetes in the late 1930s, resulted in changes to daily routine to allow nurses to administer injections before the patient's breakfast time.

Although medical and technological advances brought many positive changes to nursing in the home, some of the retired nurses interviewed felt that they undermined the basic ethos of nursing care by increasing the nurses' caseload and reducing visit time with each individual patient. This argument is discussed further in Chapter 8. Here, we focus on the practical implications of technological progress on the daily routines of district nurses.

DRESSINGS AND EQUIPMENT

We see later in this chapter how changes in means of transport affected the district nurse's daily work. However it is relevant here to point out the restrictions placed on the nurse in terms of what she could carry with her. If travelling around her district on foot or bicycle, the nurse's bag had to be packed with care and considerable forethought (see Figure 6.1). If she were to forget an important item or run out of essential dressings, lotions, and so on, this would entail a long walk or cycle back to base. The equipment and materials available to her, shown in Figure 6.2, required a considerable amount of resourcefulness and improvisation even in the first two decades after the NHS Act. For example, the instruments on this trolley setting still had to be sterilised for five minutes before and five minutes after each procedure, and swabs and dressings had to be cut up and baked in a sealed container such as a biscuit tin in an oven to sterilize them. This process effectively increased the time taken per visit considerably. The nurse's daily workload and nursing techniques had changed dramatically in all but the most remote areas by the 1970s. By then, sterilised packs from a CSSD,

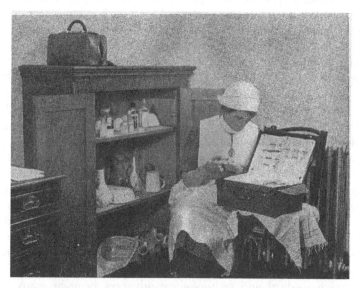

Figure 6.1 District nurse preparing her bag for the day's visits. Image from E. M. Day (Ed.), *Cassell's Modern Dictionary of Nursing and Medical Terms* (London: Cassell and Co. Ltd.) (1939): p. 90. We acknowledge the author and Cassell Plc., a division of The Orion Publishing Group Ltd. (London), as the Publishers; unfortunately all our attempts at tracing the copyright holder of the image proved unsuccessful.

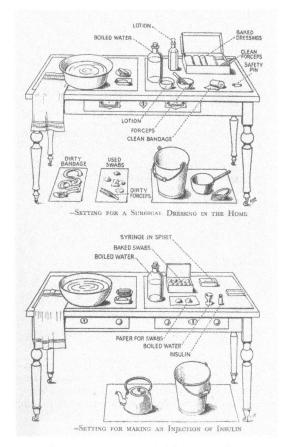

Figure 6.2 Equipment required for a dressing and giving an insulin injection, c. 1948. From E. J. Merry and I. D. Irven, *District Nursing: A Handbook for District Nurses* (London: Bailliere, Tindall and Cox, 1948): facing p. 116. As neither Elsevier nor Lippincott, Williams & Wilkins have been able to recognise copyright ownership of these images, we regret that we have exhausted all lines of enquiry in trying to establish the true copyright owners.

disposable sterile rubber gloves, prepacked lotions and syringes, and a vast array of new materials and devices were being provided. The contrast between equipment used before and after the introduction of CSSD is suggested by the comparable requirement and layout shown in Figures 6.2 and 6.3 for exactly the same nursing procedures. The system and problems were explained by many of the interviewees; for example:

> I used to go the day before, I mean, the first visit, and I'd say, "Now, have you got . . . how are you fixed for a bowl? Separate little bowl," was a big thing. "Have you got a bucket?" "Yes, yes." "And soap and some flannels," you know, the usual things. If they hadn't, they'd go

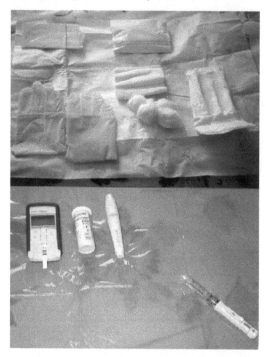

Figure 6.3 Equipment required for a dressing and giving an insulin injection after introduction of CSSD and disposables. Courtesy H. Sweet, private photographic collection. Thanks to District Nursing Sisters Sandra Crofts and Wendy Lloyd Sweet for these photographs and for their insightful contributions on this subject.

and buy something, you know. I used to go and buy it myself sometimes. Many times. Anyway, so . . . that's all geared up, and they're all kept in the corner of the room, all those things. And they'd get me a kettle boiling, there was no hot water. Got no taps, from the taps, very seldom. And so you'd start off from scratch. So, in other words, you spent a lot of the time preparing, for what you did with the actual patient. And the same with dressings. [. . .] Well, you see, today, it's all pre-packed. Steriles, autoclaved. Well, in them days, we had to ask for the milk saucepan to boil our syringes in. Yes! And I used to get old biscuit tins, scrounged from neighbours, lining with baking paper. I'm talking about dressings now, post-ops, and . . . I had to show the wife, or the patient who was capable, to . . . they used to get a prescription from the doctor for a roll of cotton wool, a big roll, and a packet of gauze, which you had to cut and do your own thing. So I'd cut them one out, to show them how to do it, and to give the patient something to do, to roll the cotton wool, cut the swabs up, pop them in the . . . in the biscuit tin, and explain to the good lady, "Could you put them in your . . ." they were all gas ovens in those days, "in the gas oven, for 20 minutes, with the lid off." Well, of course, when you went the next day, they'd done very well, thank you very much, but they were all black![2]

Similarly a description of an injection (the requirements for which are shown in the bottom half of Figure 6.2 and contrasted in Figure 6.3) was explained in this way:

> It was all ready for you, as a rule, you'd get them all organised. But you'd use one of their little saucepans, fill it with water, put water in, and we had a bag, you know, a proper bag with all the instruments in, and syringes, glass syringes, and then came the plastic ones eventually. But needles had to be boiled, because they were used time and time again. And so you had to wait a good five minutes, five or ten minutes, boiling it, before you start. You do your injection, you clean everything out and wash the . . . you dried them with the cloth that you have, put them back in your bag. So, in other words, you could be 20 minutes, or 25 minutes in a house, to give an injection. Whereas today it's in and out.[3]

This last point is contrary to the initial theory behind the development of CSSD, which was that time saved in boiling instruments could be devoted to better bedside nursing, thereby freeing the nurse to spend more time with her patient.[4] However, these developments dramatically changed the more technical nursing tasks, obviating the need for time spent on rudimentary chores. Early textbooks describe procedures such as dressings, douches, poultices, and fomentations, and even home surgery,[5] on a step-by-step basis. Syringes had to be disassembled and boiled for five minutes in a saucepan in the patient's kitchen together with (nondisposable) needles, placed in a separate egg cup and all put back together, and the procedure had to be repeated after the injection had been given. Old cups, saucers, small pudding basins or pie dishes, biscuit tins, jam jars, and washing bowls were commonly requisitioned from the patient's kitchen together with newspapers, towels, and rags.[6] Consequently, the change to preprepared, purpose-made equipment, dressings, materials, and so on, also represented an important modification in professional image from one that incorporated a considerable amount of time carrying out a form of culinary domestic work (cooking dressings, boiling instruments, and cleaning saucepans) to one that was technicalised and medicalised through association with modern surgical practice.

Seemingly simple changes in materials available to the nurse also had a considerable effect on the most basic practical work; for example, care of the incontinent and bed-bound was greatly simplified by the introduction of disposable incontinence pads at the end of the 1960s, as one nurse described:

> We'd no disposable . . . sheets . . . not sheets . . . they used the rubber protective sheets on the bed, which had to be washed and dried. . . .

Things were acquired. There were commodes, of course. And then we were just beginning using the inco. sheets, and you had to say how many general nursing care you'd got, of course, Matron knew really, and we were allowed three a day for these patients, and we were told they were 3d. each! Old money! And we had to be careful how many we used. It's only these underneath them. When you think of it, three a day. But that was because they were new coming out, and before that, of course, they just used the draw sheets and they were washed. So the family were involved a lot more.[7]

Changes in materials used for dressings, particularly in the second half of the century, demanded regular updating of the nurse's knowledge and understanding of wound care. As new lotions, gauzes, suturing, and dressing materials were introduced, patients could be sent home from the hospital following more complex surgery. Different lotions and materials were deemed appropriate for cleaning and covering different types of wounds. For example, a varicose ulcer would require a completely different treatment regime from a wound following abdominal surgery or trauma, where the standard application of warm water, lint, and gauze had previously represented a one-size-fits-all approach. Patients and their relatives were therefore no longer considered capable of changing dressings, and equally outside the experience of the GP this became recognised as part of the specialist knowledge of the district nurse. However it did require that she carried more with her as the range of separate preprepared packs, dressings, gels, lotions, and so on, and simultaneously her expertise in this aspect of practice, steadily expanded. This also led to more research-based approaches to practice. Wound-care progress, for example, was recorded using Polaroid or digital photography, enabling accurate ongoing assessment of response to treatment.[8] Early dressing packs were standardised and contained a full set of metal scissors, forceps, and gallipots, together with gauze and dressing sheet and cotton wool. Before prepacked sachets, all liquids used for dressings were transported in bottles. The resultant increase in dressing materials needing to be carried by the nurse together with larger items such as prepacked urinary catheters and drainage bags, syringes and needles, incontinence pads, disposable enemas, and an increasing amount of related documentation, all contributed to the need for motorised transport.

PILLS, POTIONS, AND INJECTIONS

This period was one of continuous change for the nurse's daily caseload and work routine, as outlined in the final Annual Report for the East London Nursing Society written in 1968.[9] The nursing superintendent described in her report a heavy caseload containing a high percentage of elderly patients yet noted a general trend since 1957 toward a decrease in work, which she attributed to "tablets replacing insulin injections and similar changes for other conditions previously requiring injections" (mercurial diuretics, antibiotics, steroids, etc.) with 1967–1968 showing the first significant increase in patients and visits for ten years. She commented that improvisation had become "less part of the nurse's job than in the past," although the provision of disposables and other nursing equipment was proving more costly. The disposal of dressings also became a growing problem for the Public Health Department as people no longer had coal fires to allow convenient and immediate incineration. Interestingly, Miss Clewes stated that in her view, responsibility for care of the elderly was "not expected of the family to the same extent" and concepts of rehabilitation were becoming increasingly important but were possibly more time-consuming than bedside nursing had been. She noted that the districts of Stepney and Spitalfields had high rates of mental illness and alcoholism and an increasing drug problem. Finally she reported that the introduction of male and married nurses to the association's staff and the increase in specialised knowledge were important recent changes. According to Ramsay, infectious diseases had been the main problem encountered in this area until fairly recently and the population had more than halved between 1901 and 1968.[10] She noted that in 1933, with the introduction of insulin injections, the workload increased with a twenty-two percent increase in the number of visits with a corresponding fall later when self-injections were introduced. Sulphonamides and antibiotics were partially responsible for the fall in infectious diseases together with (inter)national immunisation programmes.[11] Tuberculosis nursing in particular was a major feature of urban district nursing before the war, yet by 1960 many of these skills were virtually redundant.[12]

Many of the district nurses interviewed referred to a fall in the tender loving care (TLC) of informal care and in particular, that provided by neighbours and relatives of patients. At the same time there was a rise in expectations from biomedical care provided by the new NHS and what was felt by the nurses to be an unreasonable understanding of patients' rights. Some of these changes were therefore not perceived by the nurses as heralding total and absolute progress but were viewed in a more mixed and realistic light. For example, a nurse writing in 1958 claimed:

> Discoveries of new drugs have done more than anything to change the aspect of nursing and in many cases injection therapy has replaced bedside care. This has also brought problems. Many nurses have suffered from dermatitis. The adequate sterilisation of syringes has been difficult to cope with and there have been many breakages . . . In some areas arrangements are made whereby all syringes issued to district nurses are autoclaved.[13]

In addition, the vast array of drugs introduced from the late 1950s onward increased the number of patients—particularly psychiatric patients and the elderly—who could be cared for in the community rather than the hospital, and by 1961 most tuberculosis sanitoria were closed.[14] Many terminally ill patients were nursed at home. This therapeutic revolution in so many fields of medicine combined to increase the pressure on the community as a whole, with "care in the community" coming to be seen as an excuse to offload care onto the informal carers and under-resourced district nursing service.

Postwar Britain saw a transformation in the housing of the working classes particularly in urban areas, such that by the end of this period many houses had bathrooms and inside toilets, and domestic appliances were becoming increasingly common with a resultant raising of (expected) standards of hygiene and cleanliness.[15] In addition, furniture such as the old feather beds and low, deep armchairs were gradually replaced by modern designs. These changes had important implications for the district nurse in reducing the heavier and more time-consuming aspects of her work, simultaneously cutting down patient-contact time.

DEVELOPMENTS IN TRANSPORT

These developments, together with increased use of cars to get around larger districts, also contributed to an increased caseload, and consequently less time spent with individual patients. A superintendent of District Nursing and Midwifery training in Plymouth remembered that by 1970, "most [district] nurses were trained, all lived out, all had cars or use of a Council car, all had telephones."[16] Transport technology certainly made a considerable difference: The move away from pedestrian or bicycle to motorised transport in urban areas, and from the donkey cart or the tricycle to motorbike or car, enabled the district nurse to cover a wider area in less time. Cars gradually became more readily available, but several nurses mentioned the unreliability of their cars, as did a nurse who worked in a rural area of East Sussex in the 1950s and 1960s:

> I did have a car when I went to Lewes to begin with, but I did have to empty every night, you know the radiator, and swing it in the morning, it was good going out in the night doing that, you know! It was quite hard actually, but they did produce a new one after the snow had gone. They were very good about cars, in the South East actually, they did change them quite frequently. There came a spell, eventually, when you were allowed to have your own, but it was a bit too late for me.[17]

The LCC was able to provide twenty-five cars as early as 1951 for nurses in the Central London Associations,[18] which was remarkably early for an urban area, whereas in Lancashire the "corporation" cars were described as the "worn out vehicles that nobody else would, or often could, drive."[19] By 1977 most of the difficulties had been largely overcome and the car had

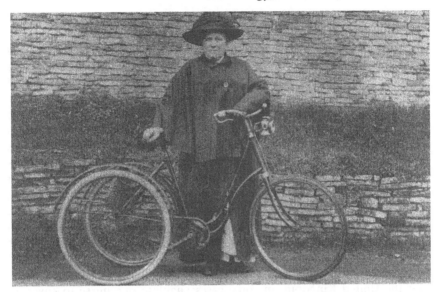

Figure 6.4 Mrs. Grey, rural village nurse-midwife, c. 1905. From Cynthia O'Neill, *More Pictures of Health* (Oxford: Meadow Books: 1991): 58. The reference there is "(Courtesy of Photocare Laboratories, Kingham)." We acknowledge the author and publishers, but unfortunately all our attempts at tracing either Ms. O'Neill or the copyright holder of the image have proved unsuccessful.

replaced the bicycle in most urban as well as rural areas, as Monica Baly described:

> Nowhere have changes been more marked than in the community [. . .] High hospital costs have promoted research into how hospital equipment can be converted into "do-it-yourself" home kits, and machines that were once the wonder of hospitals are now found as standard portable equipment in the back of the district nurse's car. But often the district nurse will have to do treatment in cramped conditions without proper plumbing, and in an emergency there is no bell to push.[20]

In one of several articles in the *QNM*,[21] the "Ivy" Motor Cycle was recommended by Nurse Mary Williams, a Queen's Nurse at Llandaff, South Wales (£50 cost compared with 22 guineas for the McKenzie motorbike). She described it as "easy to handle and most reliable" and noted that in one year she had ridden 8,000 miles although this might not have been all on district work. In her case, the DNA committee paid the insurance and contributed toward running costs. By 1928, in the Gower district, two Queen's Nurses were reported to be riding motor bicycles "which will be a great help in this very scattered district"[22] but Stocks noted that this was not evenly distributed nationwide and that "on Exmoor a Queen's Nurse still visited her patients on horseback in the late thirties."[23] Some nurses worked and lived together in pairs and were provided with a small cottage and transport varying from a bicycle to motorbike or car depending on the size and geography of the district to be covered (see Figure 6.5), whereas in towns a bicycle or mixture of pedestrian and public transport were common until the private car became more ubiquitous in the 1970s.[24]

The QNI's National Survey[25] carried out in 1934–1935 perceived the increased introduction of the car in rural areas as a major enabling factor in regrouping nursing districts and thereby reducing the need for more nurses in those areas. In 1938 this was reiterated in the QNI report to the Interdepartmental Committee on Nursing Services,[26] in which the QNI stated that "A gradual change in public opinion has taken place in recent years owing to more general demand on the part of the public for skilled nursing care, the use of the telephone and better transport facilities. This has resulted in the requisitioning of the services of Queen's Nurses by quite small districts with populations numbering 1,000 or even less."[27]

By 1938 it was estimated that 1,600 cars were in use by DNAs throughout the United Kingdom, in some cases enabling one nurse to cover an area previously covered by two nurses. This underlines the very different experience between a nurse or nurses working singly or in pairs in the rural environment and those living in nurses' homes, working in the urban setting, and traveling much shorter distances either on foot, bicycle, or public transport. However, this meant that the urban workload was

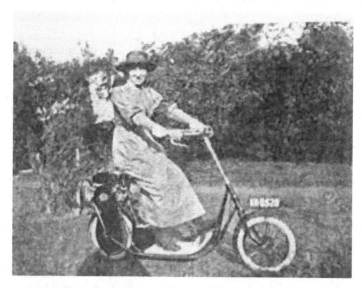

Figure 6.5 Nurse Radburn on her motor scooter. Photograph from "Swanscombe District Nursing Society" *QNM* XVII:3(1920): 49. Reproduced by kind permission of the Queen's Nursing Institute.

often extremely heavy as described by a nurse who trained in London in the 1930s:

> Oh yes, in the mornings, must have been around eight o'clock, we congregated down the basement, round a big table, and the Supervisors were there. They took us out for a few days to get to know the area, and then you were allocated your work, well, lots of it you knew, because of previous days. And there were insulins every morning. There were so many. All the tenements, a lot of walking! (Prompt: You were walking? You didn't have a bicycle?) No, not in London. No bicycle, no. But we trotted out with our bags, everybody going to their own area. And then we'd come in for lunch . . . but I think it was around about five o'clock you started on the evening visits.[28]

We have shown that geographical isolation made rural district nursing a particularly difficult undertaking and distinct in many ways from the urban situation. Combined with harsh winter weather it could become treacherous at times. Just getting from one patient to another in rural or remote areas often required great physical endurance. Hence, travelling tales are a feature of district nurses' stories and are often told with nostalgic pride (see Figure 6.6). Nurses used all sorts of transport aside from the usual bicycle, bus,

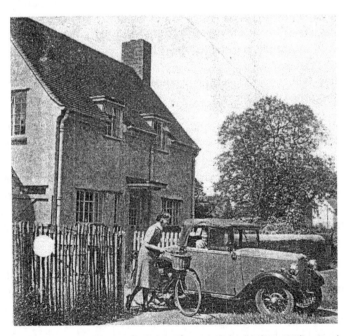

Figure 6.6 Nurses setting out. From QNI recruitment leaflet: "Why not become a Queen's Nurse? A worthwhile career" (c.1947): 2. Reproduced by kind permission of the Queen's Nursing Institute.

car, or walking. One nurse who worked in a rural area spoke of travelling to confinements during thick snow on a horse-drawn sledge.[29] Another who worked in a city recalled the brakes being removed from her motorbike while she attended a case.[30] However, such behaviour toward the nurse and her property was unusual. On the contrary, the public were generally aware of the amount of travelling the district nurse's job incurred and invariably she would be given a seat on a bus or have her bag carried up tenement stairs for her:

> Mind you everybody looked up to the Queen's. If you got into a bus even an old buddy would offer you a seat and I would say, "No thanks, but if you take my bag." "Oh what a weight," they would say when you put the bag down on their knee.[31]

People often tried to help the nurse with transport. Local garage workers would rescue nurses whose cars had become stuck in mud or deep snow, boatmen remained on call to ferry nurses to and from patients, bicycles were designated by locals for the nurse's use, and in particularly inaccessible parts farmers offered the use of horses and carts. However, nurses had their preferences, and not all offers of help were welcome:

> And then one day, at dinner time, the back door went, and here's the man with a motor bike. And I said, "What are you doing with a motor bike?" He says, "It's for you." "Well," I says, "you can take it away" I says, "I'm not putting my leg over that."[32]

One nurse who covered several islands recounted a memorable journey highlighting the island nurse's reliance on local boatmen:

> Mull, the island of Aird, these were two islands I went to. Iona had quite a population, perhaps about a hundred or less than a hundred, but I didn't have to go very often. Aird, on the other hand, was served by a ferry boat complete with oars—the Iona one was an engine . . . But it was quite a responsibility going to a confinement in these areas. The doctor was old, not very robust, and I remember on one occasion, the tide was very low and we couldn't go over, so the ferryman had to take us over on his back, piggy back over to the island.

> The sea could be quite boisterous between Mull and Iona, but the ferryman had a great reputation, they would never take the boat out if it was going to be really dangerous, except in the very direst of emergency. I remember going over once [and] there was a blanket put over my head you know, they said to keep me from the sea, but I know it was to keep me from seeing the boat going up and down in case I'd be petrified.[33]

A series published in the *Nursing Mirror* in 1948 followed a Superintendent's summer visit to her nurses in the Western Isles and featured lengthy descriptions of travel by boat, plane, foot, and pony and trap, with scarcely more reported on actual nursing matters:

> One night last winter Nurse received an urgent call to Grimisay. It was blowing a gale then, but the boat, the boatman and the Nurse braved it to the other side, and a message was sent to Hector to meet Nurse with the trap at low tide. Nurse was delayed, and when she got to the appointed place Hector had gone. (His horse had grown too restive). So nurse had to fight her way home in the dark on foot, struggling along in her oilskin and rubber boots, shining a torch and trying to avoid the rocks and the quicksands. It took her four hours, but she made it![34]

COMMUNICATIONS TECHNOLOGY

Digby noted that in the United Kingdom, "widespread adoption [of the telephone] amongst doctors began to occur mainly after 1900."[35] Although this was rather later than in the United States, it was still long before U.K. authorities considered it to be a necessary tool for a district nurse. District nurses who worked during the interwar period therefore described the main method of contact as word of mouth and recognised it as an accepted part of living and working within a community.

In practice, except where there were larger numbers of district nurses living at a nurses' home staffed during working hours, communication was achieved through a combination of a slate or message board left outside the nurse's front door to say where she could be found (see Figure 6.7), written or verbal messages sent from the patient or doctor, and messages left during the daytime at a central location such as doctor's surgery, chemist shop, or post office. It is obvious that this also made interprofessional communication less feasible, particularly in the rural setting. For example, a district nurse working in rural Hertfordshire in the late 1930s explained:

> I was the first nurse in that village—they'd had a "handy-person" there before ... They [the patients] sent someone for you—I always had a slate outside the door and they'd leave a message ... this was before they had the telephones ... they hardly ever had doctors! They said we knew more about it than they did, you see! They were practically your family.[36]

As well as increasing her sense of professional isolation, this arrangement simultaneously reinforced the nurse's position within the community and even at their beck and call. It effectively limited the degree to which she could plan her working day as she had either to return home or to check at

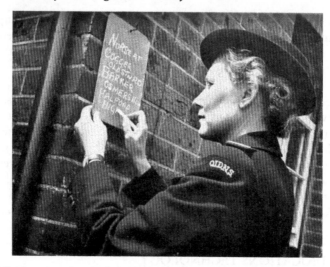

Figure 6.7 Nurse's message slate, traditionally left outside her front door. From a publicity flier for E. J. Merry and I. D. Irven, *District Nursing: A Handbook for District Nurses* (London: Bailliere, Tindall and Cox, 1948).

a message point regularly during the day. Nurses remember the discomfiture of having to ask patients with a telephone if they could use it to check for messages, or contact the GP or hospital. Mobile telephones and computers represent the most recent advance along this continuum, bringing more effective and efficient delivery of care and underlining the enormous contribution this particular technology represents.[37]

Between 1932 and 1935, a QNI-led campaign to have telephones provided for district nurses noted in its final report addressed to the Postmaster General: "It would be possible for the utility of the nurses to be greatly increased by taking advantage of modern inventions."[38] In their view, the best way of organising DNAs was to provide a nurse with a motorcar or motorcycle and to install the telephone in her house. It added, "There was not enough work in some places to keep a nurse fully occupied, but she could not be moved as she must be at hand for midwifery cases. The provision of cars and telephones would enable the nurses to be centralised and would reduce the number required."[39] This, it claimed would be an economy of approximately £12,000 per annum for rates of county councils and substantial savings for nursing associations. In response to their questionnaire-led inquiry intended to inform this campaign, a nurse wrote that if a nurse were provided with a telephone, "She would be able to work much more usefully with the doctors, since she attended cases sometimes not seeing the doctors for days, not knowing when they will call, nor they, when she will visit the patient."[40] The Postmaster General, however, did not consider this to be such an essential requirement and although a concession was granted to DNAs, it was not until the postwar period that district nurses themselves were provided with telephones and a telephone allowance as standard practice.[41]

However, as with changes in forms of transport, the improvements in communications also had a negative impact on the nurse's workload. To be readily accessible to patients and colleagues raised expectations and encroached on private life. Unlike the married GPs whose wives often defended their husband's private life at the front door or on the telephone,[42] in many cases district nurses had no gatekeeper and could therefore be more easily called on day or night, especially where nurse-midwives were concerned.

CONCLUSION

The period from 1919 to 1979 covered by this book was a period of considerable technological development, both in transport and communications technologies and in the field of pharmaceuticals, materials, and disposable equipment. These developments affected the daily work undertaken by district nurses and their workload as much as—if not more than—that of the hospital nurse. The combination of more efficient lines of communication and modes of transport, combined with a vast new array of pharmaceuticals, materials, and so on meant that district nurses were increasingly expected not only to cover a larger geographical area, but also to see more patients per day. In all but the most remote islands, time to pop in for a chat with patients and their relatives to check up on them became less practicable, contributing substantially toward a change in that relationship within the community.

Pharmacological developments, particularly the introduction of antibiotics and sulpha drugs in the mid-twentieth century, made a dramatic difference to the work and experience of the entire primary care team, not least that of the district nurse. Certain aspects of her training, such as fever nursing, became virtually redundant as infections became easier to control, and widespread infant and child immunisation programmes were adding to this change.[43] Simultaneously a rapidly expanding knowledge base was demanded as the market was flooded with new drugs under a confusing array of proprietary and generic names. The nurse was expected to learn these names, together with dosages, possible side effects, and contra-indications, at a time when district nurse training was severely compromised. Nevertheless, the district nurse's need to adapt to changing technologies was essential both to carrying out her daily work and to maintaining and improving professional status, as discussed in the next chapter.

7 Generalists and Generals: District Nursing Professionalisation

Professional society is based on merit, but some acquire merit more easily than others.[1]

District nursing has been referred to throughout this book as a sub-profession of nursing with frequent reference to its complex professional relationships, in particular, those with other members of the community-care team: the HVs, the midwives and village nurse-midwives, and the GPs. This chapter examines the meaning and implications of *profession* and *professional*, particularly as applied to district nursing and the district nurse working in the community health care context, and how this might relate to a wider nursing and medical field. It explores the contested roles that were outlined chronologically in Part I before going on to highlight what this suggests about the changing perceptions that differentiate the generalist and specialist, and what this reveals to us about the hierarchy of related professions.

Although hospital nursing increasingly gained recognition as a *profession*, particularly after the Nurses' Act (1919), the district nurse to a considerable extent appears to have retained a more *vocational* image for at least the subsequent thirty years. In contrast, over this same period the GP was most commonly a male practitioner and until the NHS Act came into force his practice was owned and managed by him as a business, having moved away from being perceived as a trade in the early nineteenth century to a "respectable" profession.[2]

Why did the professional image become so highly prized above other descriptions such as vocation, trade, or occupation? To begin with, these last two imply elements of lower status, combined with subservience or submissiveness, which tend to be associated with skilled but traditionally lower class-based work. Occupations can be differentiated from professions by looking at the method of regulation; that is, the self-regulation through peer review and an internal control mechanism of the latter as opposed to external controls used in regulating the former. Freidson, among others, referred to the professional system as "collegiality."[3] Vocation, on the other hand, implies a quasi-religious calling often associated with amateur enterprise in which material gain and organisation as a recognised body have low priorities compared with the sense of spiritual fulfilment.[4]

WHAT IS A PROFESSION?

Profession implies a set of values and judgments recognised both nationally and internationally. Identified by Giddens in his seminal work *Sociology*,[5] these are briefly summarised here, before considering how nursing meets with them as a profession. The first of these relates to a profession's autonomous regulation and control and (to a large extent) internal accountability incorporating the significance of a standardised training, qualification, and registration to professional identity. Accountability also implies the policing of "professional" behaviour of registrants; that is, accountability to a self-regulating body such as the GMC for medicine, the Bar Council for Law, and the GNC (later becoming the UKCC and since 2002, the Nursing and Midwifery Council) for nurses.[6] The second of Giddens's professional prerequisites is that of autonomous practice. Taking medicine as an example, this includes ownership of the client, particularly in the public sector, and control of positions of social and economic power in the market. This might include keeping "irregulars" out of public offices,[7] and maintaining a large degree of control over regulating ethical practice and malpractice. Although autonomy of practice applies in a similar way to most professions, that of nursing and other health-related professions often seems weaker, operating as it does in such close proximity to that bastion of professional autonomy, medicine. Larkin referred to this as "occupational imperialism,"[8] which is discussed in more detail later.

Third in Giddens's list of qualities separating the professions from non-professions is that of public recognition and respect. The professional is perceived as the gatekeeper or bridge between elite knowledge and skill base and the lay public. It is this expertise that is marketed rather than the *trading* in material consumables such as medicines. In turn this creates a professional relationship with the patient or client that combines authoritative power and a strict code of confidentiality and ethics, with professional distance. In Foucauldian terms,[9] medical discourse has come to represent an authoritative body of knowledge that has permeated society both through ideas and beliefs and through a powerful set of social and political institutions. Finally, inter- and intraprofessional recognition and respect are seen as significant professional attributes. This usually signifies power and status linked with specialisation rather than generalisation. Larson[10] referred to this as "exclusive cognitive identity" necessary both for creation and subsequently for exploitation of the market. Whereas a common educational experience created group solidarity within the medical profession, beneath this there lay a complex professional hierarchical system of "cooperative competition"[11] and prestige of specialties, teams, and institutions.

Both Davies and Witz[12] added a further characteristic, which is that a profession is traditionally male-dominated. The medical, legal, and clerical professions all carry this tradition, which despite twentieth-century inroads by women remained top-heavy with men at the beginning of the twenty-first century. As a result, nursing and midwifery sit uneasily here and might have been perceived more as vocations or occupations or semiprofessions throughout the period under discussion here. Stacey wrote of the inadequacy in trying to express concepts for understanding how women fit into the workplace, introducing the category of semiprofession. She saw this as encompassing:

> tasks which, like nursing, are undertaken in both the private domain (unpaid) and in the public domain, where they are paid at market rates depressed because they are "women's work." The confusions which abound in the analysis of professions can be related to this conceptual lacuna and result in such awkward notions as the "semi-professions," not only an unhelpful concept but insulting to those (mostly women) in the occupations so labelled.[13]

The notion of a continuum ranging from manual occupations to recognised professions such as law and medicine, as proffered by Wilensky,[14] implies that there is no definite division between an occupation and a profession, and that an occupation can be more developed professionally in one area than another. In reality, the values and judgment used to define nursing in any debate over its professional status are constantly changing. This is necessarily so, as nursing has and continues to adjust to developing specialisms, medical practice, developments in surgical and medical technology, social and economic change, and the bureaucratic control of power.

Bellaby and Oribabor, discussing the "contradictions within professionalism," applied Johnson's approach to help understand the position of nursing within the health professions. This approach places "professionalism within the relation between the producer of a service or goods and the consumer" and considered that "the establishment of a profession depends upon external factors—breaking loose from the patronage of consumers, gaining a monopoly over a sphere of practice and establishing the means to defend it (usually a law), freedom from intervention by third parties—and internal factors—means of socialising and disciplining members."[15] Their discussion is centred on the professional development of the hospital nurse and points to the fact that the framework within which nurses worked had been established and was largely controlled by the medical profession, whose ideology dominated the hospital and placed doctors in the role of gatekeeper defining the needs of patients. Bullough explained that "In the process of emerging as a profession, an occupational group tends to delegate many of the more mundane tasks to other groups or individuals."[16]

This concept can be applied both to occupational imperialism demonstrated by doctors delegating downward to nurses, and to subgroups of nursing seen within its hierarchical construct, particularly with the emergence of the Enrolled and Auxiliary nurses. Similarly Jewson described the process of medicalisation from person-oriented to object-oriented through institutionalisation and the development of an authoritarian medical profession.[17] This process is described as being multicausal and includes a range of changes. Jewson cited some of these changes as being in medical patronage, the perception of the patient, perceptions of illness, and changing roles and tasks of the doctor. With the introduction of specialisation and reductionism through anatomy and pathology, and later through the development of laboratory science—in particular, cellular biology—the doctor came to be seen as a medical investigator in a science-based medicine (based on research, diagnostics, and therapy). The professional distance between practitioner and patient was therefore increased as "a ritual mode of differentiation between the established and the outsiders."[18]

Marks compared the doctor–nurse relationship to the "power relations of the archetypal Victorian family: [using] the analogies of father–doctor, mother–matron/lady nurse, servant–paid nurse, child–patient."[19] These ideas that seeped into the language of professional curing and caring were based on stereotypical features of masculinity and femininity and the embedded notion that caring was women's work and an extension of their "essential" nature. Attitudes toward male district nurses described in Chapter 8 suggest they were similarly underrated—if only temporarily so—in the mid-twentieth century. In the male environment of the services there was no alternative, and in the psychiatric institutions they were required for their brawn, but in the more domestic sphere of community nursing, men were relegated as professionals.

The resultant separate spheres doctrine was undoubtedly used to advantage by some women in establishing their positions in a heavily class-influenced nursing hierarchy. Nevertheless, nurses were professionally subordinate to the monopolistic male medical authority until the mid-twentieth century (and arguably beyond). Bynum described how the emergence of nursing as a profession in the late nineteenth century, despite becoming increasingly diverse, had at its focus "the hospital," where nurse training schools were located and younger trainees were "initiated" into particular duties and skills, rather than in the community.[20] Walby et al.[21] conveniently presented the perceived importance of these three models of professional autonomy as either having complete professional autonomy or having only partial autonomy, but representing the patient's advocate[22] in a symbiotic yet subservient relationship with the doctor, or as totally subservient and obedient "handmaidens of medicine."

After consideration they rejected both the idea of subservience and of complementary professions. Instead they pointed to two models of professionalism acknowledging the possibility that they are gender generated or culturally differentiated. These, they claimed, were reflected in their distinctive modes of professional organisation, particularly evident in the pre-1972 situation, and continued in a modified form well after this date.[23] For a GP this would have implied taking direct responsibility for his or her own actions. Even within a medical team where a patient might be referred to a senior colleague, this does not bow to the bureaucratic model, and was increasingly so in general practice. For a district nurse, however, being professional suggested accountability to others for his or her practice under guidance of rules and hierarchical monitoring procedures. This did not mean that doctors were not to be held accountable to their professional body, more that there was a subtly different understanding of that body's role and the mode of intervention, based on historical precedent as well as their own professional autonomy. Central to this is the gendered professional ideal that implies individuality, objectivity, and mastery of knowledge, particular science-based skills and techniques based on formalised training that placed the doctor in a privileged, detached, and controlling position over the patient, whereas the nurse was held in a supportive and multifarious role, attending merely to physical and emotional needs. Rafferty described nursing as "caught in a contradiction in so far as it provides the necessary support for medicine to maintain its dominance, thereby perpetuating the subordination of nursing to medicine."[24] Nevertheless it should be noted that since the 1980s nursing has been moving toward the autonomous model of medicine, whereas medicine has become more accountable to the patient as consumer and to medical audit.

If we apply these concepts to the district nurse's developing role, she occupies what has been stereotypically represented as a vocational, maternal, or semidomestic dominantly female role, as a generalist, located outside the hospital institution, concerned more with the caring than the curing of her patient (and until the NHS Act [1948], largely supported through the voluntary sector rather than by local authorities). White[25] saw this as critical to the isolation of particular sectors of the nursing profession at least until the Rushcliffe pay agreements of the 1940s. In contrast, the arrival of qualified district nurses and midwives reduced the GP's workload (particularly from the mid-1920s) with less time spent by the GP at the bedside, thereby creating a move toward the surgery list and prescription pad and a professional disposition that was becoming more clinical and less holistic or domestic.[26]

However, it was not quite so clear-cut within community nursing (i.e., outside the hospital's medical domain) where an increasing degree of perceived autonomy was attainable and where the more rural or remote the practice, the less apparent might be the medical or nursing supervision. In addition, where the district nurse practised a more holistic form of caring encompassing a wider range of roles, the mundane tasks would have been less clearly differentiated from the more glamorous or challenging ones than might have been the case in hospital nursing. Therefore, where the practitioner and the patient were outside the institutional setting, many of these object-oriented aspects were either greatly reduced or made virtually irrelevant.

THE DESIRABILITY OF PROFESSIONALISATION
AND OF PROFESSIONAL STATUS TO NURSING

As society became increasingly secular and consumer oriented, the development of a profession became the means by which the market took control by restricting competition. Considering the financial relationship between doctors and patients in the process of professionalisation, Digby pointed to medical professionalisation as more than a "simple power relationship in which doctors increasingly dominated their clients."[27] Medicine's struggle for autonomous control of the market and of the patient throughout the nineteenth century can be perceived as one against all "unqualified" practitioners with scientisation of medicine as a central theme. The characteristics of the profession that promoted exclusivity and protection of status through a closed-door society supports this concept, effectively replacing a diffuse range of approaches to sickness and healing, with this dominant biomedical approach. This located both professions within a social- and consequently gender-structured, hierarchical, and patriarchal system, both professions being at their most sensitive formative stages at a time when lack of female suffrage and internal professional disunity weakened the nurses' position still further. In addition, this placed greater value on the treatment and cure of acute illnesses and less on longer term management and cure of the elderly, chronically sick, or mentally ill.

This early clash of views was documented and discussed in detail by Katherine Williams,[28] who based a chapter on references from an article published in the *BMJ* by an unknown author, which is then compared with one by Margaret Breay,[29] published in the *Nursing Record and Hospital World*. In this comparative study, Williams made an important point concerning professionalisation. To the section of the nursing community supporting registration, represented by Miss Breay, selective recruitment of suitable—and by implication, female—students, combined with a "modern system of [hospital, apprentice-style] training and educating" were the essential "first principles" that would raise the professional status of the nurse and "it is upon the principle of Profession that the public identity of nursing should be settled." In contrast, the medical view expressed in the *BMJ* article cited suggests that some doctors would prefer nursing reform to be limited to reform of selection procedures only, with the aim to increase the "womanly character" or feminine attributes associated with caring for the sick, while retaining the position of employment as "ward-maid."

This represents an oversimplistic view of medical and nurse theorists at the end of the nineteenth century. For example, Mortimer argued that the private nurse was in quite a different position, possessing far greater autonomy of practice in some circumstances, working in close proximity with doctors in others, and as colleagues rather than as competitors.[30] It would be reasonable to assume that other nurses working outside the constraints of the hospital might also have experienced a similar, albeit diluted, feeling of independence. It would also seem reasonable to believe that some more enlightened doctors would have welcomed skilled and educated nurses rather than ward-maids, appreciating that they could be trusted both to care for and to educate their patients, albeit under their own terms. Nevertheless, this discussion is important in underlining the recognised significance of skilled independent practice by both nursing and medical professions, despite the fact that professional autonomy was not highlighted as an important characteristic of professionalisation until 1933, when Carr-Saunders and Wilson wrote *The Professions*.[31]

A paper presented by the Deputy Medical Director, Central Council for Health Education, Dr. Dalzell-Ward, in 1957[32] attempted to establish the meaning of profession and the reason and need for professional organisations with particular reference to those involved in medicine and nursing. He based this initially on the need for a contractual relationship that would create confidence in the practitioner, stating that this must include possession of "qualifications obtained after recognised training, which will be a guarantee to a client" whilst taking personal responsibility to the client as an essential to this. In his view it followed that this also involved the need for a professional organisation that was neither a guild nor trade union, and yet involved maintenance and promotion of professional status (presumably from within), through provision of a service to that part of the community that needed it. Therefore he claimed that a "profession exists primarily to serve the community" and "should not further its own interests for its own sake, but only in so far as this is necessary in order to serve the community." This is rather an altruistic definition compared with the more self-interested rationale put forward in this and previous chapters; however, the boundaries between altruism and enlightened self-interest can prove difficult to define in reality.

However, being a professional might be measured using alternative or additional criteria. Society often recognises a person as having professional rather than occupational status, but the criteria used to make this distinction are quite obscure and amorphous. In 1937, Miss Wilmshurst, the General Superintendent of the QNI, referred to the freedom and independence experienced by a (Queen's) district nurse, and particularly to the possibilities for district nurses to:

> have homes of their own, for instance. It is a joy to every woman to have her own home. [. . .] "This freedom" is not, to her, a catch phrase: it is an ever-present condition of her life. Frequently she has a car. What other working woman dependent on her earnings can have a car so early in her career? Of course her car is for working purposes, but the office clerk, clinging to her strap, will probably never know the joys of handling a car at all.[33]

These were the standards against which she was measuring district nursing as a professional career for a single woman, for whom the opportunities were largely limited to office work or teaching. Several oral history inter-viewees similarly offered office work or teaching as the main alternatives they saw for themselves in the 1940s and 1950s. Three had actually worked as secretaries, one as a cashier, and another as a teacher, prior to training as nurses. For those who reached supervisory or nursing officer status, the pay and conditions of work that might appear unfair and male dominated over half a century later appear to have been accepted with little question, and the potential opportunities of travel, managerial experience, independence, public respect, and material things such as a car, telephone, and the possibil-ity of home ownership, marked the district nurse out as a professional per-son. As more women were able to aspire to these symbols of status, a fall in the social prominence of the district nurse seems unsurprising. In addition, the district nurse's standing within the nursing profession as a whole fell for a while following the NHS Act (1948).

In 1943 in a lecture explaining the possibilities of an NHS in the postwar reconstructing of health care provision, Dr. Balme described the difficulties created by nursing not being a "closed" profession. By this he meant one in which training centres set a fixed high standard and the title of nurse was reserved for those whose qualifications admitted them to the Register. He described five categories of nurse practising in the community, from the SRN (who might be a Queen's Nurse or district or private nurse), a par-tially trained nurse or nurse-midwife, a school-leaver prior to starting gen-eral training acting as a Probationer at the local cottage hospital, untrained village women who "specialised" in the care of bedridden folk (referred to as "good practical Nurses"), and finally children's nurses or nannies. With the war there was the addition of Auxiliary Nurses, British Red Cross and St. John's Ambulance Nurses.[34] and Assistant Nurses who later were given a recognised training and became State Enrolled Nurses.[35]

In the community situation few nurses openly questioned the GP. From being relatively independent practitioners in the mid-nineteenth century, despite their royal charter and patronage and the powerful backing of the Queen's Institute, district nurses were answerable to, and under the direc-tion of, GPs by 1900, a position fiercely defended in some instances by local branches of the BMA.[36] However, it is significant that it was the HVs rather than the district nurses who eventually managed to establish a far more equal and autonomous professional relationship despite their appar-ent marginalisation and the later threat from social workers. Hart[37] partly ascribed this to the lack of a preconceived public image. The Women Sani-tary Inspectors' Association, which preceded the Health Visitors' Associa-tion, was formed as early as 1896, but unlike district or hospital nurses, health visitors did not have an earlier public image to hamper their profes-sional development.

From a national viewpoint, the World War II marked an important water-shed in the professionalisation process, with a substantial increase in the number of nurses employed at Ministry of Health headquarters, including the creation of a Nursing Division and appointments of nursing officers for general public health as well as for hospital nursing. It was felt this gave nursing "a voice in formulating policy affecting it, and not as one which, as hitherto, has had its problems presented chiefly by the Medical Profession."[38] At the grassroots level there was also a move from within the QNI to have a greater say in the running of the profession through the formation of the Queen's Nurses' League in 1942 and its subsequent regional and national meetings and conferences.[39]

The NHS Act marked a move away from voluntaristic control and employment and to uniformity of pay under the Rushcliffe and Taylor salary scales and compulsory inclusion of all nurses employed by local authorities in the Local Government Superannuation scheme.[40] Nevertheless, as was shown in Chapter 4, these advances were of little value with regard to the critical issues of professional organisation: training and self-regulation of district nurses, which received low priority from government. The result of this was that grassroots employment and supervision of district nurses fell largely to the office of the MOH. Kratz claimed the Working Party that was set up in 1953 to look at the training of district nurses was "at the behest of local authorities and their medical officers of health"[41] and that this influenced the findings that "only little additional preparation was required" for SRNs and none for SENs, a fact supported by testimony from several interviewees who were employed and expected to learn on the job. A comment in the *Royal Society of Health Journal* expressed the economics of the situation: "It remains to be seen how many authorities will consider it desirable or will be able to insist that their district nurses have some special training, especially in view of the fact that a district nurse with special training at present earns £10 per annum more than a nurse who does not have such training."[42] Interprofessionally, even following NHS reorganisation in 1974, some district nurse sectors came under hospital nurse management, whereas others were under the community-based control of HV directors of nursing, either scenario continuing effectively to bar district nurses from direct participation in their own management, policymaking, and implementation. This was eventually addressed in 1979 with the Nurses, Midwives and Health Visitors Act, which was responsible for reconstituting the Panel of Assessors for District Nursing Training.

A further concern was the introduction of home help, auxiliary nurses, and SENs to community nursing (see later) and the title home nurse to encompass all grades of nurse working in the community and was also used to describe care provided by voluntary organisations such as local branches of the British Red Cross and St. John's Ambulance. Concern was expressed "for proper distinction between the amateur with an elementary knowledge of basic principles, that enables her to look after a sick relative or neighbour, and the experienced, fully trained, professional district nurse."[43] This emphasises the importance of professional (as opposed to amateur) status. The editorial continues, "A general practitioner would not expect to

be called 'home doctor' because he visits patients in their homes. [. . .] To
refer to a district nurse as a 'home nurse' is just as illogical."

GENERALISTS OR SPECIALISTS?

Writing a series of articles to *The Times* in 1926 Dr. Shadwell, an MOH and
member of the QNI executive council commented:

> Of all the multitudinous forms of social service carried on today none is
> more real and practical, yet more unobtrusive, than what is called dis-
> trict nursing. Little is heard of it, and many readers probably have only
> a vague notion, if any, of what it is . . . The sick nurse is the doctor's
> assistant and ally, universally recognised to-day as indispensable, and
> the district nurse in particular is the assistant and ally of the general
> practitioner, who practises among the sick poor. She shares his work,
> the importance of which is becoming better understood and appreciated
> than it used to be . . . The public have a curiously exaggerated idea of
> the extent and value of specialism . . . But the modern general practi-
> tioner is an all-round specialist, if one may use the expression, and his
> assistant . . . the district nurse must be one, for in her sphere there is no
> specialism; she must take the cases as they come, medical or surgical,
> acute or chronic . . . It is as necessary for the nurse as the doctor, and
> in some respects less easy. He comes and goes and wields an authority,
> which she does not command, by virtue of his position. Her relation
> is more intimate and homely . . . But that gives her a unique influence
> equally free from patronage and officialism, both of which are generally
> suspect and often resented.[44]

The notion of the modern GP as an all-round specialist seems something
of a contradiction in terms and yet district nurses and hospital nurses
alike recognised that a generally (but hospital-only) trained nurse "should
undergo special training in district nursing by specialists in this branch of
her work before she commences work on the district."[45] Clearly, certain
aspects of the work differentiated between the specialised techniques and
demands (seen as specialist) and the broad mixture of patients and their
illnesses to be nursed (viewed as generalist).[46] In particular this article specified the need for more initiative than in hospital nursing, emphasised the
ability to improvise in less than ideal surroundings, and placed the weight
of increased responsibility as among the specialist facets of district nursing.
Other articles emphasised the educative, public health role of preventative
medicine or early symptomatology of disease or terminal care management
at home, in a similar light as specialist aspects of district nursing practice.
  Burnham described medical specialisation as having grown "out of the
proliferation of knowledge and technology that called for physicians to limit

their focus so as to have a deep competence in a restricted field"[47] (i.e., expertise). Similarly, in making the case for recognised and standardised training, a special group set up by the RCN Executive Committee noted that HVs and midwives were both required to undertake specialist training before being allowed to practise. In their view it was equally necessary for district nurses to fulfil a similar postregistration requirement because of their particular responsibilities in supporting whole "families in the crisis of illness" or in the special demands of clinic or school nursing, and taking into account the growing "complexity and volume of work undertaken."[48] In addition, they felt that the increasing trend toward "a community health team, able to provide comprehensive family care" and the desired "close co-ordination of the hospital and community services" could be better achieved if community nurses were "adequately prepared." Explaining what this implied for the proposed training curriculum, the report itemised aspects such as awareness of the district nurse's distinctive educative role, understanding the social services available for patient and family, awareness of particular socioeconomic and emotional implications of illness at home, together with instruction in presymptomatic diagnostic procedures, adaptation of hospital techniques for community practice, and preparation of the student "for her role as a member of the family health care team within general practice."[49] However, like the GP it is significant that generalisation was often considered inferior to specialisation by their respective hierarchies and that training was confined to hospital practice with the community aspects not reaching the compulsory teaching curriculum in either profession until the mid-twentieth century.

The postwar period is therefore seen as one marking considerable changes, particularly in interprofessional relationships. First, the doctor was being forced to become a team player particularly through his role in the primary health care team. He was seen to be losing autonomy and becoming increasingly answerable to a more critical and litigation-minded public, handing over management to practice managers, and devolving much of his previous role (including some prescribing) to practice and district nurses. In addition, an increasing trend toward alternatives to biomedicine had found a market-led response by the GP in particular to embrace homeopathy, acupuncture, osteopathy, and so on. Similarly, district nursing from the 1970s was embracing specialist areas of nursing such as terminal care, stoma care, diabetic care, or respiratory care, either combined with general district nursing or working alongside specialist nurses working in the community.

The integration of these specialisms within the general field of district nursing was met with varying degrees of success, with some nurses seeing this development as a direct threat, encroaching on their professional territory or diminishing their status.[50] Similarly, the widespread introduction of practice nurses in the 1970s was felt to be removing some of the more interesting aspects of district nursing work such as running clinics, doing minor surgery with GPs, and giving vaccinations or doing dressings for the more ambulant patients able to attend the surgery. At this stage practice nurses were often SRNs with no specialist training and employed directly by the GPs, and so presented something of a threat to the district nurse in several ways—coming between district nurse and GP, undermining her status, and taking away her more ambulant, easier cases.

Through changes in administration and the move to GP attachment, a better channel of communication was established between members of the primary health care team. This, together with other studies, suggests that although the team approach brought members of the primary health care team together to work from the same physical environment and gave them opportunities for better interaction, in reality they continued to work alongside one another rather than together as an integrated team.[51] Nevertheless, day-to-day practice was increasingly based on negotiation and exchanges of ideas between nurses and doctors were becoming a more common feature than subservience. In general the district nurse was becoming a more interdependent practitioner at patient level. Perhaps the final word on this should belong to the oral history interviewees. We were bemused by the responses of district nurses and GPs to questions about interprofessional relationships, which were almost invariably "We always got on very well," and rarely indicated the existence of tensions or conflict. Personal experience confirmed that this was not always the case and reminded us of the "silences" that alerted Gittins to unspoken problems in some of her oral histories.[52] Closer enquiry revealed that where there were personality clashes or professional disagreements, the solution on the part of the nurse was often to take evasive action and avoid that particular doctor if at all possible.[53]

Attempting to ascertain exactly what the district nurse perceived necessary to make her a professional led to some quite different observations. In particular, the relationship with the patient was seen as a professional one if there was a degree of business-like detachment or what might appear to be impassiveness on the part of the nurse; for example:

> I mean, there have been patients, you know, that's complained about me as well. Well, there was one particular one, and . . . Ted and Mary, and, of course, Mary had multiple sclerosis, she was ex-nurse . . . the man she was living with, this . . . with Ted. Well, he's had every nurse in St. Helen's crying. Everybody's come out of that house and said, "I'm not going back again." And he used to then . . . sometimes he would phone up and he would say, "I am not having Sister Skepper in this house again." And I would walk in the next morning, and I would just say, "Good morning, Ted. Did you have a good night?" But, you see, I always went in exactly the same every day, because I'm not a moody person, I don't take umbrage. You tell me, "Get lost!" well, you know, I'll just go back in the next day . . . And I really do think that you've got to keep that being professional with patients, because . . . I have got

to tell you off if need be. You know, if you're not pulling the weight, really, so I . . . and when I went in, I always introduced myself as "Sister Skepper," you know, so I did . . . although I was very kind to patients, I was still, you know.[54]

Being professional was a term applied not only to particular skills and practice, but also to professional behaviour, which incorporated the code of nursing ethics. However, what was considered unprofessional behaviour ranged from criticising the doctor in front of the patient to rather less obvious failings such as spending too long talking to the patient or relatives (i.e., not keeping a professional distance).

By the mid-1970s nursing was beginning to move toward the longer, university-based, training bearing more similarity to the medical model with post-registrational specialisation (including district nursing and community specialisms) becoming the trend. Professional nursing skills were becoming more easily defined, identified with technical expertise and associated with formally acquired knowledge. Gender balance was also changing during that decade. More men entered the mainstream nursing profession and, significantly, reached the higher levels more quickly than women (averaging 8 years against 18 years from qualification to nurse manager[55]) and there were more women entering the medical profession, although, in contrast, they remained noticeably absent at the upper levels. As might be expected, district nursing attracted fewer men than hospital acute nursing, although numbers had risen considerably in the thirty years of accepting men into this field. This might be partly explained by the fact that for promotion to senior jobs, midwifery was a prerequisite, and until the mid-1970s this was an area closed to men.

CONCLUSION

The professional image of nursing as judged against the opening key characteristics appeared no longer in doubt by 1979. District nurses had become by then, like their hospital counterparts, more closely associated with the medical model and the team aspect of health care,[56] losing much of their communitarian image. With changes in hospital policy, particularly relating to reductions in inpatient length of stay,[57] the job was becoming more demanding in knowledge of medical and surgical advances as a nursing science. Corresponding changes in the terminology associated with current nursing procedures such as reflective practice, nurse prescribing, and patient care plans, were soon to mirror this. A question remains to be asked: how far could this paradigm shift in nursing values allow the district nurse's professional role to be extended toward the "curing," specialist-focused medical sciences and away from the gendered social limitations of the more holistic and generalistic "nursing art" of caring?

1919 to 1979 was a period during which district nursing saw a pendulum swing back and forth between professionalism and managerialism, with the professional model emphasising the educational and theoretical foundation of nursing combined with self-regulation. The managerial model pulled in a different direction, following the hierarchical system of levels or grades of specialist-trained, basic-trained, and untrained nurses, allowing for some degree of non-nurse management to oversee practice or patient care. Throughout this time period, there was a continual struggle to achieve parity of status with other nurses in the community and with medical colleagues largely through striving to establish an "autonomous knowledge base."[58] Although it would be oversimplistic to suggest an either–or scenario, as the emphasis clearly drifted between the two models rather than totally embracing one or the other, this does provide a useful approach for understanding the changing situation in which district nurses had to live and work. The issue of reconciling professionalism and caring skills and "the frustrations of nurses who say that the system does not allow them to nurse"[59] is highlighted by the dilemma of extended, technicalised roles that continue to the present, often resented as money-saving paramedical skills and the placing of responsibility by time-pressed doctors onto nurses without adequate training or appropriate financial recompense. It created a dilemma for nurses in the community as in hospitals, attracted by previously "forbidden fruit" in the form of technical skills that reduce patients' and nurses' waiting times for harassed GPs to perform tasks clearly within the nurse's capabilities. At the same time, accepting these extra duties added significantly to workloads and feelings of being taken advantage of by medical colleagues and management.

8 Language of Caring:
Care and Nurses' Lives

Here we look at how the concept of caring underpins ideas in nursing. With reference to debates on nursing services we see how definitions of care can be used as pragmatic, political tools to shape government policy. This entails a delineation of nursing tasks and personal care. Testimonies show that nurses of the past were not ignorant of this distinction but that it did not impinge on what was for them an intuitive understanding of nursing practice. Commonplace understanding of nursing is inseparable from a notion of caring but within this relationship the term *caring* is itself nuanced by the context in which it is used. In current policymaking, for example, it is imbued with political significance, sociologically it often serves feminist argument, and for individuals it can help to bind professional and personal identity. The latter holds true for many of those interviewed for this book, but in the professionalisation of nursing the indivisibility of nursing and caring has been unpalatable. The history and sociology of the professions has informed contemporary thinking on the relationships among caring, nursing, and femininity and presented theories that help to disentangle one from the other. Adopting this perspective, nursing commentary has increasingly tended to shy away from traditional holistic notions of caring, in the pursuit of an image for nursing that conforms more to professionalism and associated biomedical treatments of illness, rather than to comprehensive responsiveness.

Nursing care was a ubiquitous phrase in oral testimony and one often underpinned by moral and spiritual values. Similarly, marriage and motherhood were viewed as inherently caring roles but were not compatible with a career in nursing. They also reinforced traditional notions of femininity that resonate throughout nursing history. With due consideration of Davies's seminal work on the gendered nature of organisations we suggest that past district nurses managed to balance a sense of professionalism and a feminine, caring ethos with relative ease. By looking at a few individual cases we explore the place of these values in the concept of nursing care. In a brief examination of the way in which both male and female nurses recount their experiences, we see how the language of care has been modified to reflect a more contemporary perspective and how the nurse–patient relationship became increasingly framed more by a professional ethos than a personal one.

NURSING CARE AS A POLITICAL EXPEDIENT

That the definition of *care* is a contentious public issue has been evident in recent debates over the levels of support the sick and elderly should be offered by the state. Responding to the Commission on Long-Term Care (1999) the New Labour government in Westminster drew on a distinction made between nursing care and personal care. Although the Commission recommended that nursing and personal care be funded out of taxation and be free at the point of delivery, the government agreed to fund only nursing care and "only that given by a qualified nurse, as opposed to a healthcare assistant. Personal care, such as help with washing, using the toilet, eating and dressing, would still be subject to means tests."[1] This distinction between personal and nursing care can be seen as a tactical manoeuvre by the government on two counts: One, it appeals to the psyche of the highly qualified nurse keen to protect her professional status, thereby inviting her support; and two, it lays the ground on which the government might hope to reduce its financial responsibility for health care. As pointed out by Sir Stewart Sutherland who led the Commission, this means that those elderly people requiring long-term personal care at home might have to pay for it themselves while those being cared for by nurses in hospitals will be given this care free of charge.

People suffering from dementia, such as Alzheimer's disease, where personal care is often the only treatment, are much more likely to be cared for in the community and therefore, in line with government policy, are more likely to be subjected to a means test and its outcome. An elderly person suffering from a long-term illness requiring hospitalisation and nursing care would not undergo a financial assessment and care would be given free. Not only does the decision by the Westminster government inspire a sense of injustice—why should one be open to financial penalty according to which illness one falls victim?—but it also draws into sharp relief the shifting boundaries of care and its use as a political and economic expedient.[2] The Scottish Executive approached the matter in a manner arguably more profligate than egalitarian, stating that, in Scotland, all care for the elderly, both personal and nursing care, would be provided free of charge. This was regarded as controversial, with critics claiming the scheme would be inherently problematic to implement and expensive. Although costs have indeed been higher than expected, the policy has brought benefits, notably in raising debate on the quality of care at home and in supporting informal carers.[3]

This debate over long-term care for the elderly is undeniably a political issue concerned more with economic prudence than the philosophical nature of care. It is a working definition for the reshaping of government responsibility to serve financial ends. Its intention apart, logically this distinction rests on categorising the tasks that health care workers carry out for and with their patients according to two different kinds: personal tasks and nursing tasks. This strategy suggests that the patient can be separated from his or her illness, that personal care and nursing care are given in quite different situations and are focussed on separate aspects of the patient. It is arguable whether this is a perception of the patient or a definition of care that enters into the daily reckoning of district nurses today, but testimony suggests that to question care in this way did not occur to district nurses in previous decades. Without exception, all those interviewed for this book emphasised the district nursing they practised as a caring activity. They did this unashamedly and with some degree of personal conviction that what they called care is not necessarily what the term means for present-day district nurses and their managers. This calls into question the conception of care that drove district nurses of the past and how it relates to that of present-day district nursing practice.

DEFINING NURSING TASKS

Throughout the period between 1940 and 1999, there was a distinct shift in attitudes to non-nursing tasks and discussing this with interviewees has helped to shape both the experiential and ethical landscape of past district nursing that they portrayed. Almost all elderly nurses interviewed, most of whom retired in the 1970s or 1980s, spoke of "non-nursing care" as a feature of the past and not the present. Although we remain sceptical of this (the few younger nurses interviewed who were still working in the 1990s also interpreted their nursing responsibility with reference to patient need as well as, and independently of, nursing skills), the prevailing narrative of the past is one of the selfless nurse responding equally to nursing and social need.

With the development of health and social care services since the 1970s, the range of people providing home care has increased throughout the country. Since then, more routine bedside nursing tasks, such as bathing, dressing, and feeding have been delegated to lesser qualified auxiliaries, paid or unpaid carers, leaving the nurse free to exercise her clinical nursing skills in more technical tasks. Now, as a complement to home nursing, nurses with specialist training deliver nursing care in the home for specific conditions or provide palliative care to the terminally ill, home helps undertake light housework and shopping, "tuck-in" services check up on the elderly and infirm in the evening, and social workers offer advice and practical help with a range of financial and social difficulties. Hence, tasks that were once discretionary but often perceived as a moral obligation for the district nurse are now the legitimate responsibility of other services. Most district nurses of the past undertook as a matter of routine what are now regarded as non-nursing tasks, but testimonies also show that there were differing attitudes toward this practice:

> You were a Jenny-a'-thing. And the people needed you and the help that they needed was very often not entirely all nursing. I mean they

wouldn't have any breakfast, they wouldn't have had a cup of tea, their fire wouldn't have been put on. Now of course that's changed.[4]

Despite the perception that this had changed, one younger district nurse who was still practising in the late 1980s suggested that the nurse's response to patient need might not have changed dramatically; that it was not uncommon for her to carry out simple domestic tasks for a patient, such as replacing a light bulb, but that, strictly speaking, she should not have done this.[5] Whereas in the past such things were done at the nurse's discretion (and were very common), in more recent times nurses have been told explicitly not to do them. This is influenced largely by a concern to maintain a high professional status for nursing as well as insurance considerations regarding liability if the nurse were to be injured while performing a non-nursing task, the latter underlining the current concern to detail nursing duties more formally than in the past. However, the point is made that district nurses of the past tended to respond in a personal way to patient need, continued to do so until the very recent past, and presumably often still do regardless of regulations.

In rural or island districts the relative isolation of patients could mean the nurse staying with a patient for days either through the need for personal care or through the effects of bad weather. One Shetland nurse told of a winter midwifery call to deliver a baby in a lighthouse. A snowstorm isolated the house and she was stuck there for five days until the nurse of the adjoining district informed the authorities, who then sent out a snowplough to clear the nurse's way. While there, she was able to attend to the mother and help look after the newborn baby, giving the mother an unplanned but appreciated degree of support. Whereas weather conditions impacted on the district nurse's work in rural areas, housing conditions and poverty were more pertinent factors in the city.

Many an urban district nurse's work was informally extended as they tried to help patients with financial or social problems. One nurse recalled organising a repayment scheme for a family to help them out of a spiral of debt. For others, understanding and adaptability were crucial in households where basic material goods were in short supply:

> You learned to be very adaptable. Patients probably wouldn't be able to give you what you were asking for, you might have to wait weeks before they would see a relative that would buy, say basins and facecloths and towels like that . . . But you could be adaptable. And we always kept bits and pieces in the nurses' home . . . sheeting and that sort of thing . . . you couldn't even get a piece of newspaper in some of their homes, but you, it was nothing to put a newspaper in your bag.[6]

Nurses of all districts recall efforts to alleviate difficulties beyond the call of their nursing duties either by confronting patients' problems directly or notifying the nursing superintendent:

It was a farm cottage out the town, he was a farm worker . . . the baby was born . . . and the bed was soaking wet . . . and I said to the husband we'll need to get another mattress . . . when we lifted the mattress it was maggots under it . . . so I just phoned Miss D. [Superintendent] and she got in touch with the medical officer of health. I couldn't be responsible if that woman gets an infection.[7]

By the mid-1970s the range of health and social workers in the community had become wider and brought with it greater accountability. Professional boundaries were more closely guarded and all staff were obliged to respect procedures for dealing with patient and client needs. For nurses who had been used to both identifying and fulfilling the needs of their patients in a direct and personal way, this new bureaucratic approach to need was felt to be heavy-handed and laborious:

Until the change-over in '75 . . . we could do some of the social work and everything, . . . but then, when that change took place, you were told definitely that . . . if you wanted any social work done or anything like that you applied to the appropriate department, you didn't do any of it . . . I found it was quite good when you could really do everything yourself . . . It didn't take so long to happen . . . if I felt I wanted something done for the welfare of somebody, I wanted it done, not two or three weeks hence.[8]

I found it frustrating . . . in fact I overstepped it an odd time . . . One of the times, there was somebody and there was nothing happening and I contacted the appropriate department and I got into trouble . . . I was carpeted more or less and told that it wasn't my job to do that sort of thing, that it was social work department . . . and the head of the social work department had been in contact etc. etc. . . . so please do not do that again.[9]

Generally, the district nurse's concept of nursing was one that supported the inclusion of non-nursing tasks in her remit. It was an accepted part of the nurse–patient relationship that the nurse would care for the patient in this holistic way. There were, however, some dissenting voices on this matter:

I found that a lot of the people, I think, were thinking back to the days before the National Health Service where they had had private nurses and things like that, and felt that when you went in to do something in their house, that you had unlimited time to just do anything, and spend any amount of time. And they could be right time wasters. Just that they could be awkward and slow you up in doing things, and ask you to do odd bits and pieces that's really, unless you were rude, you couldn't refuse to do. But you felt that it was taking advantage. . . . I've been asked to clean the bath, handed the cloth and asked to clean the bath. But unless I knew the circumstances . . . were such, I refused to do [it], because I told them that was not my job to clean baths.[10]

Well, making maybe cups of tea and stuff like that, you know. And occasionally lighting a fire . . . I didn't tend to do an awful lot that was beyond nursing, because it's something I disagree with, very strongly, that the nurses, that people expect the nurses should be everything. Why? You know. I mean, other carers could have been in and the doctor could have been in, or anybody, and they wouldn't ask them to light the fire or anything, so why? And then, well, of course, you did it because they put you in an awful position, you couldn't leave somebody . . . Well, it was very difficult to say no. But, I learned after a while to be a bit more, strong willed about it. Because, you know, it was ridiculous.[11]

The undertaking of non-nursing tasks was something that featured significantly in the interviews. For most of the nurses interviewed, undertaking non-nursing tasks was considered to be a defining characteristic of district nursing and one of the things that differentiated past from present definitions. Although one younger nurse spoke of still doing non-nursing tasks in the 1980s, the perception among elderly retired district nurses is that this was something of the past. Those who did not easily agree to doing these tasks used phrases like "that was not my job" or compared themselves to "other carers and the doctor" who were less likely to be asked to do them. Here the practice of district nursing described as a job suggests that it is one that can be defined by the inclusion or exclusion of given tasks. For the majority who incorporated non-nursing tasks as essential to their definition of district nursing, the whole process of nursing tends to be seen in terms of their relation to patients as opposed to either colleagues or to clearly delineated professional tasks. Although current thinking has erected clearer professional boundaries around the nurse's duties, it has been more difficult to retrieve a concept of care from traditional ideas of gender and morality.

GENDER, CARING, AND MORAL GOOD

The activity of caring viewed as the sphere of the "ideal woman" has persisted at some level since the nineteenth century:

Medicine and Nursing came to be seen as complementary activities in the sense that if nursing was feminine, medicine was masculine: the nurse was the ideal woman, the doctor the ideal man. His intelligent, active, pragmatic qualities were appropriate for the aggressive treatment of disease but not compatible with caring.[12]

In the Nightingale era this notion of care assumed a heightened significance as central to the concept of the ideal woman and the spirit of nursing. Even today it continues to define the moral basis of nursing as a moral good. What has changed is the definition of the ideal woman and the degree to which caring enters into this definition: "From history it can be learned that the objective of care for the sick requires certain virtues . . . such virtues do not merely derive from attitudes, preferences or feelings, but are embodied in universal moral principles."[13]

The discussion here is largely based on the oral testimony of retired district nurses. As might be expected, then, it relies predominantly on the testimony of women and so gender-based theories of care must be considered. However, a few men were also interviewed and later in the chapter the experience of one of them who trained in the 1940s is outlined briefly. Of particular interest is the similarity between his approach to district nursing and those of his female counterparts. First, we show how some elderly district nurses conformed to traditional notions of nursing by portraying their work as a feminine occupation, describing nursing care in terms of a maternal or spiritual activity.

NURSING CARE AS MOTHERING

As we have seen, in many districts, particularly in rural areas, the district nurse was a central figure. If she was a triple-duty nurse in a single district, as many were, she was on call day and night and involved in the major life events of her patient community. She was often asked for advice before the doctor, confided in on personal matters, and could be instrumental in helping to alleviate the worst effects of poverty. The repeated use of the term *general nursing care* in interviews suggests that all-encompassing care was understood and unquestioned as a basic standard of all nursing activity, that a fundamental principle of district nursing was the idea of caring as a personal and a holistic activity. For these women, nursing as essentially caring became a part of their personal identity as much as their professional one.

Adopted as a raison d'etre, nursing care, defined in this way, blurs the boundaries between professional and personal identity, bestowing a femininity on the carer that might otherwise have been difficult to express in conventional terms. In the environment of professionalisation prevalent since the 1980s and mindful of the need to counteract discriminating paternalism, this notion of care linked to femininity carries pejorative implications and remains a recurrent irritant to those keen to influence the professionalisation process.

One district nurse likened nursing care to the mother–child relationship, a metaphor of care that has been viewed as particularly unhelpful to the professional status of nurses:

Well, I, what would I say was the greatest change? . . . I think, when I started nursing, the care of the patient, no, the caring like a mother to a child, you know, that sort of caring, and you did things that perhaps you didn't need to do.[14]

This notion of nursing care as a form of mothering reflects a traditional image of nursing characterised by nurturing and lack of authority. It has been discussed elsewhere as one that places nurses in a relationship to the doctor where she is necessarily subservient and sometimes justified as so "for the sake of patients."[15] As shown in earlier chapters, subservience to doctors was not as evident in community nursing in the 1940s to the 1970s as it was in the hospital ward during the same period. District nurses were more likely to work independently of the GP rather than in subservience to him.[16] Furthermore, this independence and relative autonomy in their practice was coupled with a degree of authority derived from their status as skilled and knowledgeable people, professional people within their community. This being the case, subservience was not a necessary relationship. On the contrary, a clear distinction between nursing and medicine was crucial to the district nurse's unique identity and autonomy and one still keenly guarded even in retirement: "All dressings, or general care of the patient—that was yours . . . Medicine's them, that was his function, not yours."[17]

Having experienced a rapid growth in technology, burgeoning professionalisation and complex organisational changes in the course of the last 50 years, caring described by retired district nurses as a maternal relationship simplifies the nature of their work by use of what was an unchallenged metaphor for a particular generation. For those who worked as district nurses in the mid-twentieth century, there was little tension between the notions of mothering and caring, in theory if not in practice. *Mothering* was understood as looking after the well-being of families, in particular children, and doing so with relatively little physical support from the male members of the family, and on a twenty-four-hour-a-day basis. It also implied that the well-being of these specific others was the first priority of the mother, coming before thoughts of career or self-fulfilment from other external sources. So, for the district nurse, involved with whole families as well as individual patients in the patients' homes, working long hours on call both day and night, with minimal direction from the GP or supervisor, the mothering metaphor, defined by the culture of their time, continued to have more resonance for them than it did for the ward nurse working within an authoritarian hierarchy where the doctor still dominated and nurse–patient contact could be subordinate to hospital routine. It must also be remembered that the mothering metaphor, as used here by retired district nurses, operated in a time when the character of patients and the nurse–patient relationship was different. Mothering implied not only love but gratitude, and this was something that would have been read into the behaviour of patients both before the NHS and in the subsequent two decades. Where the habit of deference might have obscured a critical opinion in patients, it is nonetheless undeniable that in these decades patients were less well-informed on matters of health and medicine and so less well-equipped to demand defined standards of care and treatment. Patients were much more likely to succumb willingly to the knowledge of the nurse and to her care.

One might argue that patients were *subjected* to the care of the nurse and that the mothering metaphor merely obscures an insidious culture of control operating within a set of moral norms, but this would be to underestimate the complexity of both care and control in which "control can imply care, just as care can imply control."[18] On the contrary, nurses themselves were subjects of contemporary notions of femininity that imposed certain social values. Nursing as mothering appealed to such a sense of femininity and we suggest that it is this, rather than the subservient relationship to the doctor implied by Kuhse, that the claimed maternal relationship of district nursing might point to.

MOTHERHOOD AND MARRIAGE

Of the district nurses interviewed, many married, took time off to bring up young children, and returned to work after some years. A few married and were at some stage widowed but a considerable number remained unmarried. At a time when motherhood framed femininity, those who did not marry might well have used other caring relationships as expressions of their femininity. Many of them became the principal carer for elderly parents. Indeed, the QNI was particularly cooperative in this respect by providing nurses' houses that would accommodate parents or by giving the nurse extended unpaid leave to care for sick relatives. By looking after a parent, by mothering the parent, the daughter could be redefined as a motherlike figure. Femininity, though of a more sterile form, was assured and publicly accepted.

For those who neither married nor had a family to care for, the community substituted for the family and provided the means for expressions of femininity. Whereas a feminist analysis now rejects the notion of nursing as mothering (and for very good reasons), this was not available to those working at the time who were locked into a society that valued femininity over professionalism and even saw them as opposites. District nursing seen as an extension of family life allowed women to bridge the gap between the two concepts in a plausible and logically coherent way. That this is no longer acceptable should be regarded as reflecting a shift in the sociology of nursing rather than the active, retrospective imposition of a contemporary position by individual women that might itself be subject to revision and correction in the future. In short, the mothering metaphor is just that, a metaphor. District nurses did not mistakenly believe they were the maternal spirit of a community but could find, at that time, no alternative socially acceptable metaphor.

CARE AND SPIRITUALITY

For some interviewees, "care" was also spoken of as an expression of love, more specifically, Christian love. Religious faith was something spoken about in most interviews and the majority of interviewees professed a Christian faith. For some this was influential and helped them to come to terms with the reality of mortality, which they confronted at close quarters on a regular basis. For others it was a motivating force that spanned the distinction between life and work. One who felt this way was Miss Lamont.[19]

Miss Lamont was born in 1913 and developed a desire to nurse from an early age, influenced by a couple of spells in the hospital as a child and the acquaintance of a district nurse as a young girl. At seventeen, too young to enter general nurse training, she secured a place in a tuberculosis sanatorium where she was dressed in a uniform, was called "nurse," and trained in the care of tuberculosis patients. As a young woman her social life was typically simple compared with today:

> Well, we didn't have a lot of entertainment . . . But we didn't know that we were missing anything. Oh, there was lots of girls that would go a lot to dances. I was never, I liked it, but I wasn't, it wasn't a priority with me. I liked church things, and I liked, I liked going to church. I wasn't over burdened with that [kind of] thing, but I used to like to go to church things . . . You went to the pictures, you went to visit your relatives, and you went walking.[20]

From the sanatorium, Miss Lamont went on to complete her general training in Birmingham and in 1942 she joined the army, travelling overseas in 1943. Her experiences as an army nurse in wartime were both frightening and funny and although her friendship with men was limited by regulations, she enjoyed as full a social life as conditions allowed:

> They were all colonels and captains. Well, we were lieutenants. You weren't allowed to go with men. You couldn't go out with a private. And so you made your own enjoyment . . . Oh, it was very pukka. And you had to be very careful also, cause a lot of these men were forever telling you their wives didn't understand them, that kind of thing, you know.[21]

After the war Miss Lamont trained in midwifery, which introduced her to domiciliary work. Having previously eschewed district nursing as inferior she then decided to do her Queen's training, completing it in 1948, and took up district work in the Borders area. Although unqualified as an HV, Miss Lamont acted as a triple-duty nurse but remained unpaid for her health visiting duties. Miss Lamont gave many examples of how her patients confided in her and called on her before the doctor and how she was invited to give out prizes at the local school or take part in a local quizzes, all indicating her sense of belonging to the community and their willingness to accept her as part of it. Miss Lamont never married because, as she said, "I have never met anyone I would like to have given up my work for." Such was the custom of the day that the inevitable choice between marriage and work was not one she challenged at the time.

Miss Lamont was also a woman who placed great faith in her religious belief. The Church was a focus for social interaction and she was regularly involved in its functions including the Women's Guild, but the Church was more than a social focal point. Miss Lamont recalled how her Christian faith crept into her daily life and how she viewed this as an integral part of nursing:

> And I used to say, before I went out on a case, cause the Lord's not far away from me, you know, he's just there, and I'd say, "Well, don't go away Lord, I might need you, you know, just stick around." And when I left a case at night, I used to say, "Be there till I come back, you know. Keep her alright." . . . And, without my faith, I don't know if it would have been the same.[22]

Faith was important to Miss Lamont both as a motivating principle and as a support to her in her nursing. In this sense, nursing care, for Miss Lamont, was something that sprang from spirituality. The term *spiritual care* is often used in another sense; as the "making of arrangements for the provision of patients' spiritual needs" where *spiritual need* is defined as "a lack of any or all of the following which are required to produce spiritual well-being: meaning, purpose and fulfilment in life; the will to live; belief and faith in self, others and God."[23] Miss Lamont also practised spiritual care in this sense.

> One old lady [a terminally ill patient] that I went to, she wouldn't have a bath, she wouldn't have anything. She was stinking to high heavens . . . And eventually when I got going with her, and was able to bath her and got her nice and clean, one day she said to me, "Will you do something for me? Will you read to me?" And I said, "Yes." But it was the 139th Psalm, and I never forgot it. And I read it to her. And after that, she used to say, "Will you read to me today?" And I'd say, "Yes, five minutes, just give me five minutes." Right. And she used to say then, "You're my guardian angel."[24]

Ross outlined how the dualist philosophy of the scientific era has characterised medicine in the twentieth century rendering "illness, suffering and death meaningless."[25] She went on to suggest that "the goal of nursing is . . . to assist them [the patients] to achieve inner harmony from which will emanate self-healing. This can be achieved through the "caring" action of the nurse who is required to be sensitive in order to nurture faith and hope in the patient."[26] A sense of hope in the face of illness or death was something important to Miss Lamont and something she took the opportunity to nurture where the patient expressed faith: "But I wasn't out to convert them all. That wasn't my job to convert them all. But I like to think that they had a hope."[27]

Although the testimony of Miss Lamont reflects the importance of spirituality in the lives of the majority of district nurses interviewed, it must be stressed that she was one of just a few who spoke candidly and at length about her faith and the role it played in her manner of nursing care. For many others, their Christian faith played a less central but nonetheless influential part in their life and work.

The defining of nursing care in terms of either a maternal or spiritual activity is not well accepted today, the emphasis now being on professionalism in nursing rather than personal qualities. However, this presents a dilemma as what is practised and what is valued by nurses is challenged by a professional ethic already constructed according to what is sometimes seen as a gendered masculine model. Hence, notions of caring as expressions of maternalism (i.e., essentially feminine) or spirituality (i.e., personal rather than professional) encompassed in nursing activities are driven by qualities of compassion, sensitivity, and intersubjectivity. They are not easily absorbed into contemporary professional thinking that inherently values technical skill, detached objectivity, and self-esteem.

Celia Davies, writing about nursing, set out a landscape of gendered identities that feeds into the construction of gendered organisation and institutions and goes on to suggest that the structure of *professions* is also influenced by "cultural codes" that privilege the masculine values of separation and autonomy over the feminine values of attachment and connectedness. As she suggested, "to bring the terms profession and care together is more than a step in semantics."[28] Davies outlined the difficulties for nurses in adopting both this professional ethos that devalues caring, but also the equally difficult construction of a "new professionalism" if it cannot acknowledge and resolve the cultural baggage of that old masculine model. We would claim here that, at least in retrospect, district nurses managed this synthesis very well. However, there is a tension between perceptions of past and of present district nursing held by elderly district nurses that, we believe, is embodied in their emphatic placing of caring at the centre of their work. They value their skill and training as nurses and accept a position within their communities that they liken to the teacher, minister, or policeman; they assume their status as a professional but they use the word infrequently.

On the surface, the integration of nursing care and nursing professionalism is not problematic for them, but we have already seen that, in the employment of the mothering metaphor, there was a perceived need to recover a feminine identity through notions of care, which suggests that this could not be found easily in the concept of professional open to them. This suggests that the concept of the gendered professional outlined by Davies did encroach on their thinking and that there was a distinction to be made between caring and nursing in the professional sense, a distinction that reiterated a masculine–feminine divide. However, it is important not to conflate masculine and male or feminine and female in the discussion of nursing care or professional ethos; masculine and feminine are concepts that do not necessarily correlate with the physical attributes of male and female. To help avoid this, the next section looks at two different approaches to district nursing each described by males, the first by a nurse working predominantly in the 1950s to the 1970s, and the second by a nurse working in the 1990s. Although caring remains a central tenet of each nurse's work, their approach to practice is expressed in different terms that imply a different cultural understanding of masculinity, care, and professional nursing.

MALE DISTRICT NURSES

Although there have been male district nurses for more than fifty years, their numbers remain disproportionate to the number of qualified male general nurses. In 2005 male nurses accounted for ten percent of all nursing and midwifery staff but only two percent of district nurses throughout Scotland.[29] District nursing had always been regarded as a woman's job, but at the end of World War II this changed as the service suffered a recruitment crisis. At this time some men returning from the services who had acquired paramedical training in the Royal Army Medical Corps (RAMC) wanted to continue this work in civilian life. This was encouraged, and given their experience, they were offered a shortened period for general nurse training as an added incentive. The QNI accepted its first male nurse into training in 1947 and although take up was slow at first, by the end of 1951 189 male nurses had trained as Queen's Nurses throughout the United Kingdom. After twenty years the figure had risen to 423 in post, which was nearly five percent of the total number of district nurses.[30] Male district nurses were barred from midwifery and attended only male patients, leaving them effectively excluded from promoted posts.[31] However, they were often specifically sought after in areas with large numbers of patients requiring heavy lifting.

Apart from concerns about possible prejudice from colleagues and patients, obstacles that male nurses had to overcome included a reduction in salary during training, having to find and pay for lodgings in one part of the country while in many cases keeping a wife and family elsewhere, and having to cover a larger working area than their female counterparts because they were only permitted to visit male patients.[32] One of these men entered Queen's training following his marriage to a Queen's Nurse, herself undergoing midwifery training at the same institution. She described their subsequent difficulties:

He did Queen's and the Queen's pupils sat on that table—all the training staff sat on the middle table and the Pupil Midwives sat on this table. So he sat over there and I sat over here. And any marriage that can last out six months because as you will appreciate I was on call most of the time, we were never allowed to lock our bedroom. We were offered a double post in Torquay and we had to sign an agreement that I would not get pregnant for three years.

Harold had an enormous problem in Torquay because the Queen's training home, it had a maiden lady in charge and she did not want a man . . . and she actually went and saw people and told the patients that she had this man coming, only men, because of course there was no question at all of him going anywhere near women . . . She said if you don't like him and you don't want to be nursed by a man you tell me, we'll put in a written complaint and we shall get rid of him. But he was very, very skilled and within a month doctors were ringing up and saying "I've got a man I want Mr. Diamond to go and see. Can you please arrange for Mr. Diamond to see this man as soon as possible?" But she was livid, she was furious.[33]

These and similar examples strongly suggest that male nurses experienced a difficult transition stage, facing prejudice from some quarters before being accepted as district nurses, in many ways mirroring the prejudice experienced by women entering general practice medicine several decades earlier. For many years, career development for male district nurses remained blocked, as this usually required a midwifery qualification, whether for entrance to health visiting or for promotion to supervisory level. Where women GPs had defended their right to treat male as well as female patients,[34] it was not until the mid-1970s that these gender barriers began to be broken down for male nurses working in the community.

One of the first male district nurses in Britain, Mr. Orr[35] was drafted into the Royal Army Medical Corps (RAMC) in 1940. After an initial period of training (basic army training plus first aid followed by a course in a hospital) and an initial posting in Britain he was then sent out to Italy.[36] Male RAMC personnel and female nurses worked closely together at this time and Mr. Orr had great respect for the female nurses he met. On being demobbed in 1947 he was keen to continue in nursing and immediately applied for nursing training, admitting that "had I not been in the army I would never have thought of it. It certainly did sow the seeds of my future." He was readily accepted for training and found no difficulties working or associating with the female nurses. Influenced by his experiences during the war, he opted for district training. He was accepted to the QNIS headquarters at Castle Terrace, Edinburgh, where he spent six months in district training as one of only two male nurses. With the exception of midwifery (and being lodged separately from the women), Mr. Orr's training followed a similar pattern to that of female district nurses, consisting of practical district placement and clinical lectures.

Mr. Orr took up his first post in Greenock, an industrial town on the coast west of Glasgow where the main employment was in shipbuilding and marine engineering. Here, a male district nurse to complement the group of female nurses already covering the districts was specifically requested and Mr. Orr's post there was secured even before he took up his training place with QNIS. Greenock was organised into various nursing districts plus one additional male district that covered the whole area. So, when a case required heavy lifting or the catheterisation of a male patient (female nurses did not do this), Mr. Orr was called in. In this post Mr. Orr worked with all the Greenock GPs. His workload was similar to any other district nurse involving work with diabetics, the acutely ill, tuberculosis patients, long-term or terminally ill patients, stroke patients, bladder cases, changing dressings, delivering painkilling injections, and treating bedsores and ulcers. Mr. Orr continued to work in Greenock until retiring and was a pioneer in the development of the night-nursing service there.

As one of only a few male interviewees, Mr. Orr's is a somewhat solitary voice, but one that concurs with the female perspective regarding the caring aspects of nursing. It is interesting that although his interview had some characteristic differences to those with women (e.g., he tended to take more control in the interview situation) he shared the same perceptions of the nature of nursing and used the term *care* in much the same way as his female counterparts; that is, almost interchangeably with the term *basic nursing*:

> In my day it was mainly the patient, contact with the doctor, the relatives, environment, all of that thing carrying out more basic nursing than it is today and these days there is so much sophistication . . . the only thing is I think there's a tendency to get away from the basic nursing.[37]

He went on to describe basic nursing in the following terms:

> Basic nursing is making the patient comfortable, spongin', bedbathing, prevention of bedsores, helping to become mobile again, this sort of thing—feeding, nutrition, oral cleanliness, em, things that really make the patient, give them a feeling of well-being, and eh, help them on the road to recovery. An awful lot of those things have to be forgotten now, I don't blame the nurses because there's so much of other things to do.[38]

Mr. Orr's description of district nursing duties is echoed throughout the collection of interviews. Similarly, Mr. Orr spoke of his relationship with the doctors in the same way as female interviewees. He considered GPs to be less remote in the past. Although there was no formal structure for case discussion with the nurse, "You could go and knock the door and explain the situation to them" [the doctors]. He might have disagreed with a doctor's suggested treatment on occasion, but he felt that he could reason with them on this issue and deferred to them on matters of diagnosis. Like many nurses, Mr. Orr found his relationship with doctors in the district to be relatively free of conflict. Where a clear distinction between the medical and nursing role was identified and observed by both parties, cooperation prevailed. This not only prepared the ground for successful healing but also for professional individuation and development. However, Mr. Orr found it difficult to distinguish between nursing and social care, calling it a "grey area" where the nurse used to just do it all. On housing matters, where a patient's housing conditions adversely affected health, he felt able to contact the MOH who could then influence change. Above all, Mr. Orr was a man who invested a great deal of energy and value in his work. Given the few male nurses spoken to for this book, formally and informally, it cannot be said that Mr. Orr represents a typically male perspective. Nevertheless, it would be remiss not to note the lack of a male voice in district nursing and include it where possible.

Mr. Orr's experience was not wholly untypical among his male contemporaries nursing in the community. However it contrasts with that of a male nurse working in the late 1990s, in particular, that of Mr. Peterson. When we spoke to Mr. Peterson in 1998 he had only very recently come with his young family to take up a post on a remote Scottish island. Although not described as such, Mr. Peterson was in essence a triple-duty nurse combining nursing, health visiting, and midwifery. No formal interview was undertaken with Mr. Peterson, but he expressed his views during an impromptu conversation, which, regrettably, was not recorded.[39] Nevertheless, it revealed an approach to district nursing that stood in sharp contrast to that of previous district nurses on the island. One of those, a woman who had previously occupied the post for more than ten years and remained resident on the island, had been interviewed.[40] It also betrayed a different attitude to that of Mr. Orr.

In conversation, both Mr. Peterson and the retired female nurse referred to the differences in their respective approaches and these were also evidenced in their practice: The older nurse had worn her uniform when visiting patients, the younger one, Mr. Peterson, did not; the older one had accompanied the doctor on his rounds when he came to the island, the younger one did not; the older one adopted a proactive approach to her patients, the younger one only responded to calls. What the retiring nurse saw as keeping in touch with her community of patients, Mr. Peterson tended to see as "nannying" people. It must be borne in mind that the situation on this island is quite unique. It is very remote from the mainland and the weather can be extremely harsh. The island has always had a very small population and everyone is known to everyone else. Until the advent of commercial flying, the island was linked to the mainland only by local boats that delivered supplies. Today it is served by a small plane running a daily schedule, but this is frequently cancelled due to unfavourable weather conditions, even in the summer months. The island has never had a resident doctor and in the 1970s, when the retired nurse was working there, the doctors from the main island visited only twice a year or in the case of emergencies. Although a sense of community was crucially important to both styles of nursing, and accepted as a necessary approach to life on such a small island, Mr. Peterson made a distinction between the community and the individual with regard to caring:

> Nursing is about caring for individuals and communities. In terms of community practice I had a strong focus on community development and individual empowerment—with the individual taking responsibility for their health/care.[41]

To exemplify this he told of an elderly man with diabetes who was required to take a blood sample on a regular basis to measure his blood sugar levels. When Mr. Peterson came into post the patient had a little red notebook (provided by "the nurse") in which the nurse wrote the blood sugar reading after she had carried out the finger prick blood test. Mr. Peterson explained that this practice of the nurse taking control of the blood monitoring had gone on for a very long time and was typical of the way things were done on the island:

> I then arrived and taught the gentleman how to carry out the test for himself! I do not think this was an attempt to distance myself from him or as a way of "getting out of doing work" and I still visited and had contact with him . . . I found the islanders *very* dependent on the services of the nurse and I saw that as a bad thing—I moved them on to the notion that they should have their own first aid supplies in their homes so that if they cut their finger then they could apply a plaster etc. instead of calling me.[42]

While on the island, Mr. Peterson focused more on the promotion of health and increased awareness as well as offering a listening ear or counselling "with a small *c*," and noted that much of his work related to "emotional or psychological support—often a much more draining and difficult service to provide." On the question of his "maleness," Mr. Peterson felt completely accepted as the island nurse:

> The island did not appear phased by my "maleness" and we had four pregnant women on the island while I was there—and I supported and was involved with all age groups and a multitude of problems . . . As a man I do not believe that women have the monopoly on care—but accept that there are differences. I am sure [the retired nurse] would have happily put a patient's hair in rollers or whatever—I wouldn't, simply because I would not know how![43]

Eventually, Mr. Peterson found the professional isolation, the twenty-four-hour availability of the nurse, and a perceived lack of support from his employers very demanding, and after only two years he decided to leave for a post elsewhere. In contrast, the retired nurse had come to the island in 1973 with her husband and three children on the basis that they would probably stay for a year or so. Such was the family's attachment to the island, they stayed on. She was given dispensation to act as HV and took her additional training in health visiting in 1976 and 1977 and retired as island nurse in 1986. Thereafter, she continued to work as relief nurse when required and has remained living on the island.

Looking at district nursing on this island is interesting because it exemplifies the experiences of male and female nurses working in similar circumstances as well as those of an older and younger generation. As we saw earlier, with reference to non-nursing tasks and social welfare, Mr. Orr recalled how the nurse would just "do it all." He also recognised a distinction between past and present district nursing that he characterised as being a difference in "basic nursing care" defined in holistic terms. In these respects Mr. Orr's ethos of district nursing was closer to that of the retired female island nurse than the younger man, Mr. Peterson. This suggests that the difference in approaches of the two island district nurses might owe less to direct gender influences than to a nursing ethos changed over time. However, bearing in mind Davies's discussion of cultural codes, this ethos must itself be subject to gendered influence, whether masculine or feminine.[44]

THE LIMITS OF CARE

It has been noted elsewhere in this book that the view of nursing as a holistic process was crucial to the definition of nursing for many interviewees. This is reiterated in the frequent use of the terms *basic nursing care* or *general nursing care* when referring to the kind of care that was frequently given but required little or no nursing expertise. As we have seen, district nurses in the past regularly undertook what might today be regarded as non-nursing care, which could include all manner of tasks relating to bodily health and social or domestic well-being "Filling forms, mending heaters sometimes if there was no heater in the house—my attitude was that if there was anything I could do to alleviate medical problems, then I did it."[45] Similarly, just listening to people was part of basic or general nursing care: "To me it's not just bathing people, it's hearing their stories."[46] The following quotes suggest some of the many ways district nurses illustrated their understanding of basic nursing care:

> It was mostly elderly people that we had, with strokes and that sort of thing . . . we used to give them general nursing care . . . Tender loving care.[47]

Well, say you've got a dying patient. Well, obviously you're going to have to give them nursing care . . . that means attending to the whole patient. Seeing that everything about them's as comfortable as you can make them. So that's left to you.[48]

You had what you call a general nursing care. That was, you went in in the morning, washed your patient, maybe gave her a bath or washed her down, made the bed, tidied . . . watched for bedsores . . . But it was a case of keeping people clean and giving them a little bit of your time. Listening to them while you were doing the job. Finding out their little troubles and all that.[49]

Listening went beyond the patient, reinforcing the holistic nature of general nursing care:

Well, you would very often spend a long time in somebody's house, maybe just chatting to their carer, you know, having a cup of tea, chatting to their carer as a, in a supportive role. And that would just all come under general nursing care.[50]

From these descriptions of care as something inclusive, the nursing practiced by Mr. Peterson on the island district, where he said that much of his time was spent offering a listening ear, can be seen to fit the traditional model of basic nursing care. However, when considering the collection of testimonies as a whole, there is a sense in which the traditional model of nursing care in the district is sometimes conflated with social care where the nurse just did it all. Yet we see that Mr. Peterson was not prepared to take things to that extreme, preferring, where appropriate, to instil a sense of personal responsibility in his patients. It might be argued that this contemporary conception of nursing care not only sharpens the definition of the nurse's role, but also confers an active, participatory role on the patient, that it is empowering for both parties. Is this empowerment of both nurse and patient an integral part of holistic care?

The following quotes are taken from the 1995 *Assessment of Need for District Nursing* conducted in the West of Scotland and involving interviews with district nurses practising in the 1990s. They suggest that district nurses today still face situations where the caring needs of a patient might go beyond nursing tasks. In theory, nurses adopt a holistic approach to care, but time constraints mean they frequently have to delegate social tasks to untrained or lesser trained staff. "Thus assistance with care where need is due to frailty or lack of informal support rather than medical illness is deemed social need and referrals received for such care are considered inappropriate."[51] In practice nurses find it difficult not to offer support:

I feel it's difficult to separate—people usually come on with nursing need initially, like a knocked leg needing a dressing, then you find they haven't had a bath for three or four years and you get involved with that and can't stop.[52]

Bathing, putting out daily medication, installing eye drops, keeping an eye on someone, making tea and peeling potatoes were all given as examples of care given which does not represent the district nurse's idea of nursing need.[53]

Here, nurses' involvement in two distinct forms of care, nursing and social, is a problematic issue. The quotes suggest that present-day nurses feel a personal obligation to undertake general non-nursing tasks but regard this as conflicting with their professional outlook. Where past district nurses tended to accept a definition of nursing care that did not have a clear boundary, this is currently perceived as a dilemma. Not only did past district nurses accept such an inclusive definition, but most have now built it into their professional, and in many cases their personal, identities. Hence nursing care extends to include anything that they found themselves taking on. The mere existence of the *Assessment of Need* reinforces the fact that in the present day, defining the bounds of nursing care is an issue requiring discussion, resolution, and formalisation.

CONCLUSION

In the context of this book, district nurses of the past appear to have placed a distinctly higher value on the caring aspect of their work than they credit to today's district nurses. Listening to them it is difficult to resist the notion that district nurses of the past somehow cared more. In contemporary discussions of gendered ethics, the distinction between medical care and the kind of care so long attributed to nursing, and represented here as a defining character of district nursing, has been perceived as an acceptance of subservience to the doctor; a pejorative assessment betraying a lack of professional identity and autonomy. Why then do district nurses who have been shown to be both independent in the face of the doctor and keenly aware of their professional skills, use this distinction so readily? Is it that the attribution of caring by those nurses is a retrospective justification for the acceptance of conditions that do not now fit into the contemporary model of district nurses as skilled professionals, far less into the modern notion of ideal womanhood? Does this mean that district nurses of the past were not professional in their approach to nursing, or that their brand of caring was indicative of an unsophisticated understanding of their social and professional status?

The contemporary concern over professional status is also reflected in the different use of language used by Mr. Peterson and by the older nurses. What Mr. Orr's generation might refer to as "looking after" a patient by providing "basic nursing care" in a proactive way, Mr. Peterson described as "nannying." Mr. Peterson also used the language of official documents and theories of nursing, including phrases such as *individual empowerment*, and *monopolies of care*. This different use of language supports the argument that nurses of the different generations think about and express ideas of nursing care in quite different terms; that the nurse–patient relationship is, more and more, defined by the terms of professionalism rather than those of person-centred caring. We would argue that district nurses of the past were not caught up in notions of caring and professionalism as conflicting concepts. Rather, they viewed district nursing as a unique opportunity to express both in the one activity. Perhaps this betrays a very naïve understanding of the relationship of gender to both, but it is one that the district nurses represented here still hold true. At least in retrospect, district nurses of the past were confident in their definitions of care and managed the synthesis between care and professionalism very well.

Writing in the twenty-first century, Kelly and Symonds stated the importance of community nurses being able to articulate what they mean by *care* and that "nursing potential may be lost if nurses themselves persist in a reluctance to define what they mean by" it.[54] They also noted that current discourses within primary health care might have served to curtail the caring activity of community nurses, effectively ensuring that their activity, now, is more medically than socially oriented.[55] This curtailment facilitates a clear distinction between the social and the scientific or technological; the personal and professional identity that, it seems to us, precludes the very kind of personal integrity expressed by a previous generation of women through their work.

It seems clear then that the concept of *care* can be both problematic and divisive. However this is not the way the women of this time used it. Many of them were unmarried, childless, and geographically remote from original family relationships, and relied on the essential quality of their work (i.e., the connectedness of care) to confer family status. Given the role of family in the construction of female identity, the relationship of care that defined work was also essential in their construction of a personal identity. Hence, the working life of these nurses was psychologically intertwined with their social (in this context, their private) life. Care, then, was not divisive but a cohesive concept.

9 Portraits of a District Nurse

The power of nursing imagery in producing a powerful stereotype to the public through a variety of media forms has been considered by a number of historians, but usually in relation to hospital rather than community nursing.[1] District nursing represents one of the earliest home visiting services and it has developed as one of the most prominent in the public perception of community nursing. As an integral part of community nursing, it is subject to the same dilemmas regarding its function, direction, and focus. Unlike the practice nurse, the learning disability nurse, or the community mental health nurse, we have seen that the district nurse has a long tradition and history that influences the perceptions of colleagues, patients, and district nurses themselves with regard to their professional role.[2] Furthermore, despite (or perhaps because of) the reorganisation of district nursing services since the 1960s, the image of district nursing has been questioned publicly with particular reference to changes both in practice and nurse–patient relationships. In this chapter we therefore consider the district nurse's changing professional role through a number of representations in films and television. We compare these images with the more official views projected through textbooks and recruitment leaflets, asking how they reflect the public and private spheres dichotomy.

In 1913, Miss Paget[3] referred to Florence Nightingale's vision of nursing as "not destined for all time merely to wait upon disease but to be the handmaid of preventative science," seeing the role of the district nurse as central to this. She warned that "If district nurses, those who go into the homes of the people up and down the land, who are the links in a great chain of endeavor, will not rise to the occasion, this big task will fall to others, less well trained for it." She also cited Nightingale's conception of the nurse as a "health missioner" rather than an "angel smoothing a pillow" and the image of the "ideal nurse in the business-like figure of the modern woman who, armed with a sanitary certificate and a determined spirit in addition to her nurse training and her hospital cloak, is adding an intimate knowledge of drains, an intense antagonism to the house-fly and a healthy dislike of illness to her nursing equipment."[4]

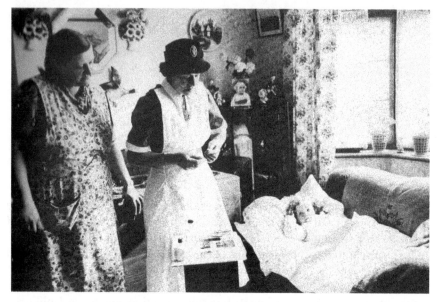

Figure 9.1 A Queen's district nurse, mid-twentieth century. "Rotherham Home Nurse." Photo by Haywood Magee Image #71279885 (RM) 5 November 1955. Copyright licence purchased from Hulton Archive.

This is a powerfully evocative image, yet the Briggs Report,[5] written sixty years later, perceived Florence Nightingale's role as being the creation and perpetuation of this ministering angel image but with no mention of these other aspects of the district nurse with a mission for sanitising society. The Report acknowledged that there was a class element in the traditional imagery that encouraged the vocational/quasi-religious theme of "dedicated" women, serving the patient without consideration of personal monetary gain, supported and guided by a hierarchical and strongly authoritarian structure. The image still surviving in the 1970s was, according to Briggs, presented through both the media and nursing recruitment literature. An example of this is taken from a speech made by Lady Salisbury at the opening of a district nurses' home in Watford: "The district nurse needs special qualifications, not only of skill and independence and presence of mind, but a constant sympathy and real unselfishness, and almost a cast-iron constitution." She referred to the home as "a centre of ministry to the health and comfort of the sick," where they could, "relax from their angel status to human beings."[6] Two of these representations are shown in Figures 9.2 and 9.3, each presenting a totally different image of the nurse: first as unprofessional "Gamp," and second as nurse dressing a child's leg—even the latter must have been posed for the camera although it appears less obviously constructed than the two cartoons.

At the other end of the spectrum, Dickens's caricature of nurses Gamp and Prigg[7] provided a caricature of the worst kind of district nurse and was

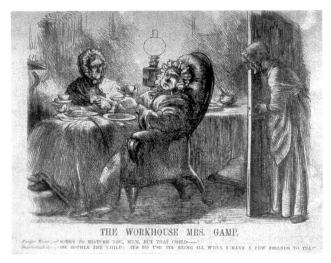

Figure 9.2 Cartoon of "The Workhouse Mrs. Gamp" *FUN* March 31 (1866).

a powerful image in the campaign for nursing and social reform. This was such a compelling image that it has endured for more than a century-and-a-half and is still easily conjured up by the public and professionals alike when illustrating the undesirable characteristics of a nurse behaving unprofessionally. A possible side effect, however, is that this image has sometimes obscured reality to the dis-service of the mass of excellent and devoted informal carers and unqualified nurses while promoting the professionalisation of nursing. The image of the district nurse has not always reflected reality:

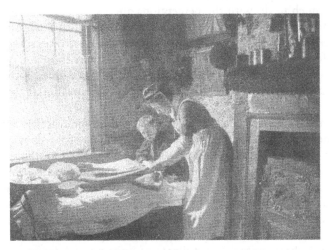

Figure 9.3 District nurse attending young child, c. 1920. Source unknown. The authors have made every effort to trace the original holder of reproduction rights for this image without success.

"A lot of people . . . still see us as matronly ladies who go round and have cups of tea with old dears." The reality, increasingly but not universally, is that district nurses are highly-skilled practitioners carrying out complex procedures once undertaken only in hospital.[8]

This quote from *The Guardian* suggests that there is a public perception of district nursing that is rooted in a now outdated stereotype, the same stereotype that shaped popular media characterisations of district nurses such as the motherly Anna in the television drama series *Where the Heart Is* or the comic, dominating, and somewhat raunchy Gladys in *Open All Hours*. Among health professionals, district nurses seem to be consistently misrepresented in television portrayals:

> There is no shortage of current television programmes which seek to portray up-to-date role models of general practitioners (GPs), consultants, hospital nurses of all grades, hospital managers and even the relatively recent role of the practice manager; however, if a community nurse is portrayed, it is usually a district nurse, whose role has not been updated since the 1940s.[9]

In the pursuit of a unified discipline for community nursing, such media stereotyping is viewed as counterproductive but it betrays an attitude that can also be found within the profession itself:

> "*Community nursing is all about caring for the sick.*" This idea has much to do with the traditional nurse image, the origins of district nursing, and the perpetuation of stereotypes via the media. Perhaps it also has much to do with the perceptions and expectations of other caring professions and consumers of care i.e. society . . . This belief may also be perpetuated by some community nurses who have resisted political and professional pressure to adopt a health-oriented approach and assume responsibility for empowering others. They have opted rather to fulfil the traditional nurse role, attempting to preserve familiar territory.[10]

Poor communication seems to be the root cause of many misunderstandings about the role of the district nurse, not only between professional colleagues, but also with the public. In an article written in 1928, outlining the decision to set up a League for Queen's Nurses, a comment from Miss Wyatt, County Superintendent for East Sussex noted, "Our status in the Nursing World is often questioned and misunderstood. Some of us have been pained by a recent article which appeared in a leading Journal giving a very misleading account of the training and work of Queen's Nurses."[11] She then called for tighter control over tidiness of uniform and dress, stating, "The general public often judges a nurse's work by her personal appearance." A similar comment was made to a meeting in Cardiff at which "Mrs. Thomas

Evans ... referred to the prejudice that once existed in the minds of the public against the District Nurses, and said that that feeling had now died out largely because of the tact, efficiency, and devotion to duty shown by the Nurses themselves."[12] In other words, the public was coming to recognise that district nurses presented a more dependable and presentable and thus more professional image.

OFFICIAL IMAGERY: TEXTBOOKS
AND DOCUMENTARY FILM

We first consider the changing image of the district nurse presented by official sources such as nursing textbooks, advertisements, recruitment leaflets, and documentary films produced either by the QNI or government before moving on to look at the unofficial voice of the media. One of the earliest pictures of district nursing was presented in the best-selling series of books by Martha Loane (1852–1933), a Queen's Superintendent who worked first in London and later in Derbyshire and Portsmouth. She was a prolific writer and social commentator, having produced at least six books and numerous published articles including many in the *QNM*. We look at just one of the most relevant of her books, here: *The Queen's Poor: Life as They Find It in Town and Country*.[13]

As with most of Loane's books *The Queen's Poor* was based largely on the author's own first-hand experience of nursing what she termed "the decent poor." There is considerable anecdotal material—a style commonly used by her contemporaries and popularly received—much of which is presented as if it were oral evidence, but which the historian has to treat with caution. Loane anticipated our concern with the reassurance that "every anecdote including the apocryphal ones ... was genuine ... they have been written down exactly as they were uttered."[14] Drawing on her district nursing registers, time-record, and casebooks, she discussed a very eclectic mix of subjects. These ranged from health and welfare policy and her own views on proposed legislation to the complexities of marital relationships, commenting on levels of violence and drunkenness, and on treatment of children, plus commonly held attitudes toward religion, education, nutrition, and even use of language and behaviour toward nurses. Although only two chapters deal directly with district nursing, there is much witting and unwitting testimony concerning health care, standards of living, perceptions of health professionals, and prevailing social attitudes. The role and professional and public images of District Nursing Superintendent and District Nurse are vividly revealed, and Loane's first-hand experience is evident in detailed descriptions of the considerable pressures, demands, and difficulties of working in both urban and rural areas of extreme poverty. Much of her work would be best described as sanitary and health education plus basic midwifery, but the illnesses she and her nurses commonly dealt with encompassed tuberculosis, epilepsy, respiratory diseases including pneumonia, congestive cardiac failure, blindness, paralysis, and terminal illnesses, where often the best they could offer was comfort and some pain relief. In her books she exposed occasional abuses of the district nursing system aimed at providing nursing care specifically for the "sick poor in their own homes" and drew attention to serious failings of the Poor Law revealing inadequacies and injustices in both institutional and outdoor relief.

Admittedly it can be difficult to gain such insight about public views of nursing from nursing textbooks, but occasionally they do reveal something of changing professional self-images when viewed over a period of time. The earliest textbook dedicated solely to district nursing was by Mrs. Dacre Craven,[15] first written in 1888, and subsequently revised and republished as *A Handbook for Queen's Nurses* in 1924 with two further editions in 1932 and 1943.[16] The first edition included the advertisement shown in Figure 9.4—not included in subsequent editions—for E. and R. Garrould, who

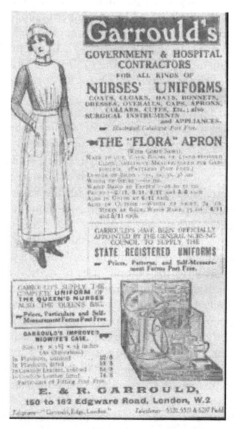

Figure 9.4 Advertisement for nurses' uniforms and bags. From "Some Queen's Superintendents," *Handbook for Queen's Nurses* (London: QNI, 1924): Front cover. Reproduced by kind permission of the Queen's Nursing Institute.

were suppliers of Queen's uniforms and bags as well as hospital nurses' uniforms. The picture shows a "Flora" apron suggesting an attempt to use the Nightingale image to attract the nurse to this product. For district nurses, by 1924 there was usually a £10 annual uniform allowance included as part of the emoluments to their salary, but it is significant that before 1948, district nurses would have been responsible for providing, laundering, and maintaining their uniform, unlike their counterparts in most hospitals.

The main additions to the 1943 third edition of the handbook are chapters on "The Routine Responsibilities of the Queen's Nurse," "Clerical Work and Equipment," and appendices that contain suggested additional reading, specimen forms, and a pull-out chart of infectious diseases and their characteristics. This reflects a change in emphasis toward increased administrative bureaucracy and a more scientific approach in contrast to the image of handmaiden implicit in the earlier advertisement.

District Nursing[17] by Merry and Irven was published in 1948 and was the first standard textbook for district nurses intended as both a training manual and reference text. Its front cover (shown in Figure 9.5) presents quite a different image of the nurse from that in Figure 9.3. The nurse is

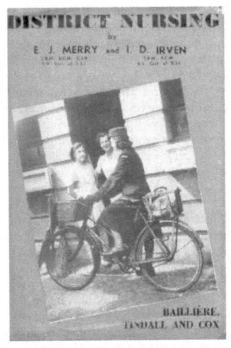

Figure 9.5 Front cover of a 1948 textbook. From E. J. Merry and I. D. Irven, *District Nursing: A Handbook for District Nurses* (London: Bailliere, Tindall and Cox, 1948): Front cover. As neither Elsevier nor Lippincott, Williams and Wilkins have been able to recognise copyright ownership of these images we regret that we have exhausted all lines of enquiry in trying to establish the true copyright owners.

shown in a more casual pose, in an urban setting, on her bicycle and wearing a modern, more practical uniform. She is apparently communicating with members of her community but has an air of comfortable self-assurance and a genial professional air of cool authority and expertise that is maintained throughout the book as the desired image. The contents expand on some of the information in the earlier handbooks, but add detail on "Techniques of District Nursing," "Nutrition and Food Values," "Public Health Legislation and Vital Statistics," "Record Keeping and Statistics," "Social Insurance," and an appendix that includes "Operations in the Home" and "The National Health Service." The nurses shown in the numerous photographic plates are all Queen's Nurses and many of the plates, along with the text, stress the educative role of the nurse. In some, patients are shown looking up at the nurse reverentially, reinforcing this new-found relationship.

Between 1932 and 1949 there were a number of documentary films produced relating to district nursing and midwifery,[18] but there were very few after 1950.[19] There were also several recruitment brochures produced by the QNI.[20] These presented the most immediate images of district nursing to the public and were either made for the purpose of nurse recruitment or for fundraising on behalf of the QNI. The brochure from 1960 is packed with photographic images. These present the selection, training, and examination process, and show midwifery and health visiting training as an important part of the QNI commitment, emphasising new attitudes within the profession by including male as well as female district nurses and State Enrolled as well as State Registered Nurses. Likewise, a broad multi-ethnic mix is suggested by several of the pictures, and reference is made to post-registration refresher courses, research, surveys, and conferences, and in particular to the William Rathbone Staff College. The overall message seems to be to make the nursing profession aware of the continuing role being played by the QNI in raising the professional status of district nursing as a modern, diverse, and specialised sector of nursing.

Friend of the Family is an unusual film, having been commissioned by the QNI but paid for by the South African Gift Fund, in 1949.[21] The technical advisor was the Education Officer of the QNI, and the three nurses were acted by three Queen's Nurses. In addition, a GP also acted the part of a GP doing an emergency tracheotomy. It is said that the main purpose of the film was to show the work of the district nurse "to the public at home and abroad, and to the special audiences of nurses or potential nurses whom it might interest." Locations were carefully chosen "to show slum areas, better class houses, country village and wild rugged coastal scenery."[22] The storyline is based on a planned reunion of three district nurses five years after training together. Despite the technical accuracy, the film seems contrived, with prominence given to the more dramatic side of the job such as delivering twins at a home birth, resuscitation of an attempted suicide, and attending an injured fisherman on an island, following which the nurse is drowned. The nurse is presented as dedicated and selfless, but the variety of settings and of tasks undertaken—together with the need for ingenuity and initiative—echoes the breadth of experience expressed in numerous oral histories, autobiographies, and QNI records referred to throughout this book. The overlap between fact and fiction in the imagery presented through this film is therefore extremely potent as can be seen by the realism of Figure 9.6, with a real nurse tending a patient in a real location, although the patient is an actor and the action is make-believe. The tender intimacy of the nurse–patient relationship seems to be the intended image with the patient posed to look adoringly up at the comforting, supportive, yet authoritative nurse and (on the whole) supporting the claims made by the Briggs Report. The film was originally only expected to have a life of three years but was still being shown a decade later.[23]

Unfortunately many of the early films are not currently accessible for viewing, but two that have been successfully copied by the National Film Archive for viewing are wartime Ministry of Information films. The first, *Nurse*,[24] is a general nursing recruitment film that opens with a picture of and quote from Florence Nightingale presenting the profession as founded on "a noble tradition of sympathy and skill." This certainly plays heavily

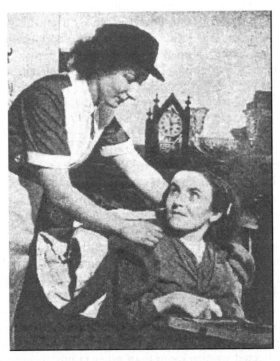

Figure 9.6 Film still from *Friend of the Family*: "The District Nurse visits one of her patients." From J. Cunningham, "The British District Nurse on the Films," *South African Nursing Journal* (May 1949): 40–41. We have made every effort to contact the holder of reproduction rights for this image without success.

on the imagery complained of by Briggs. Although student nurses are shown learning anatomy, physiology, Latin, and medical terminology (a subject generally associated with the medical profession), the film also shows cookery, bed-making, bandaging, and dressing techniques, and the overall picture is presented as both strongly female oriented and highly vocational. District nursing is introduced by the image of a plaque outside the East London District Nurses Home displaying the foundation date (1868). The narrator states, "Those needing skilled attention are the words on the board and from these headquarters nurses are sent on their healing mission making a kindly enquiry or passing a cheery moment with those who know and love her well. Her work is among the poor and needy, her skill is for those who seek it." A shot of a rural district nurse stresses that "she is everything from doctor to health visitor" and that "evacuation has added to her duties."

The second of the two films, *District Nurse*,[25] opens with the comment, "This film is about one of those women who are sturdily carrying on their peacetime jobs in spite of wartime difficulties: the District Nurse." It is set in the rural Southwest of England and follows an elderly triple-duty Queen's Nurse from a home confinement to a call-out by the GP to a farm accident to a sick evacuee child and finally to the welfare clinic. Her relationship with the doctor appears formal and rigid. This professional demeanour is also exhibited with her patients, but suggests a social distance created through an air of authority on her part rather than an uneasy relationship. In both films, the missionary-like, selfless image is stressed, and the work is presented as a valuable wartime contribution. The film was shown later on television and was felt by the QNI to be "particularly suitable for career programmes at school and showing to hospital nurses and general audiences."[26]

The BBC TV documentary programme *Mustn't Grumble*[27] used a mixture of clips from earlier documentary film footage and oral history to provide a vivid image of the impact of the "Health Bus" in Merseyside that provided mobile, direct access to health care for those living in deprived areas of Liverpool and that was particularly aimed at women. The opening discussion between a midwife and a district nurse centres on problems of health care access for women and especially poor, single parents. The nurse commented, "They have no time to be ill . . . they have to just soldier on." Both saw early health care provision being predominantly for the male working population, added to which there were few women doctors. They stressed the problems arising from a combination of modesty and taboo such as gynaecological and sexual problems, violence, and a high maternal mortality and morbidity rate, explaining that networks of women friends and neighbours provided the main source of help and advice, together with home manuals on health problems. The effects of cramped, damp, and unsanitary surroundings were felt to have affected women more than other family members, as they had to spend the most time exposed to them.

The doctor was often "too expensive" at 6d per visit and this point was reinforced through images of the slums of Liverpool and Birmingham from a

Public Office of Information film on public health. Both midwife and district nurse commented on the problems of infestation with lice, fleas, and house mites, and in providing a layette for new babies, before describing the problems in procuring abortions and getting family planning advice, commenting that home versions were used such as Epsom salts. The remainder of the film is devoted to explaining the development of family planning clinics. The images presented through this documentary were of the poverty of the slums and, although justifying the need for the mobile clinic, the community's dependence on the nurse and midwife was implicit throughout, as was the lack of medical provision for many women prior to the NHS. In particular, the images tied in very closely to those provided by one interviewee who described her experience while training as an HV in Liverpool:

> Most of the houses in Liverpool that we went to had no facilities for . . . washing, and hanging the washing out. They just had yards, didn't they, you know? . . . and a brown sink in the back kitchen, and a cold water tap. But the Wash Houses, they had in various areas round Liverpool—and for the women, it was a day out, really—they used to put all their dirty washing in a pram, and push it up to the nearest Wash House, take their own soap powder with them, and . . . I think . . . I can't remember how many sinks there were . . . there might have been as many as 14 or 15 sinks, and they had the hot water and everything, and they took their own powder. And I remember, Tide had just come in at that time, and they wouldn't let them use it, because they thought it was wrong for the sinks. . . . Because, you see, people didn't have washing machines then. They were just beginning to come out at that time. And I remember the Tide, because when I came on the District, as a Health Visitor, an awful lot of women had dermatitis on their hands then, and they all said it was due to the washing powders, the new ones that were just coming out.[28]

Like the nurse and midwife in the film, she also commented that two of the major problems she encountered when first working in Liverpool and St. Helen's in the 1950s were infestation of the heads with lice and impetigo in children, as it had been for the nurses in Bacup thirty years earlier.[29]

NOVELS AND TELEVISION DRAMA: THE UNOFFICIAL VIEWPOINT

Well-researched fiction can provide valuable testimony when viewed with the appropriate degree of caution. The images presented through fiction can reveal something of the popular imagination for which it was produced, which in turn can add a better understanding of the sociocultural factors involved in the conceptual configurations that form "the play of mediations between the ideals, practices and institutional formations of professional nursing at any one time."[30] On a more cautionary note, however, fiction cannot be presented in historical research as providing an accurate, objective, or dispassionate view and might occasionally contain misleading factual errors. Fiction in the form of books, film, or television drama often presents a populist opinion, lacking in perspective, and imposing a contrived or politicised view of the present onto the past. With few supporting documents it is difficult to measure their popularity or effectiveness, or even to know who watches or reads them. Nevertheless, through the witting and unwitting testimony they might contain, there will often be some form of social comment underlying the narratives and it is this we will be looking for in the final section of this chapter.

In the case of a novel or screenplay with a nursing or medical bent there might be some insight to the role of the professionals seen through the eyes of the author either representing or questioning the dominant ideology. *The Citadel*[31] by A. J. Cronin (1896–1981) is one such case. Cronin was a Scottish novelist who graduated in medicine from Glasgow University in 1919. In 1921 he took up general practice in South Wales and spent some time investigating occupational diseases in the coal industry, being awarded the MD degree (University of Glasgow) in 1925. *The Citadel* is, to a considerable extent, based on his personal experiences as a GP and is largely set in 1920s South Wales. The midwife and later the nurse are both portrayed as older women, rather in the Gamp style, with little medical knowledge, and with their practice rooted in folk remedies and familiarity rather than professional training and modern scientific method. The short episode in which Nurse Lloyd is depicted is nevertheless essential to the ensuing story. She has dressed a serious scald with a dirty carron oil dressing and is unwilling to carry out the orders of Dr. Manson (the young assistant GP) with tragic results for the patient. His first communication with her is a tactful and carefully worded note left in a sealed envelope at the patient's house. His attitude toward her is polite and respectful and it is the nurse who is confrontational, acting unprofessionally by arguing in front of the patient. She is described as a local woman having twenty years of district nursing experience. Her experience and familiarity attracted the patient's loyalty, and he then transferred to another doctor's list so that the nurse would continue to treat him. It is noteworthy that medical colleagues are presented by Cronin as those ultimately responsible in allowing the nurse to continue with the wrong treatment and are repeatedly depicted as acting unprofessionally or lacking in current practice and scientifically based knowledge. The underlying message is the importance of professional conduct and of the biomedical scientific model. Cronin appears to have no time for folk-remedies or for medical or nursing practitioners who do not fit into this ideal.

Another novel, also set in the 1920s in a Welsh mining town that is depicted as similarly poor and unhealthy is *The District Nurse*[32] written by Hugh Miller in 1984. The following year it was developed into a memorable BBC TV (Wales) series: *District Nurse*, in which Nerys Hughes played Queen's Nurse Megan Roberts.[33] District Nurse Roberts, the district nurse of the title, is portrayed as a young, unmarried district nurse with a highly professional outlook, working under the watchful supervision of the GP with whom she must battle for professional recognition, simultaneously having to compete with the untrained village nurse who has lived and worked in the town all her life. She gets around on foot or bicycle in mountainous terrain. She is Welsh speaking, although she is not from North Wales, and her patients are mostly miners and their families, with the majority of her work being public health, educational and preventative practice, nursing industrial injuries, assisting the doctor, and a bit of school nursing thrown in for good measure. Unsurprisingly, the menial nursing tasks such as the run-of-the-mill daily dressings and bed baths, rarely (if ever) feature in the book or television series. Although it inevitably takes a retrospective view, the relationships between Queen's Nurses, GPs, and village handiwomen suggest that the arrival of a newly qualified Queen's Nurse in such an insular community must have been similarly challenging in reality.

A different emphasis was presented by the BBC TV drama series *Angels*, in which a contemporary view was portrayed of student and newly qualified nurses at a fictitious London hospital, St. Angela's. Two episodes featured the nurse in the community. The first, "Health Visitor,"[34] focused on the trainee health visitor's role in community health care, whereas the second, written by Paula Milne (the script editor to the series), was entitled "Walkabout,"[35] and concentrated on the district nurse. Both had suitably qualified nurse advisors as part of the credited research team. These two episodes are surprisingly refreshing, as they tend to explore the less stereotypical image of the nurse while being less spectacularly dramatic than later hospital drama series. Hallam noted that the series *Angels*, through this socialist realist format, "quickly established itself as a popular favourite among young and old female viewers because of its strong female characters and positive portrayal of feminine values," and referred to "a new 'authenticity' that was critically acclaimed for showing a more realistic view of nursing life."[36]

At the centre of the "Health Visitor" episode were issues such as the heavy workload of the hands-on district nurse compared with the more social working hours, but less formulaic approach of the HV, whose work was shown to be equally demanding but difficult to define. In one scene the student and her supervisor have a case discussion with the GP, the setting being a health centre, within an atmosphere of cooperation that surprises the student. The supervisor stresses, "We work with the doctors, not *for* them." The rather unsubtle psychological coercion used by the student HV to persuade a difficult client into sheltered housing, however, detracted from the credibility. There were similar shortcomings in the "Walkabout" episode, which followed a student nurse on her community placement with a district nurse, yet there were also well-researched insights into professional autonomy as well as differences between community and hospital experiences that fell directly into line with those expressed in oral histories. One such example was the district nurse's comment at one point that, "on district there are no textbook answers like on the wards, no procedure book to run to when you're in doubt" and she underlines that they are the visitors in the patients' homes. She describes hospital nursing as "secure and comfortable, performing the same daily chores without conscious effort but with loss of initiative and independent thought and your own hidden resources." Instead of the usual emphasis on the rewarding nature of nursing work, the stress is on the "revealing aspect" of seeing how some people live, underlining the challenging and stressful aspects to district nursing.

The social aspects addressed in both episodes take prominence, but the images portrayed are of student nurses and postregistration students struggling against overwork and inadequate pay in a challenging learning curve. There is a distinctive bid for public sympathy for the nurses emerging from *Angels* that portrays the complexities of the social and ethical dilemmas faced in community health care. Hallam, in her study of media, culture, and professional identity in nursing, criticised the choice of a London teaching hospital for the *Angels* series, rather than a less prestigious provincial general hospital, and the lack of attention paid to current issues such as the RCN's stance on industrial action and restructuring of the profession.[37]

CONCLUSION

The visual image, pen portraits, and media representations of the district nurse can all be extremely potent whether used for the purpose of recruitment, fundraising, political or social reform, public information, or purely entertainment. They can combine as a number of stereotypes to construct a symbolic identity by the media or from within the profession itself. Nurses are especially aware of this imagery and what it is seen to symbolise, as demonstrated by the attention this topic constantly receives in online nursing history discussion lists, the popularity of photographic collections, and the inclusion of pictures of nurses in uniform in most nursing histories.[38] From within the nursing profession and from outside in the public and media domains, this imagery and the stereotypes held within it are influential in the values and beliefs encoded by them that distinguish between various members of the community health care team, for example, in distinguishing male and female aspects or medical and nursing roles that go to make up concepts of professionalism and vocationalism.

10 Discussion and Conclusion

Summers described a paucity of sources relating to nursing in the domestic environment.[1] Although concerned primarily with the nineteenth-century community nurse, her comments about the obscurity of these practitioners were equally relevant to the district nurse of the twentieth century. In the use of oral histories, personal testimonies, and written autobiography, this book has gone some way in challenging that state of affairs. Wherever possible, its aim has been to recount the actual experiences and work undertaken by district nurses.

> There is a documented lack of clarity over the direction and focus of community nursing that raises significant issues. To address them Goeppinger suggested that certain questions were implicit: What are the goals of practice? At what levels do community nurses practise? What roles are particularly salient? In what settings do community nurses practise?[2]

That these questions are not easily answered suggests that a "singular definitive concept is not just elusive, but non-existent."[3]

Given this quandary over professional definitions and focus it seems an appropriate time to investigate the historical roots of current perceptions of community nursing. To do this one must have a clear understanding of what community nursing entails. Baker et al. highlighted the wide range of practitioners this service encompasses including district nurses, HVs, health-authority-employed treatment room nurses, practice-employed nurses, community psychiatric nurses, community midwives, and school health service nurses.[4] This list, to which could now be added numerous other nurse specialists, gives some indication of the fragmentary nature of community nursing and illustrates the difficulty in providing a singular definitive concept. One way of addressing this difficulty might be to examine community nursing for its continuities, but this, too, is a difficult task as the historical roles of many of the various services are themselves under-researched. Alternatively, specific community nursing services can be examined for their own internal continuities and fractures in studies that would provide a greater understanding of nursing work within the community. Such studies would eventually contribute to the wider question of definition of the community nursing concept in general, and it is this approach that has been taken throughout this book. We have sought to record what constituted the nature of district nursing for those who worked in the United Kingdom during the twentieth century through the perceptions of those who practised. To this end we must acknowledge the contradictory nature of memory that is both frail and compelling, incomplete and yet acute. This book therefore offers a perspective that like all historical narratives is shaped by the conditions of its production.

The twentieth century saw the waxing and waning of the QNI from the height of its powers as a voluntaristic association responsible for overseeing training, examination, and subsequent regulation of a large percentage of the district nurses working in Wales, Scotland, and England. By the 1960s it had redirected its remit toward research and development, relinquishing the postregistration training by placing greater emphasis on refresher courses and management training. Since 1975, the QNI has fulfilled its obligations through an awards programme that provides both funding and professional support for nurses administering community nursing projects, and running a series of seminars and conferences relevant to community nursing policy and practice. Furthermore, it continues to provide welfare support for elderly and infirm district nurses. For the district nurses themselves, the NHS Act meant a move to employment that was no longer subject to the uncertainties of charitable collections or voluntary subscriptions, or in the case of Queen's Nurses, to the bureaucratic and authoritarian control of the QNI and district associations. However many who had enjoyed the experience of living and working in Queen's Nurses' homes and training centres regretted their loss. The loss of influence of the QNI also marked a reduction in professional status and pride in the title of Queen's Nurse, as well as the loss of an important support network. For some interviewees, the diminished role of the QNI reflected the prevailing shift in home nursing away from traditional practice toward what they perceive as a depersonalised approach to patient care; that is, an approach that shows less consideration to the patient as a person than as a case for treatment. Depersonalisation within the nurse–patient relationship is one of the central themes to emerge from interviews although it might be regarded with a degree of scepticism given that a number of interviewees are now closer to being the recipients of home nursing care than the givers of it; the view from the other side of the fence inevitably alters perception. Notwithstanding, the relationships forged by nurses of the past were crucial, not only to the way they practised but very often to the way they lived and the way they review their lives today.

Organisational changes that occurred within the century were substantial but the impact of the NHS, although discussed in every interview, was rarely singled out as uniquely significant in itself. However, it gave rise to more emphatic discussions on the changing technologies and organisational structures that came in its wake. The transition from working in geographical districts to attachment schemes or health centres was definitive for all interviewees and difficult for many.

The difference between urban and rural districts is a theme that has run throughout this book. Nurses in either setting were aware of the different experience each entailed. Rural nurses were often more isolated but involved in their communities, whereas urban nurses tended to encounter home conditions and poverty involving them in more non-nursing tasks. Hence both situations affected working relationships and the scope of the nurse's work. Even though large numbers of people still live in isolated areas, improved transport and communication have made nurses, doctors, and hospitals more readily accessible to patients than ever before. At least, that is the theory. Interviewees argued that the district nurse has become increasingly invisible and remote. A home outside her area of work that she owns and has chosen for herself has replaced the association or council house allocated to her in the district; the surgery has taken over much of her working time and even in the city, the car has removed her from the public path. In terms of availability, elderly district nurses regard this as a poor substitute for the local walking nurse in her instantly recognisable uniform who could be stopped on the street. In their view, the nurse no longer belongs to a district whose boundaries are shared by her patients in common geography but to an abstract district defined by the administrative requirements of GPs and their practices.

1900 to 1979 also marked a period of change in composition of district nursing as a workforce from one that has been shown to have a rapid turnover of unmarried women in many posts, and with older nurses preferring rural nursing and younger ones concentrated in the urban areas, to a more stable and mixed workforce including men and married women staying in posts for longer periods. The introduction of men into district nursing was clearly accepted by some colleagues better than others, but the fact that some perceived them as a threat might be indicative of the uncertainty and lack of professional security just below the surface at a time of considerable change. Nurses' autonomy also underwent considerable changes during this time. Perhaps most obvious was the change from practice under a lay committee with infrequent supervision by QNI inspectors (in the case of rural Queen's Nurses) or tight supervision by QNI superintendents (in the case of urban Queen's Nurses). This transferred to local government control and reduced levels of supervision all around. The move into team practice and GP attachments resulted in increased accountability and more direct line management. There was also a considerable change in the nurse–patient relationship over this period that indirectly affected nurses' perceived autonomy. In 1900 the main aim of district nursing was to provide nursing care for the sick poor. Assessment of ability to pay was often left to the nurse's discretion, although she remained answerable to the GP for treatment and care provided. During the 1920s and 1930s this remit widened through Provident and other subscription schemes to include any patients who were willing to contribute.

From 1948 the district nurse cared for anyone and everyone under the pro-visions of the NHS but with the nursing care becoming solely the province of the nurse and progressively less intervention coming from the GP. By 1979 few district nurses, except in very remote areas, combined nursing with midwifery, school nursing, or health visiting, so that the nurse's work in rural areas was no longer so dissimilar to that of the urban district nurse. In fact, many no longer lived within the districts in which they practised by the end of the 1970s. This had a dual impact on the role and image of the rural district nurse: areas instantly doubled in size as district nursing for one area was taken from the midwife by the district nurse, and simultaneously, loss of midwifery dramatically reduced the broad community focus of her daily work to a more specialist one. It has not been part of the scope of this book to look at the midwifery role of district nurse-midwives in any depth, but this particular transitional period deserves further study.

By the late 1970s and 1980s developments in community health pol-icy were also beginning to force a number of fundamental changes in role, workload, and working day or routine, constantly redefining the nurse's job description and changing the relationship with other health care profes-sionals. He or she could no longer remain as autonomous, especially with specialist nurses such as community psychiatric nurses, stoma-care nurses, and Macmillan or Marie Curie nurses, increasingly present, whereas daily liaison with practice nurses and GPs was becoming essential.

Changes in hospital nursing practice also made their impression. With shorter inpatient stays, some hospital nurses complained of lack of continu-ity and experience reducing the degree of job satisfaction, whereas district work was becoming proportionately more fulfilling. Oral history interview-ees always commented on this aspect of community work as high among their reasons for leaving hospitals, together with the freedom of general nursing that gave the opportunity to care for patients of all age groups and the variety of medical and surgical conditions encountered as well as the pleasure (and challenge) of nursing patients in their own homes.

The balance of specialism within generalism has proved a difficult one to address. With medicine still holding many of the aces, the room for negotia-tion over extended roles was (and arguably still is) limited. This was dem-onstrated by the power held by the GPs first in avoiding the team approach, and later in pushing it forward when it appeared more advantageous. Nev-ertheless, doctors' control over patterns of work and division of responsibil-ities in the community remained less straightforward than in the hospital.[5] As Dr. Hockey, a prominent campaigner for specialism within generalism, commented:

> A GP is considered as a specialist in his own right because he is a general practitioner, but a general nurse is always considered to be of less value than a specialist nurse . . . I think we're educating in the wrong way. . . . In the past the well qualified district nurse was out on her rounds doing

bed-baths for old women and the less well trained practice nurse was doing what was considered to be the prestigious aspect of practice and she was close to the doctor physically so he would confide in her and get her to help him with technical tasks and all the rest of it—and she became more prestigious than a better qualified district nurse.[6]

GP attachment and the team approach had obvious advantages in terms of improved communications interprofessionally, but this and similar comments made by other district nurses interviewed suggest that some of these were offset by the introduction of the practice nurse as Dr. Hockey indicated in this quote.

There were also practical and ethical concerns expressed about intraprofessional difficulties relating to continuity of care and the interests of the patient, including patient advocacy. A study that looked at the intraprofessional team working concluded that "there are multiple ethical problems to address in team-working, and that mechanisms for discerning moral issues, patterns of communication, self-scrutiny and conflict resolution are substantially under-developed at the present time."[7] This study suggested that one alternative might be to assign responsibility for overall nursing management to one member of the care team as care manager to ensure that "the patient has a spokesperson who is well placed to steer a course through them." The loss of the QNI county superintendent of district nurses in 1948 effectively removed some of the peer review and internal controls, which had been one of the strengths of that system in regulating and maintaining a high standard of care. Subsequently the move from geographical community-based district nursing where the nurse was "our" nurse to the GP attachment where he or she became "one of the" district nurses might have increased some aspects of efficiency of care provision, but might have reduced inadvertently the more holistic characteristics of care provided.

There are a number of areas either not covered or only touched on in this book, yet deserving of further consideration. First, legislation since the 1960s has been considerable. This has been referred to only briefly, as this work was not intended to be a political history of community health legislation. This marked a period of intensive reassessment of community health care with numerous official studies, inquiries, and reports resulting in a stream of legislation. Equally it has not been possible to look in detail at the effects of changes in policy toward community health care, nor the effects of a dramatic surgical and technological ascendancy on changing patient demands. The rising expertise of specialist community nurses and the introduction of the practice nurse and nurse practitioners into community health have also received only brief attention. Likewise, it would be interesting to draw some comparisons with overseas developments in district nursing; for example, was there a one-way or two-way sphere of influence and how were similar problems dealt with elsewhere? Work done in the United States suggests there were many similarities, with the biggest of these being the problem of caring for the elderly and chronic sick. Their lack of adequate finances created a stumbling block that repeatedly brought down an otherwise effective home nursing service on each attempt to re-establish it.[8] Similarly, work undertaken in South Africa demonstrates a racially and culturally defined system of community care provision in which the nurse might find herself in the position of culture-broker, although her district area would be considerably greater and medical contact much more physically remote than for her British counterpart.[9]

The overriding feature of this research has been the individuality of the nurses, which often comes through vibrantly in inspectors' reports, oral histories, photographs, films, and autobiographies. Many show a strong degree of independence and adaptability in tackling harsh and often unpleasant working conditions—from the descriptions of QNI Chief Superintendent Amy Hughes to the lowliest of village nurse-midwives—that enabled them to draw on innate resourcefulness and initiative to handle the most difficult situations. Their mobility of practice throughout the interwar period was one of the surprises of this research, upsetting the stereotypical image of district nurses staying in one place throughout their working lives. They were largely women from working-class backgrounds[10] (although not invariably so), which makes their determined bid for professional status and autonomy particularly remarkable when set alongside a much more powerful, largely male, established medical profession.

Bearing in mind the emphasis on the professionalisation of this nursing specialty it is significant that at the time of writing, a steering group of the RCN has been preparing a definition of nursing led by Professor Dame June Clark, intended to cover the whole range of nursing and to be used "to influence policy, to determine skill mix, to inform resource management, in job-description, in legislation, and in many other ways."[11] Part of the underlying rationale to this has been concern, "to be able to distinguish between professional nursing and the nursing undertaken by other people," and therefore to establish a particular knowledge base for nursing. The need to be recognised as a profession remains as strong as ever, with professional tensions or conflicts of interest never far below the surface as the main motivation. However, the latest report from the QNI and English National Board for Nursing was ominously entitled "District Nursing: The Invisible Workforce."[12] It revealed continued concerns about the role of the district nurse, workload and caseload management, education, and "a workforce which clearly feels under-resourced, over-burdened and lacking in support. Serious variation in service provision across the country, confusion about the district nurse's role and the impact that the lack of visibility has had on patient care, are strong messages which cannot be ignored. District nurses see themselves as members of an unseen and unvalued workforce who provide the bulk of care outside hospital settings." It has been the intention of this book to address this invisibility and to provide a better understanding of the historical background to some of these issues.

From the oral histories we have identified two distinct aspects that divide the second half of the twentieth century. The first reflects the experience of district nursing in the 1940s and 1950s with an emphasis on long hours, isolation, travel and transport, medical and pharmacological developments, and the professional isolation of district nurses. The second refers to changes that took place in the 1960s and 1970s to do with the organisation of district nursing and focuses on interprofessional relationships, the development of health centre working, and GP attachments. The later years, the 1980s onward, did not feature strongly in the interviewees' stories, probably because either they had retired by then or they came at the end of their career when they were less able or willing to take on and adapt to change. It might also be argued that we are not yet distanced enough from these years to assess and reflect on the effect of the changes within them and this also might account for the lack of focus on the years after the late 1970s. We have tried to record what they felt was important to include in an examination of district nursing during their working years and how it has changed since that time.

For these nurses, district nursing is not something consigned to memory; it is something that continues around them and often affects them and their friends and family in a personal and direct way. So, in recalling their working life, not only did they tell stories of the past, but implicit in these were observations and opinions of the service today. However, many of them continue to assess current district nursing, judge it, and expect from it, according to an internalised definition they developed as young nurses and this must be borne in mind. It must also be acknowledged that their perceptions of both past and present district nursing could have been altered by encroaching old age and, for many, the personal experience of ill health. Their narratives of nursing work are constructed within this framework. What this book is based on, then, is not simply a collection of stories of how things were, but stories that are at the same time illustrations of how these nurses think things have changed, stories already selected for the way they illustrate difference and change. Essentially, they are stories that bind the past to the present. District nurses interviewed for this book who lived and worked through the 1940s, 1950s, and 1960s regarded themselves as a privileged generation of nurses in a time of significant change, and it is for this reason that oral testimony was considered such a valuable resource.

Arguably the most radical change, the transfer from a voluntary to a statutory service, occurred in the middle of the twentieth century and was within the direct experience of a small number of interviewees who remembered their early working years under the local nursing associations. With their roots in nineteenth-century philanthropy, these associations reflected an organisation of home nursing based on social hierarchy and class distinction at the management level. However, this was mitigated to some extent by the affiliation of most associations to the QNI where standards in nursing care, the training curriculum, and the well-being of their nurses was as much the concern of the appointed committees as was exploiting social status in the collection of funds. Although the QNI Councils comprised the great and the good, the district nurse trainee's daily contact was with nursing superintendents on nursing matters. The interests of the QNI allowed and encouraged a sense of professionalism and a specific identity as a Queen's Nurse (a title no longer conferred by 1970) and most interviewees proudly referred to themselves as Queen's Nurses even although their contact with the QNI during their working life might have been infrequent. This continuing affinity with the QNI as opposed to the nursing associations and despite its diminished role since the 1970s, might be viewed sceptically as a nostalgic attachment to the past, but it also suggests that the QNI embodied a particular kind of district nursing that is not recognised in today's service. It was this kind of nursing, influenced by the QNI, that interviewees identified themselves with rather than the QNI per se. Although it can also be argued that it represented an outdated kind of district nursing, nevertheless, it is one that remains definitive for a generation.

What emerges here then is the possibility that definitions of district nursing, like anything else, are contingent and derive relevance and meaning only within a given context or culture. Even the term *district* is a misnomer now because district boundaries no longer apply to the nurse's area of work. Thus the term *district nursing* is determined by other factors implicit in its title and is subject to interpretation. Just as the regimes in wards fifty years ago would not be tolerated by general nurses today, nor would the conditions endured by past district nurses in QNI training homes. Although they were criticised by those who trained there, in the 1940s and 1950s these conditions reflected a general culture in which thrift, authoritarian control, deference, and obedience were relatively unquestioned. Elderly retired Queen's Nurses experienced a radical change in this culture over several decades and so the QNI can be appreciated as a powerful marker of difference not only between past and present district nursing, but in society in general. A second marker of difference was interviewees' experience as young people living through World War II. This was something certainly unique to their generation and momentous in its impact both personally and in terms of the social changes that followed in its wake. It is interesting that these two experiential landmarks were quickly established in the interviews, locating interviewees' sense of place and identity in a particular cultural milieu.

Professional isolation could be compounded by the social isolation experienced in having a distinctively professional role within a small community. There were often personal adjustments to be made when settling into a new community in which district nurses had to live as full members but within which they were privy to the crucial confidences of so many others. District nurses working in rural or remote communities, or even in small town districts, sometimes found it difficult to form close friendships within their districts and many relied strongly on maintaining family ties. Hazardous weather dogged the working life of rural nurses in wintertime and for those in more remote districts, was often compounded by a lack of safe transport.

All of these aspects of district nursing serve as a reminder that Britain is not necessarily one homogeneous mass but a place that supports distinct regional differences. Under the NHS, district nurses might have benefited from standardisation in salary and pension entitlements but the itinerant nature of their work meant that their conditions of work were still highly dependent on the prevailing geography of their district. Internal coherence in the service was compromised by these regional variations but seen in relation to current district nursing they also suggest a certain consistency over time. For example, the unique character of the Scottish Highlands and Islands has prompted a recent revision of services and attracted the pilot Family Health Nurse (FHN) project to certain areas. Although heralded as an "alternative community health model," the FHN bears a striking resemblance to the triple-duty nurse of old. Furthermore, it is significant that in a remote Scottish island, what was essentially the triple-duty nurse still operated in the late 1990s. The triple-duty tradition, thought by most to be outmoded and long gone, has persisted in a practical sense and is currently being reconstructed in the concept of the FHN.

Following World War II and the transfer of control to the state under the NHS, change in district nursing was also imposed by the expansion of medical knowledge and technologies coming fast on the heels of postwar regeneration. Improved pharmacology replaced traditional nursing procedures in many cases and although this often brought more speedy and complete recovery to patients, it was no less demanding of the nurse. Diabetics still required early-morning injections and regular antibiotics had to be administered by the nurse at various times in the day. Only with the introduction of medication in tablet form was self-administration viable, thereby relieving the nurse of much time- and energy-consuming home visiting. Improved surgical techniques coupled with the reduction of the length of hospital stays saw home nursing of the chronic sick lessen and the need for specialised, postoperative, home nursing care increase over time. From the 1960s onward, growing numbers of patients with chronic disease were able to receive life-saving or life-enhancing surgery (e.g., from joint replacements in suitable osteoarthritis cases, to cataract removal or corneal replacement, to the transplanting of organs such as the kidney, and radical heart surgery) in hospitals before returning home where longer term postoperative care could be managed within the community if required. As these procedures have become more common, district nurses have developed appropriate skills to deal with specialised care plans in the home, and liaison between community and hospital has improved with district nurses receiving inservice training from hospital departments in specific procedures. This period also saw a decrease in home confinements, reducing the number of out-of-hours midwifery calls to district nurse-midwives. At the same time, trends in longevity produced greater numbers of elderly people requiring home nursing care. In short, this period saw a change in the types of cases the district nurse encountered as well as the skills demanded of her.

Both personal testimony and the official guidelines of the QNI have noted that *adaptability* was a recognised characteristic of district nursing. As we have seen, district nurses did not always employ the Queen's methods to the letter although their value was acknowledged. Rather, prevailing conditions in any one house influenced, if not dictated, nursing practice and nurses embraced this variety as one of the challenges of the job. They were also called on to adapt to new organisational arrangements and, for many, this was a more difficult adjustment to make. In the 1960s and 1970s nurses demonstrated that they could move into close working proximity with doctors and other health professionals; indeed, most welcomed the new opportunities this provided, viewing it as a partnership where district nursing skills would be recognised and valued. However, the imposition of new management structures in the 1970s (and thereafter under constant review) subjected district nurses to the pressures of a hierarchy and lack of local control that they were unaccustomed to and for which they were ill fitted.

On the basis of the testimonies, we have argued that district nurses of the 1940s and 1950s differed from hospital nurses of the same period and can be shown to have had an established sense of professional autonomy. A counterargument might be made that what we claim as autonomy is in fact isolation. That rural nurses, in particular, were isolated is true, but this does not negate their skill and knowledge base. They were not simply the only ones there, able to provide first aid until the doctor arrived. They, perhaps more than their city counterparts, and certainly before attachment schemes encouraged it, negotiated a sphere of work with GPs based on the definition of nursing as a unique skill, separate from and complementary but not subordinate to medicine. Isolation served to necessitate the occasional crossing of professional boundaries, but these were always within the scope of the nurse's competence, and usually undertaken with the doctor's agreement.

We have seen that district nurses earned the professional respect of the GP, in some situations enough to be trusted to effectively prescribe, and that their opinion on diagnosis was not only heeded but sometimes requested. With reference to the expansion of the nurse's role, McGuire pointed out in 1977 that "in many cases nurses are effectively making first contact decisions anyway though this may not always be recognised for what it is."[13] Yet, even among today's GPs there is still a popular perception of the past district nurse as the woman who bathed old ladies and made cups of tea and that district nurses have only recently become more competent in nursing and medical tasks. A recent study with Paisley GPs indicates this very well. When asked about the district nurses attached to their practices GPs spoke highly of their nursing skills but noted them as recent extensions to the traditional nursing role.[14] It cannot be denied that the most substantial extensions of the district nurse's role have taken place in the last twenty years in accordance with modern medical techniques, but these GPs included in their list of extended duties things commonly cited as routine tasks throughout the working lives of district nurses, urban and rural, now retired, such as caring for the chronic sick or terminally ill, treating leg ulcers, or the regular care of diabetics. Only when district nurses and GPs were brought into closer working contact through attachment schemes pioneered in the late 1960s (but not commonplace until the 1980s) did many GPs begin to appreciate the level of district nursing skills. However, this was not a chronological change. It was shaped not only by policy changes but also by geography. Where geographical remoteness prevailed, the doctor and the nurse had always tended to cooperate more closely allowing the nursing–medicine partnership to be forged, facilitating and utilising the extension of nursing skills. Ironically, in urban areas where doctor, nurse, and patient accessibility was easier, nurse and doctor often remained remote from each other (and this was the case in many city districts prior to the implementation of attachment schemes), necessary information might have been readily exchanged but understanding of the nursing role was not always forthcoming and opportunities to develop professional competency were reduced.

Effective attachment schemes relied on personal as well as professional cooperation, and scepticism or poor resources could affect success. Hence, the development of such schemes made steady but not rapid progress. It wasn't until the 1980s that cooperative working, based on attachment as the ideal model, although subject to local idiosyncrasies, could be hailed as the norm. Thus the realisation among doctors at large, of the skill and utility of district nurses was a gradual process. A notion first mooted in the Dawson Report (1920) and in early conceptions of the NHS, nurse–doctor cooperation and the primary health care team was welcomed by district nursing from the beginning but as the decades passed many felt the ideal of teamwork to have engendered an experience sullied by the fragmentation of the district nursing service and calling into question the proper role of the district nurse. Changes from the 1950s to the 1980s saw the introduction of enrolled nurses into district work taking on basic nursing tasks; the expansion of home help services providing domestic help; the development of professional social work dealing with social welfare problems; the virtual demise of home confinements making domiciliary midwifery relatively redundant; the rise in GP attachments over geographical districts, moving nurses into more surgery-based practice; and the greater specialisation of community nursing skills and the imposition of a more complex management hierarchy. Many aspects of care once held to be the province of the district nurse were now the legitimate responsibility of a range of professional and untrained workers. Any sense of autonomy that the district nurse had established was now obscured by the pressures of a team implicitly unsure of the individual roles of its members. Stripped of many of her traditional functions, the district nurse found herself not only having to adapt to change and redefine her role but, often, reflecting on the essential nature of nursing.

Under such pressure the older, traditional district nurse sought to define her practice by use of the term *basic nursing care* and this raises what was a recurring theme in interviews. Although the physical conditions of district nursing influenced the experience of nurses, a more elusive factor shaped a fundamental perception of change, the notion of *care*. This emerged as a crucial aspect of work that, for many, defined the difference in past and present district nursing. It might be argued that this distinction is based on a misunderstanding of care, characterising it as an essential, personal quality, communicated through the one-to-one encounter rather than a working philosophy. For example, a fundamental role of the district nurse is to assess the need for care and to ensure it is delivered. According to this, district nursing entails the delivery of care, but this could be carried out through the health care team, not necessarily by each individual nurse on a personal basis. However, this definition works within a very contemporary framework where the team is now well established. With a wide variety of health and welfare workers available for any one case it might even be argued that the overall prospects of care (from the patient's perspective) are magnified in today's service. Given the conditions of the past and the lack of professional colleagues working in any one district, in the 1940s and even into the 1970s it was unusual if not impossible to understand care as something to be delegated to a more appropriate person. Even in densely populated areas, the nurse, housed in the district by her local council and carrying a heavy caseload necessitating long working hours, was a familiar face among her patients. Apart from the doctor, the only health workers in the community were the district nurse, the HV, and the midwife, and sometimes the district nurse was all three combined. In the past then, a holistic knowledge of the patient's needs was more likely and care in the home was expressed as a personal and often spontaneous response to these needs. This is not an argument for the system of the past; one can imagine the case where that same familiarity led a patient to refuse the care of the only nurse available. However, it is recognition that what defined district nursing for a generation was a combination of conditions that constituted a context for nursing care that no longer exists today. That is not to agree with an underlying tone of much oral testimony claiming that district nurses of today do not care as much as those of the past; those few younger interviewees who are still practising nurses today are far from devoid of a language of care. However, their working situations now impose a compromise whereby expressions of care (both linguistic and practical) are tempered by the range of interprofessional relationships that now hold within the primary health care team. In short, the simplified one-to-one, personal contact with their patients that district nurses of the past describe might be regarded as a luxury that has been both dissipated among a team of staff and displaced by the professional, administrative, and organisational exigencies of modern community nursing practice.

It might be argued that the now-retired generation of district nurses want the best of both worlds; to be seen as devoted, personal carers with a vocation to nurse yet to be respected as highly qualified and skilled professionals. On balance, this is the achievement of those interviewed here who both uphold and challenge the old stereotype. Whether this is a distorted perception unconsciously created in reflection or a skilful integration of past and present is a matter for continuing debate. The new direction of nursing history allows us to examine the experiences of ordinary nurses, such as those represented here, and to appreciate their embracing of the gendered meaning of nursing as an active choice through which their "places within the social fabric of their communities, their neighbourhoods and their families—have emerged as equally powerful determinants of their consciousness, their roles, and their sense of agency."[15]

Endnotes

PREFACE

1. Helen M. Sweet, "An Investigation Into the Creation and Subsequent Development of the Intensive Care Unit in the United Oxford Hospitals," (Unpublished MA Dissertation, Oxford Brookes University, 1994).
2. A. Digby, *The Evolution of British General Practice 1850–1948* (Oxford: Oxford University Press, 1999).
3. See Graham Smith, *An Oral History of General Practice in Paisley: Locality and the Diffusion of Knowledge c. 1950–1990* (Unpublished project, Wellcome Trust).

INTRODUCTION

1. www.cdna.tvu.ac.uk/pnc/Oct (14 May 2002).
2. www.cdna.tvu.ac.uk/pnc/Oct (14 May 2002).
3. See a full explanation in Chapter 1.
4. The QNI organises subsidised holidays for nurses and an annual summer day gathering for all retired Queen's Nurses. It also provides a network of visitors, themselves retired Queen's Nurses, who keep in touch with those nurses now over the age of 80. The QNI in Scotland holds files on all living Queen's Nurses trained in Scotland and provides a degree of support to retired Queen's Nurses in need of help due to illness or financial difficulty. QNI records of Queen's Nurses trained in Scotland who have died are held in the RCN Archive, Edinburgh.
5. A history of the QNI is already available in M. Baly, *A History of the Queen's Nursing Institute: 100 Years 1887–1987* (Kent: Croom Helm, 1987).
6. Where the QNI for Scotland or for England and Wales are referred to specifically, this is indicated by (S) or (E and W), respectively.
7. A brief explanation of the Poor Law system is provided in Chapter 1.
8. D/N 33, 29/03/01, Oral History: Mrs. Marion Hurst (Tape 2, Side A).
9. M. Stocks, *A Hundred Years of District Nursing* (London, Allen and Unwin 1960); Baly, *A History of the Queen's Institute*.
10. District nurses caricatured in C. Dickens, *The Life and Adventures of Martin Chuzzlewit* (London: Hazell, Watson & Viney, 1843–1844). In particular these have been examined by A. Summers, "The Mysterious Demise of Sarah Gamp: The Domicilliary Nurse and Her Detractors: 1830–60," *Journal of*

Victorian Studies 32, no. 3 (1989): 365–386; and more recently by J. J. Fenne, "'Every Woman Is a Nurse': Domestic Nurses in Nineteenth-Century English Popular Literature (Charles Dickens, Mary Augusta Ward)," (Ph.D. thesis, University of Wisconsin-Madison, 2000).

11. G. Hardy, *William Rathbone and the Early History of District Nursing* (Ormskirk: G. W. and A. Hesketh, 1981).

12. See, for example, F. K. Prochaska, "Body and Soul: Bible Nurses and The Poor in Victorian London," *Historical Research* 60 (1987): 336–348; C. Davies, "The Health Visitor as Mother's Friend: A Woman's Place in Public Health 1900–14," *SHM* 1 (1988): 39–59; L. Williamson, "Soul Sisters: The St. John and Ranyard Nurses in Nineteenth Century London," *IHNJ* 2, no. 2 (1996): 33–49.

13. E. N. Fox, "District Nursing and the Work of District Nursing Associations in England and Wales, 1900–48" (Ph.D. thesis, London University, 1993); E. Fox, "District Nursing in England and Wales Before the National Health Service: The Neglected Evidence," *Medical History* 38 (1994): 303–321; E. Fox, "Universal Health Care and Self-Help: Paying for District Nursing Before the National Health Service," *Twentieth Century British History* 7, no. 1 (1996): 83–109.

14. S. Walby, J. Greenwell, et al. *Medicine and Nursing: Professions in a Changing Health Service* (London: Sage , 1994); C. Davies, *Gender and the Professional Predicament in Nursing* (Buckingham: Open University Press, 1995); J. Littlewood, ed., *Current Issues in Community Nursing* (New York: Churchill Livingstone, 1995); A. M. Rafferty, *The Politics of Nursing Knowledge* (London: Routledge, 1996). A sociological perspective is found in A. Kelly and A. Symonds, *The Social Construction of Community Nursing* (Basingstoke: Palgrave Macmillan, 2003).

15. J. Donnison, *Midwives and Medical Men: History of Interprofessional Rivalries and Women's Rights* (London: Heinemann Educational, 1977); I. Loudon, "Medical Care and the Family Doctor," *Bulletin of the History of Medicine* 58 (1984).

16. R. Dingwall, "Problems of Teamwork in Primary Care," in *Teamwork in Personal Social Services and Health Care*, ed. S. Lonsdale, A. Webb, and T. Briggs (London: Croom Helm, 1980); C. Davies, "The Health Visitor"; A. Kelsey, "The Making of Health Visitors: An Historical Perspective Part 1," *IHNJ* 5, no. 3 (2000): 44–50; A. Kelsey, "The Making of Health Visitors: An Historical Perspective Part 2," *IHNJ* 6, no. 2 (2000): 66–70.

17. E. Fox, "An Honourable Calling or a Despised Occupation: Licensed Midwifery," *SHM* 6, no. 2 (1993): 237–259; N. Leap and B. Hunter, *The Midwife's Tale: An Oral History From Handywoman to Professional Midwife* (London: Scarlet Press, 1993); S. Pitt, "Midwifery and Medicine: Discourses in Childbirth 1945–1975" (Ph.D. thesis, University of Wales, 1996); B. Mortimer, "The Nurse in Edinburgh c. 1760–1890: The Impact of Commerce and Professionalisation" (Ph.D. thesis, University of Edinburgh, 2002); L. Reid, "The History of Midwifery in Scotland in the Twentieth Century" (Ph.D. thesis, University of Glasgow, 2003).

18. Recent years have seen a growing interest in nursing history and this perspective can be seen in works on history, politics, and sociology, as well as nursing. The prestigious journal *Nursing Enquiry* now dedicates a regular edition to nursing history. Seminal works on nursing history focus on the ward nurse; see B. Abel-Smith, *A History of the Nursing Profession* (London: Heinemann, 1960); R. Dingwall et al., *An Introduction to the Social History of Nursing* (London: Routledge, 1988).

19. P. Allan and M. Jolley, *Nursing, Midwifery and Health Visiting Since 1900* (London: Faber and Faber, 1982).
20. Dingwall et al., *An Introduction to the Social History of Nursing*, 178.
21. C. R. Kratz, "District Nursing," in *Nursing, Midwifery and Health Visiting Since 1900*, ed. P. Allan, P. and M. Jolley (London: Faber and Faber, 1982), 82.
22. S. Ferguson and H. Fitzgerald, *Studies in the Social Services* (London: HMSO/ Longmans Green, 1954), cited in R. Dingwall et al., *An Introduction to the Social History of Nursing*, 197.
23. S. Walby et al., *Medicine and Nursing*; D. Wicks, *Doctors and Nurses at Work: Rethinking Professional Boundaries* (Buckingham: Open University Press, 1998).
24. Wicks, *Doctors and Nurses at Work*, 156–157.
25. C. Maggs, "A History of Nursing: A History of Caring?" *Journal of Advanced Nursing* 23, no. 3 (1996).
26. L. Hockey, *Feeling the Pulse* (London: QNI, 1966); L. Hockey, *Care in the Balance* (London: QNI, 1968); L. Hockey and A. Buttimore, eds., *Co-operation in Patient Care: Studies of District Nurses Attached to Hospital and General Medical Practice* (London: QNI, 1970); L. Hockey, "The Family Care Team: Philosophy, Problems, Possibilities," in *Ciba Foundation Symposium on Teamwork for World Health*, eds. G. Wolstenholme and M. O'Connor (London: Churchill, 1971), 103–115.
27. Ministry of Health and S. F. Armer (Chair) et al., *Report of the Working Party on the Training of District Nurses* (1955); Department of Health and Social Security (DHSS), *The State of the Public Health: Report of the Chief Medical Officer* (1970); DHSS (Cmnd. 5055), *National Health Service Reorganisation* (1972); DHSS and P. A. Briggs (Chair) et al. (Cmnd. 5115), *Report of the Committee on Nursing* (1972); General Nursing Council, *Educational Policy 1977 Annual Report* (1977); Royal College of Nursing, *Specialties in Nursing: A Report of the Working Party Investigating the Development of Specialties Within the Nursing Profession* (1988).
28. G. Larkin, *Occupational Monopoly and Modern Medicine* (London: Tavistock, 1983).
29. Davies, *Gender and the Professional Predicament in Nursing*.
30. A. Witz, *Professions and Patriarchy* (London: Routledge, 1992).
31. S. Marks, *Divided Sisterhood: Race, Class and Gender in the South African Nursing Profession* (Basingstoke: St Martin's Press, 1994).
32. E. Gamarnikow, "Sexual Division of Labour: The Case of Nursing," in *Feminism and Materialism. Women and Modes of Production* eds. A. Kuhn and A. M. Wolpe (London: Routledge & Kegan Paul, 1978), 96–123.
33. C. Davies, ed., *Rewriting Nursing History* (London: Croom Helm, 1980).
34. Abel-Smith, *A History of the Nursing Profession*.
35. H. Butterfield, *The Whig Interpretation of History* (London: G. Bell & Sons, 1963); cited in Davies, *Rewriting Nursing History*, 12.
36. J. Godden et al., "The Decline of Myths and Myopia? The Use and Abuse of Nursing History," *The Australian Journal of Advanced Nursing* 10, no. 2 (1992–1993): 27.
37. Ibid., 32–33.
38. *The International History of Nursing Journal* ceased publication in 2003.
39. S. Nelson, "The Fork in the Road: Nursing History Versus the History of Nursing?" *Nursing History Review* 10 (2002): 177.
40. C. Maggs "History of Nursing, History of Nurses: Are the Waters Any Clearer?," in *Defining Nursing History: Proceedings of the Fifth Colloquium*

for *Nursing History Research. Edinburgh, September 1999*, ed. B. Mortimer (Edinburgh: Queen Margaret University College Edinburgh, 2000), 4–7.

41. See, for example, S. Lawton et al., *District Nursing: Providing Care in a Supportive Context* (Edinburgh: Churchill Livingstone, 2000).

42. S. Dixon, "SA/QNI The Queen's Nursing Institute," *CMAC Wellcome Institute for the History of Medicine* (1998); S. Dixon, "The Archive of the Queen's Nursing Institute in the Contemporary Medical Archives Centre," *Medical History* 45 (2000): 251–266.

43. H. Burdett, *Burdett's Hospitals and Charities Yearbooks* (1900–31).

44. Ibid., 1924, 1932, and 1943 editions.

45. *Queen's Nurses' Magazine (QNM)*, 1904–1958 (later *Queen's Nursing Journal*).

46. *DN* vols. 1, no. 1 (1958) through 15, no. 12 (1973).

47. *QNJ* (1973–1979).

48. *Midwife, Health Visitor and Community Nurse*, vols. 1–27.

49. *Nursing Mirror and Midwives' Journal.*

50. For example, Stocks, *A Hundred Years*; G. Hardy, *William Rathbone and the Early History of District Nursing.*

51. J. B. McIntosh, "An Observation and Time Study of the Work of Domiciliary Nurses" (Ph.D. thesis, University of Aberdeen, 1975); E. N. Fox, "District Nursing and the Work of District Nursing Associations in England and Wales, 1900–48" (Ph.D. thesis, London University, 1993).

52. QNI Archives (1956–1965). SA/QNI Box 114 P13/1-11: Correspondence and material used by M. Stocks for preparation of *A Hundred Years of District Nursing.*

53. Stocks, *A Hundred Years.*

54. Baly, *A History of the Queen's Institute.*

55. Fox, "District Nursing and the Work of District Nursing Associations in England and Wales, 1900–48."

56. Ibid., 14.

57. Ibid., 357.

CHAPTER 1 HISTORICAL TRAJECTORIES: BACKGROUND, C. 1850–1919

1. M. Baly, *As Miss Nightingale Said: Florence Nightingale Through Her Sayings* (London: Scutari Press, 1991), 106. Florence Nightingale's emphasis on sanitary reform reflected her view that it was the essential tool for achieving Victorian health and social reform to be targeted at the domestic rather than the hospital setting.

2. Until men were admitted following demobilisation after World War II.

3. Dickens, *The Life and Adventures of Martin Chuzzlewit*; Sarah Gamp and Betsy Prig were two outdoor relief district nurses caricatured by Dickens.

4. SA/QNI Box 79 H4/1-3: Fundraising Correspondence. The QVJIN was connected by its original charter in 1889 with St. Katherine's Royal Hospital, an ecclesiastical foundation first established near the Tower of London and endowed by Queen Matilda in 1148, chartered by Queen Eleanor in 1273, and later by Queen Phillipa in 1351, who ordained among its chief purposes "the visitation of the sick and infirm."

5. Abel-Smith, *A History of the Nursing Profession* (1960), 2, claimed from census data that "as late as 1851 there were only 7,619 patients [. . .] resident in hospitals, in the whole of England and Wales."

6. J. Hawker, "Parish Nursing in Dorset 1700–1914" (Unpublished paper, 1995) differentiated between "basic" and "skilled" carers, identifying ten skilled out of ninety-nine carers in two parishes in Dorset in the eighteenth century; similarly the parochial nurse in Hanbury, Worcestershire described in Stocks, *A Hundred Years*, 92–93.
7. I. Loudon, *Medical Care and the General Practitioner, 1750–1850* (1986): 90, n.45, noted that from the mid-eighteenth century there were "a number of lying-in charities for delivering the poor in their own homes and some dispensaries also included maternity departments for delivering the poor at their own homes," claiming these were greater in number and more successful than in-patient institutions.
8. M. Chamberlain, *Old Wives Tales: Their History, Remedies and Spells* (London; Virago, 1981); and R. Hutton, *The Pagan Religions of the Ancient British Isles: Their Nature and Legacy* (Oxford: Basil Blackwell, 1991) referred to "village 'cunning-men' and 'wise-women' [. . .] operating freely in many places during the nineteenth century."
9. Dingwall et al., *An Introduction to the Social History of Nursing*, 7.
10. Founded in 1840; see R. G. Huntman et al., "Twixt Candle and Lamp: The Contribution of Elizabeth Fry and the Institution of Nursing Sisters to Nursing Reform," *Medical History*, 43 no. 3 (2002): 351–380. By 1948 these employed approximately twenty-eight nurses undertaking "charitable work."
11. Founded in 1848.
12. Prochaska, "Body and Soul," 336–348; see also C. Jones, "Sisters of Charity and the Ailing Poor," *SHM* 2, no. 3 (1989): 339–348.
13. Stocks, *A Hundred Years*, 25.
14. Two oral histories with Ranyard nurses: D/N 03, 18/07/96, Oral History: Mrs. Gladys Cruttenden; D/N 20, 12/06/99, Oral History: Mrs. M. E. Kay.
15. Burdett, *Burdett's Hospitals and Charities Yearbooks*. Entries for 1915 record 416 nurses working for the Church Army performing "evangelistic and rescue work" but "no systematic, infectious, or night nursing."
16. F. Prochaska, *The Voluntary Impulse: Philanthropy in Modern Britain* (London: Faber and Faber, 1988), 52.
17. Dingwall et al., *An Introduction to the Social History of Nursing*, 29.
18. Williamson, "Soul Sisters," 33–49.
19. A. Digby, *Making a Medical Living: Doctors and Patients in the English Market for Medicine 1720–1911* (Cambridge: Cambridge University Press, 1994), 43–44.
20. M. A. Crowther, "Medicine and the End of the Poor Law," *SHM* 38 (1986): 74–76; G. Anderson, "An Oversight in Nursing History," *Journal of History of Medicine* (1948): 417–426.
21. Abel-Smith, *A History of the Nursing Profession*, 3–4.
22. M. Baly, *Florence Nightingale and The Nursing Legacy* (London: Croom Helm, 1986).
23. "Editorial," *QNM* XXIII, no. 5 (1929): 89–91.
24. A. Hardy, *Health and Medicine in Britain Since 1860* (London: Palgrave, 2001), 19–20.
25. A. Summers, "Nurses and Ancillaries in the Christian Era," in *Western Medicine: An Illustrated History*, ed. I. Loudon (Oxford: Oxford University Press, 1997), 192–205.
26. H. W. Ackland, *Memoirs of the Cholera Epidemic in Oxford 1854* (Churchill, London, 1856), quoted in Dingwall et al., *An Introduction to the Social History of Nursing*, 174–175.
27. Stocks, *A Hundred Years*, 35–37.

28. Although prior to the 1919 Registration Act, this could mean anything from one to three years and training was not nationally regulated but varied considerably from hospital to hospital.
29. Dingwall et al., *An Introduction to the Social History of Nursing*, 175.
30. See Davies, "The Health Visitor," 39–59; J. Welshman, "Family Visitors or Social Workers? Health Visiting and Public Health in England and Wales 1890–1974," *IHNJ* 3, no. 2 (1997): 5–21; Kelsey, "The Making of Health Visitors: An Historical Perspective Part 1," 44–50.
31. P. Abbott and Claire Wallace, "Health Visiting, Social Work, Nursing and Midwifery: A History," in *The Sociology of the Caring Professions*, eds. P. Abbott and Liz Meerabeau (London: The UCL Press, 1998), 20–53.
32. Kelly and Symonds, *The Social Construction of Community Nursing*, provides a more in-depth explanation of this.
33. Davies, "The Health Visitor," 39–59.
34. "Editorial," *QNM* XXIII, no. 5 (1929): 89–91; also see, for example, Challis, "On Starting a District Nursing Association," *QNM* XIX, nos. 1 & 2 (1922): 3–4, 34–35; A. Hughes, "District Nursing on Provident Lines," *Charity Organisation Review* (July 1910); J. B. Hurry, *District Nursing on a Provident Basis* (London, 1898).
35. Stocks, *A Hundred Years*, 46.
36. Mrs. Dacre Craven (nee Florence Lees) wrote the first textbook for district nurses: F. Dacre Craven, *A Guide to District Nurses and Home Nursing* (London: Macmillan, 1889).
37. Hardy, *William Rathbone and the Early History of District Nursing*.
38. "East London Nursing Society," *QNM* XXVI, no. 2 (1933): 68–69. This society formed in 1868 and apart from a three-year incorporation with the Metropolitan and National Association (1878–1881) remained the East London Nursing Society until after World War II and was felt to have retained its own characteristics, serving 213,000 cases between 1881 and 1932 and covering the poorer boroughs of Stepney, Poplar, and the Isle of Dogs.
39. Stocks, *A Hundred Years*, 45–48.
40. "Mrs. Dacre Craven," *The Nurses' Journal* (February 1898): 16–18; R. M. Hallowes, "Distinguished British Nurses: 8. Mrs. Dacre Craven (Florence Lees). An Organiser of District Nursing," *Nursing Mirror* (December 23, 1955).
41. Ibid.
42. Stocks *A Hundred Years*, 124–130, described a confrontation between north and south and between several members of the Rathbone family. Although Liverpool eventually conceded to accept the Queen's Institute's examination system in 1909, Stocks maintained that the resentment lingered between the "emissaries from an arrogant metropolis" and the "older organisation which felt that it required no outsider from the south to tell it how to manage its own business."
43. C. Haddon, "Nursing as a Profession for Ladies," *St. Paul's Monthly Magazine* (August 1871): 458, cited in Abel-Smith, *A History of the Nursing Profession*.
44. "How the Work of District Nursing in London Began—and Continues," *QNM* XIX, no. 3 (1922): 49–52.
45. F. Nightingale, "Trained Nursing for the Sick Poor: Extracts From Letter by Miss Florence Nightingale Sent to The Times, April 1876," *QNM* XX, no. 4 (1923): 165–166.
46. C. Maggs *The Origins of General Nursing* (London: Croom Helm, 1983), 1.
47. Ibid., 30–31.

48. A. Hughes, "Answers to Correspondents," *QNM* 1, no. 3 (December 31, 1904).

49. This was succeeded in 1904 by a supplementary charter granted by King Edward VII by which Queen Alexandra became patron, at which point the Institute was no longer officially connected to St. Katherine's Hospital.

50. R. M. Hallowes, "Distinguished British Nurses: 8," *Nursing Mirror* (December, 23, 1955), quotes from the Inquiry's statistics that in London alone there were a hundred district nurses (population 3.5 million) and that "only about one third of them had any training."

51. G. Ellice, "A Century of District Nursing," *The Countryman* 94, no. 2 (1989).

52. C. du Sautoy, "Glimpses From the Past," *DN* 5, no. 11 (1963): 260.

53. C. Searle, *The History of the Development of Nursing in South Africa, 1652–1960: A Socio-Historical Survey* (Pretoria: The South African Nursing Association, 1965); CMAC: Queen's Institute Archives, Box 113, extract from an article by F. M. Roberts "King Edward VII Order of Nurses" (c. 1950).

54. R. White, *Social Change and the Development of the Nursing Profession: A Study of the Poor Law Nursing Service 1848–1948* (London: Henry Kimpton, 1978); see also Anderson, "An Oversight in Nursing History," 417–426.

55. Stocks, *A Hundred Years*, 139–142.

56. M. Grey, "Idols of Society; or Gentility and Femininity," in *Victorian Feminism 1850–1900*, ed. P. Levine (London: Hutchinson, 1874), 97–98.

57. The Medical Act (1858) contributed to the regulation of the medical profession by introducing compulsory registration—although not by "single portal of entry"—and the creation of a medical council with disciplinary powers; see Loudon, *Medical Care and the General Practitioner*, 297–301.

58. S. Walby et al., *Medicine and Nursing*.

59. Hallowes "Distinguished British Nurses: 8," noted that "Doctors bore witness to the great value of the skilled nursing provided by the Association."

60. Digby, *Making a Medical Living*, 145–147.

61. Digby, *The Evolution of British General Practice*, 25, refers to the number of "young doctors, in the decades before the state national health insurance scheme of 1911 expanded demand, were forced to become low-status 'sixpenny' or 'shilling' doctors."

62. 'A Country Practitioner' "Correspondence," *BMJ* 25, no. 3 (1899): 762.

63. QNI Archives, 1908-10, SA/QNI Box 79 H8/1: Correspondence and Minutes of meetings with the BMA re. proposed changes to the rules of County Nursing Associations.

64. Ibid.

65. J. Palmer, *Edwardian Truro* (N.p., 1994).

66. Stocks, *A Hundred Years*, 120–121.

67. Our thanks to Dr. Bradley for this information; see K. Bradley, *Friends and Visitors: A First History of the Women's Suffrage Movement in Cornwall 1870–1914* (Newmill: The Pattern Press for the Hypatia Trust, 2000), 14, 31.

68. Hallowes, "Distinguished British Nurses: 8."

69. "The Morning Round of a Liverpool 'Queen's' Nurse," *Delegates Local Handbook of Jubilee Congress* (1909), 31–35.

70. "How the Work of District Nursing in London Began—And Continues," *QNM* XIX, no. 3 (1922): 49–52.

71. "Editorial," *QNM* XXI, no. 1 (1924): 176–177.

72. M. Loane, *The Queen's Poor. Life as They Find It in Town and Country* (London: Edward Arnold, 1905), see especially Chapters VII and VIII.

73. This would have been a style commonly used by her contemporaries and was apparently popularly received.
74. S. Cohen and C. Fleay, "Introduction," in M. Loane, *The Queen's Poor: Life as They Find It in Town and Country* (reprint of first edition (London: Middlesex University Press, 1998), xxi.
75. Meetings of which were advertised in *QNM* throughout this period; see also Glamorgan County Archives and Records Office 1928–1958, D/D X 236: "Private Papers of District Nurse Ann Evans" which included a small pocket book entitled "True Morality or the Theory and Practice of Neo-Malthurianism," including details of and advertisements for contraceptive methods and appliances.
76. Loane, *The Queen's Poor*, 178–179.
77. Burdett, *Burdett's Hospitals and Charities Yearbooks*.
78. CMAC: SA/QNI.
79. QNI Archives, C., 1956–65, SA/QNI Box 114 P13/1-11: Correspondence and material used by Stocks for preparation of *A Hundred Years of District Nursing*.
80. Ibid.
81. H. Morten, *How to Become a Nurse: And How to Succeed* (3rd edition; London: The Scientific Press, 1895), 76–77.
82. Stocks, *A Hundred Years*, 82–83, 163–165.
83. Burdett, *Burdett's Hospitals and Charities Yearbooks*, 1915 entries.
84. Central Council for District Nursing in London, *History of the Central Council for District Nursing in London, 1914–1966* (London: Central Council for District Nursing in London, 1966). It was also innovative in providing a directory containing the names of more than 20,000 streets in London together with the association by which each was served, which was invaluable, for example, in improving communications between hospitals and nursing associations. Reports were also prepared by the CCDNL to review the nursing of Ophthalmia Neonatorum (1917) and infectious diseases such as measles and scarlet fever the previous year (see Central Council for District Nursing, 1916, Outline of a scheme for the district nursing of Measles, German measles, and Whooping Cough in London).

CHAPTER 2 THE INTERWAR PERIOD, 1919–1939

1. Reported in "Editorial: State Registration," *QNM* XVII, no. 1 (1920): 1–2.
2. See A. Marwick, *The Deluge: British Society and The First World War* (London: Bodley Head, 1965); A. Marwick, *Britain in the Century of Total War: War, Peace and Social Change, 1900–1967* (London: Bodley Head, 1968); M. Gente "The Expansion of the Nuclear Family Unit in Great Britain Between 1910 and 1920," *History of the Family* 6, no. 1 (2001): 125–142.
3. E. Midwinter, ed., *The Development of Social Welfare in Britain* (Buckingham: The Open University, 1994), 79, gives numbers rising from 600 to 1,335 during World War I.
4. H. Jones, *Health and Society in Twentieth Century Britain* (New York: Longman, 1994): 76–77, 84–90.
5. For example, in bringing together those responsible for the launch of the College of Nursing in 1916. See S. McGann, *The Battle of the Nurses* (London: Scutari Press, 1992), 48. Granted a royal charter in 1928, the College became the 'Royal College of Nursing' (RCN).
6. Ibid., 49.

7. H. Smith, *The British Women's Suffrage Campaign, 1866–1928* (London: Longman, 1998), 70–71, challenged the impression presented by early feminist historians such as Sylvia Pankhurst and Ray Strachey, that the equal franchise eventually obtained through the 1928 Representation of the People Act came "virtually without effort," and argued instead that throughout the interim period (1919–1928) the exclusion of these women was used as a political tool both by the Labour and Conservative Parties.
8. Abel-Smith, *A History of the Nursing Profession*, 118–119.
9. QNI Archives SA/QNI Box 115 Q6/11-22: Rolls of Affiliated Branches, England and Wales.
10. Smith, *British Women's Suffrage Campaign*, 82, referring to discussions in B. Caine, *English Feminism 1780–1980* (Oxford: Oxford University Press, 1997); P. Levine, *Feminist Lives in Victorian England* (Oxford: Basil Blackwell, 1990); and J. Lewis, *Women and Social Action in Victorian and Edwardian England* (London: Edward Elgar, 1991). This is also seen as an explicit intention among earlier medical women (e.g., Elizabeth Blackwell), but proved to be idealistic.
11. S. McGann, "Nurses Are Citizens: The Politics of the College of Nursing (UK) as a Non-Feminist Organisation in the Interwar Period," Paper given at the European Social Science History Conference, Amsterdam, 2006.
12. McGann, *The Battle of the Nurses*, 49–50.
13. "Metropolitan and Southern Counties Association of Queen's Superintendents," *QNM* XIX, no. 2(1922): 25–29.
14. See notes from WSIHVA taken at Kew in September. *Memorandum on Matters.* . . . 1926, National Archives D.2/1.
15. Cited from R. White, *The Effects of the NHS on the Nursing Profession 1948–1961* (London: King's Fund, 1985): 143–144.
16. "Association of Queen's Superintendents in the Northern Counties," *QNM* XIX, no. 2 (1922): 25–29.
17. A. M. Peterkin, *The Work of the Queen's Nurses: How They Minister to the Needs of the Sick* (London: QNI, c. 1925).
18. SA/QNI Box 114 P13/1-11: Correspondence and material used by Stocks for preparation of *A Hundred Years of District Nursing*.
19. Ibid.
20. Burdett, *Burdett's Hospitals and Charities Yearbooks*.
21. RCN Archive, QNI/A.15: *Synopsis of Proceedings at the Conference of Delegates From Affiliated Associations Held on Wednesday, 17th May 1933*.
22. RCN Archive, QNI/A.68: *Queen's Institute of District Nursing: Report of the Scottish Council. For the Year Ending 31st October 1948*.
23. Queen's Institute of District Nursing, *Survey of District Nursing in England and Wales* (London: QNI, 1935).
24. "Editorial," *QNM* XXVII, no. 8 (1935): 232–233.
25. Dorset Record Office 1918–1962, D457/5-6: "Alderholt District Nursing Association: Minutes 1918–43 and 1944–1962."
26. However, this apparent trend should be treated with some caution, as although the registers of the QNI show a dramatic rise in affiliation agreements from 1927 spread over four years, the figures actually recorded in the QNI Annual Reports show that the rise after 1931 was actually rather steeper with a marked acceleration after 1936. Figures taken from SA/QNI Box 1 B8-37, Box 2 B38-45 Published Annual Reports 1910–1947 (see Appendix 1 Graph 2.1) show this rise in numbers of affiliated associations from 1910 through to 1947.
27. For example, E. Hancox, "How We tackled the Influenza Epidemics: Sheffield," *QNM* (1919): 31–32; M. Knox Mearns, "How We Tackled the Influenza Epidemics: Leicester," *QNM* (1919): 32–33.

28. "Conference on District Nursing at Mortimer Hall," *QNM* (1919): 33–34.
29. K. E. Barlow, "The Evolution of the Queen's Nurse in Regard to the Ministry of Health," *QNM* (1919): 49–50.
30. "Editorial," *QNM* XVII, 4 (1920): 65–66.
31. R. Dougall, "Perceptions of Change: An Oral History of District Nursing in Scotland, 1940–1990" (Ph.D. thesis, University of Glasgow, 2002), included an interview with a nurse still practising as district nurse, midwife, and health visitor.
32. D. Williams, "Recollections of the RCN and District Nursing," *IHNJ* 4 (1992–1993): 25–27.
33. Hardy, *Health and Medicine*, 55, gave the numbers more than doubling during World War I "from 600 in 1914 to 2,557 in 1918." This is discussed in detail in Chapter 6.
34. "Institute News: Wales," *QNM* XVIII, nos. 2 & 4 (1921): 38, 74.
35. Digby, *The Evolution of British General Practice*, 287–289.
36. 'Nest': "Letters, Notes and Answers: Doctors and Nurses in Industrial Areas," *BMJ* 1 (March 5, 1932): 456.
37. G. Dill, "Letters, Notes and Answers: Doctors and District Nurses," *BMJ* 1 (March 19, 1932): 550.
38. 'G.P.': "Letters, Notes and Answers: Doctors and District Nurses," *BMJ* 1 (March 26, 1932): 598.
39. 'Another Devonshire GP': "Letters, Notes and Answers: Doctors and District Nurses." *BMJ* 1 (April 2 ,1932): 642.
40. S. Bartlett, "Letters, Notes and Answers: Doctors and District Nurses," *BMJ* 1 (April 16, 1932): 738.
41. Oral Testimony: D/N 18: trained SRN 1945-48 (London) then SCM in 1949 (Plymouth) before training as a Queen's Nurse in Plymouth.
42. A. M. Barford, "Letters, Notes and Answers: Doctors and District Nurses," *BMJ* 1 (April 23, 1832): 784.
43. 'Country Practitioner': "Letters, Notes and Answers: Doctors and District Nurses," *BMJ* 1 (May 7, 1932): 872.
44. "A Queen's Nurse, a Country District," *QNM* (1919): 53.
45. See Chapter 1.
46. Challis, "On Starting a District Nursing Association," 3–4, 34–35.
47. "Annual Meeting at Blackburn," *QNM* XXV (1932): 209–210.
48. B. M. Johnson, "Status and Future of the Village Nurse," *QNM* XIX, no. 2 (1922): 29–30.
49. Ibid.
50. Ibid.
51. See also E. Fox, "An Honourable Calling or a Despised Occupation: Licensed Midwifery," *SHM* 6, no. 2 (1993): 237–259.
52. 'Lethe': "A Page From an Assistant Superintendent's Diary," *QNM* XVII, no. 3 (1920): 48–49.
53. Oral Testimony: D/N 02 trained SRN 1958-62 (London) and SCM (Bristol and Weymouth) before becoming a district nurse in Weymouth, discussing training "on the job."
54. Stocks, *A Hundred Years*, 146–147, noted that 1917 "marked the first time salaried superintendents of training homes and county associations were represented on the governing body of the Queen's Institute."
55. Ibid.
56. 'Somerset GP': "Letters, Notes and Answers: Doctors and District Nurses," *BMJ* 1 (April 16, 1932): 738.
57. Burdett, *Burdett's Hospitals and Charities Yearbooks* (1925 edition).

58. A. A. Cormack, *District Nursing in Scotland: Voluntary and Statutory. Parish of Peterculter* (Aberdeenshire: Banff, 1965).
59. RCN Archive, QNI/D.4/1, Leith Jubilee Nurses Association Minute Book 1920–1933.
60. Scottish interviewees fathers' were employed in a variety of areas including, for example, shopkeeping, shipyard work, blacksmithing, crofting or farming, and managerial work, to name a few. A small number were medical missionaries or GPs.
61. E. Fox, "District Nursing in England and Wales before the National Health Service," *Medical History* 38 (1994): 303–321.
62. "Queen's Nurses' League Conference," *QNM* XXXI, no. 11 (1942): 83–95.
63. Oral Testimony: QNIT 21/2.
64. Stocks, *A Hundred Years*, 149–151.
65. See A. Hughes, "District Nursing on Provident Lines," *Charity Organisation Review* (July 1910); Hurry, *District Nursing on a Provident Basis*; also Stocks, *A Hundred Years*, 151, noted that the Provident system certainly predated the Queen's Institute, but was being actively promoted by the Institute in the mid-1930s.
66. Stocks, *A Hundred Years*, 151.
67. These grants provided toward midwifery and maternity care, tuberculosis nursing, and the nursing of notifiable diseases.
68. Figures taken from database created from Burdett, *Burdett's Hospitals and Charities Yearbooks*.
69. Oral Testimony: QNIT 13/2.
70. Challis, "On Starting a District Nursing Association," 3–4, 34–35.
71. Ibid.
72. "From the Districts," *QNM* XXIV, no. 3 (1930): 38–44.
73. Ibid.
74. "Annual Meeting at Blackburn," *QNM*, XXV (1932): 209–210.
75. Burdett, *Burdett's Hospitals and Charities Yearbooks* (1931 edition).
76. "Editorial," *QNM* XXVII, no. 3 (1934): 93–94; "Queen's Institute of District Nursing: Statistics for 1933," *QNM* XXVII, no. 3 (1934): 103–107.
77. RCN Archive, QNI/B.7: 1934-1949: *Minutes of the Advisory Committee on the Work of the Nurse Commissioners for Tuberculosis in Scotland*, provides information on the tuberculosis Nurse Commissioners.
78. A. J. Weir, *Tuberculosis in the Highlands and Islands* (Edinburgh: QIDN Scottish Branch Brochure, 1941).
79. "The 1930 Fund for the Benefit of Trained District Nurses: Report for Year Ending June 30th 1933," *QNM*, XXVI, no. 2 (1933): 77.
80. "London's Public Health" *QNM* XXIV, no. 5 (1931): 104–105.
81. M. Hogarth and London City Council, *A Survey of District Nursing in the Administrative County of London* (London: London City Council, 1931): 16–17.
82. "Long Service Fund," *QNM* XXII, no. 3 (1925): 55–56. A separate pension scheme was introduced for village nurse-midwives, and importantly the QNI defended its demand that contributions to these funds were to be claimed from associations rather than from the nurses' salaries.
83. "Institute News: Wales," *QNM* XVII, no. 3 (1920): 58.
84. "Institute News: Wales," *QNM* XVII, no. 4 (1920): 79.
85. "Institute News: Wales," *QNM* XVIII, nos. 2 & 4 (1921): 38, 74.
86. "Institute News: Resignations," *QNM* XXVII, no. 1 (1934): 54.
87. SA/QNI Box 115 Q6/11-22: Rolls of Affiliated Branches, England and Wales: Queen's Institute's registers c. 1913–1939.

88. In the case of the Ranyard nurses and some nonaffiliated associations it was built into the contract that the nurse would tender her resignation on marriage elsewhere this was a de facto understanding.
89. "From the Districts: Annual Meetings," *QNM* XXV (1932): 277–282.
90. QNI, *Summary of Evidence Submitted to the Interdepartmental Committee on Nursing Services* (London, QNI, 1938): 2.
91. SA/QNI Box 111 P6/8: Recruitment pamphlets, 1931, 1933, 1938, "Queen's Institute of District Nursing" Form T9 (4.31, 5.33, 6.38, respectively).
92. Ibid.
93. Consultative Council on Medical and Allied Services *Report of the Future Provision on Medical and Allied Services* (hereafter referred to as "Dawson Report") (1920); see also Chapter 6.

CHAPTER 3 WAR TO WELFARE STATE, 1939–1948

1. I. Irven, "District Nursing, Its Scope and Opportunities," *Nursing Times* 38 (1942): 469–471.
2. "Editorial," *QNM* XXVIII, no. 9 (1939): 252–253, quoting from the Rt. Hon. The Earl of Athlone (Chair of Enquiry), *Ministry of Health, Board of Education: Interdepartmental Committee on Nursing Services, Interim Report* (1939), 1 (hereafter referred to as "Interim Report"). The Athlone Committee was set up to look into arrangements for "the recruitment, training and registration and terms and conditions of service of persons engaged in nursing the sick [. . .] both for institutional and domiciliary nursing."
3. "Editorial: 'This was their finest hour'—Mr. Churchill," *QNM* XXIX, no. 3 (1940): 45–46.
4. M. Wilmshurst, *A Record of the Work of the Queen's Nurses during the Second World War 1939–1945* (c. 1946), 6; copy of letter dated June 15, 1939.
5. The Central Council for District Nursing in London, *A History of the Central Council for District Nursing in London*, 11.
6. Figures taken from SA/QNI Box 1 B8-37, Box 2 B38-45 Published Annual Reports 1910–1947.
7. "Experiences of a Queen's Nurse Serving in QAIMNS," *QNM* XXIX, no. 3 (1940): 46–47.
8. Edith Ramsay, *The History of a Hundred Years* (London: East London Nursing Society, 1968), 31, described making repatriation arrangements for nurses who had been visiting from Iceland and Holland, but with Danish nurses having to remain at the East London centre in Stainsby Road, "giving grand service."
9. Ibid., 30.
10. Ibid., 32.
11. D/N 17, 16/01/97, Oral History: Mrs. Evelyn Whitaker.
12. Ramsay, *The History of a Hundred Years*, 32–33.
13. "1940 and All That," *QNM* XXIX, no. 4 (1940), 70–71.
14. "Nurse Receives Honour," *QNM* XXX, no. 3 (1941): 6.
15. "Plymouth Nurses Carry On," *QNM* XXX, no. 9 (1941): 47.
16. SA/QNI Box 111 P6/16 Pamphlet: *Queen's Nurses—and What They Do* (London: QNI: c. 1945); Wilmshurst, *A Record of the Work of the Queen's Nurses*.
17. "Plymouth Nurses Carry On," 47.
18. "At a Rest Centre," *QNM* XXX, no. 3 (1941): 25, gives a description of a rest centre explaining the nurse's role.

19. "Transferred Workers," *QNM* XXX, no. 9 (1941): 45.
20. "Wartime Experiences and Opportunities," *QNM* XXIX, no. 4 (1940): 69.
21. Wilmshurst, *A Record of the Work of the Queen's Nurses*, 15.
22. Ibid., 7–8.
23. "Editorial," *QNM* XXXII, no. 8 (1943): 91–92, and subsequent articles, record the setting up of an Advisory Council by the Ministry of Labour and the issuing of the Control of Engagement Order in September 1943, which was extended in March 1944, designed to recruit and redistribute nurses and midwives to the areas of greatest shortage.
24. "Editorial," *QNM* XXXI, no. 5 (1942).
25. Hardy, *Health and Medicine*, 112–113, noted that "by the end of 1945 a total of 15,701 medical personnel had been recruited, roughly a third of the country's medical manpower."
26. Digby, *The Evolution of British General Practice*, 281.
27. Wilmshurst, *A Record of the Work of the Queen's Nurses*, 7. Also, Digby, *The Evolution of British General Practice*, 207, confirmed that during World War II there was a national improvement in maternity services resulting from the Emergency Maternity Scheme, but increased wages in the lower income bracket, together with a more nutritionally balanced diet, might also have been influencing factors.
28. Hardy, *Health and Medicine*, 112–113.
29. Irven, "District Nursing," 469–471.
30. Ibid.
31. SA/QNI Box 83 H/23: Correspondence with Ministry of Health, and statistics of cases treated, lists claims for payments for treatment of air raid casualties by Queen's Nurses.
32. SA/QNI/H23: Letter dated 23/01/1940 from Private Sec to the Minister of Health to Sir William Hale-White at the QNI.
33. SA/QNI/H23: Letter dated 25/11/1940.
34. SA/QNI/H23: Letter dated 01/05/1941.
35. SA/QNI/H23: Letter dated 27/03/1942; see also Table 5.1.
36. SA/QNI/H23: Letter dated 20/06/1941.
37. Ibid.
38. Subsequent letters asking for a response were sent in April 1942 and March and July 1943 with a reply not being received until August 1943.
39. SA/QNI/H23: Letter dated August 1943.
40. SA/QNI/H23: No signature but addressed from 28 Hollycroft Ave., NW3 and dated 15 October 1943. This letter might have been from Mrs. Beatrice Wright M.P., who seems to have taken up the case on behalf of the QNI at this time.
41. SA/QNI/H23: Letter dated 14/03/1945.
42. Ibid.
43. SA/QNI Box 81 H/13/7/2: Notes on interview between representatives of the QNI and the Interdepartmental Committee on Social Insurance and Allied Services, dated 08/07/1942.
44. Ibid.
45. Ibid.
46. "Twenty Years a Queen's Nurse" (Correspondence), *Nursing Mirror* (November 29, 1941).
47. "Editorial," *QNM*, XXXII, no. 8 (1943): 91–92, noted the recommended increases in salaries were "to date back to April 1st 1943 and it is earnestly hoped that all employing authorities will adopt them and so claim the 50% subsidy promised by the Ministry of Health towards the additional expenditure."

48. The Ranyard Association continued to provide their nurses with their own district training.
49. M. H. Dunell et al., *The Domiciliary Nursing Services* (Leicester: Taylor & Bloxham, 1943).
50. Fox, "District Nursing and the Work of District Nursing Associations," 324–332.
51. However, the associations she cited were only affiliated in 1940 prompted by problems in recruiting staff.
52. There were just nine or ten counties in England and Wales not affiliated in 1943 out of sixty-two administrative counties, including Rutland, Carmarthenshire, Wiltshire, Westmorland, and Northumberland.
53. Figures taken from SA/QNI Box 1 B8-37, Box 2 B38-45: Published Annual Reports 1910–1947.
54. "More Nurses for Lancashire," *QNM* XXVIII, no. 10 (1939): 309.
55. E. Anderson, "Queen's Nurses' League—Leeds and District Branch Report of Lecture by Dr. H. Balme on 'Post-War Reconstruction,'" *QNM*, XXXII, no. 4 (1943): 51–52.
56. "Queen's Nurses' League Conference," *QNM* XXXI, no. 11 (1942): 83–95.
57. For a more detailed discussion on NHS negotiations, see V. Berridge, *Health and Society in Britain Since 1939* (Cambridge: Cambridge University Press, 1999); H. Jones, "The Conservative Party and the Welfare State, 1942–55" (Ph.D. thesis, University College of London, 1992); C. Webster, *The NHS: A Political History* (Oxford: Oxford University Press, 1998).
58. SA/QNI Box 83 H/27/1-4: Introduction of the NHS, 1947.
59. R. W. Rave, "Annual Meeting Address to the Queen's Institute of District Nursing," *QNM* XXXVIII, no. 10 (1949): 129–133.
60. SA/QNI Box 83 H/27/1-4: Introduction of the NHS, 1947.
61. Ramsay, *The History of a Hundred Years*, 34.
62. See, for example, SA/QNI Box 111 P6/16 Pamphlet: *Queen's Nurses—And What They Do*; "A Call to Women: The Dearth of Nurses," *QNM* XXXIV, no. 5 (1945): 43–45.
63. E. J. Merry and I. D. Irven, *District Nursing: A Handbook for District Nurses and for All Concerned in the Administration of a District Nursing Service* (London: Balliere, 1948), 65.
64. M. I. Sankey, *Thank You Miss Hunter* (Crediton: Kenmar Press, 2001), 52.
65. Ibid.
66. D/N 03, 18/07/96, Oral History: Mrs. Gladys Cruttenden.
67. D/N 17, 16/01/97, Oral History: Mrs. Evelyn Whitaker.
68. Wilmshurst, *A Record of the Work of the Queen's Nurses*, 15.
69. "Editorial: A Message to Queen's Nurses," *QNM*, XXVIII, no. 11 (1939): 312.

CHAPTER 4 CHANGING PLACES, 1948–1979

1. J. Lewis, *Women in Britain Since 1945* (London: Tavistock, 1992), 68–69. Nevertheless, A. Wickham, "The State and Training Programmes for Women," in *The Changing Experience of Women*, eds. E. Whitelegg et al. (Oxford: Martin Robinson, 1982), 149–151, described the continuing emphasis being on marriage and motherhood for girls after World War II rather than on training, a point that also emerged from the Carr Report, "Training for Skill" (1958) and from the Crowther Report (1959).
2. Ibid.

3. D/N 07, 13/08/96, Oral History: Dr. Lisbeth Hockey. Dr. Hockey was an Austrian refugee who had started medical training in Gras before coming to the United Kingdom. She did her fever nurse training in London in 1938 before SRN 1939–1943, then SCM in Essex followed by QWn in 1945 in London and later HV Cert. She later became the QNI's first research officer and chaired several inquiries on their behalf.

4. D/N 26, 18/05/00, Oral History: Mrs. Elaine Parr. She trained SRN at St. Helen's from 1959 to 1962 followed, by Queen's Nurse in 1963, working for a time at St. Helen's Hospital and later becoming a practice nurse for a GP partnership in St. Helen's.

5. E. Roberts, "The Recipients' View of Welfare," in *Oral History, Health and Welfare*, eds. J. Bornat et al. (London: Routledge, 2000), 203–226.

6. Berridge, *Health and Society in Britain*, 34–41, points to services such as Meals on Wheels, Help the Aged, and a large number of charitable organisations covering particular diseases or disabilities.

7. "Memorandum on History and Work of the Q.I.D.N.," *QNM* XXXX, no. 12 (1951): 192–193.

8. "Editorial," *DN* 2, no. 8 (1959): 177. Of 145 local authorities in England and Wales, sixty-six initially elected to use the existing DNAs as their agents, and by 1958 thirty-one of these had switched to direct control.

9. Central Council for District Nursing in London, *History of the Central Council*, 15.

10. RCN Archive, QNI/B.2/6: *Minutes of Meeting of the Scottish Council, QNI Scotland*, 21 September 1948.

11. See RCN Archive, QNI/B.1/14: *Minutes of the Executive Council, QNI Scotland 1948–49*.

12. Another was Brighton, which remained a fully affiliated member of the QNI until 1974, when it relinquished responsibility to East Sussex Area Health Authority. See M. F. Gill, *District Nursing in Brighton 1877–1974* (Brighton: Benedict Press, c. 1974), 129–130.

13. D/N 26, 18/05/00, Oral History: Mrs. Elaine Parr.

14. "Districts Give Cars to County," *The Shetland Times* (October 1, 1948): 2.

15. See interview, QNIT 18/2, p. 15: 1921–1981.

16. See RCN Archive, QNI/D.2: Papers of the Comrie and Crieff District Nursing Association.

17. RCN Archive, QNI/B.2/6, p. 102: *Minutes of Meeting of the Scottish Council, QNI Scotland* (30 July 1948).

18. For example, the Bacup and Woolton District Nursing Associations in Lancashire.

19. SA/QNI Box 111 P6/20 1951: "Alphabet of Activities: Q—Queen's Institute of District Nursing," *Union of Girls Schools Record* 75 (1951): 257–259.

20. SA/QNI Box 111 P6/18, 1949: Appeal for annual subscriptions to QNI.

21. SA/QNI Box 111 P6/19, 1951: Appeal for annual subscriptions to QNI.

22. Williams, "Recollections of the RCN and District Nursing," 25–26, noted that she "felt that GPs rather than the Medical Officer of Health understood the work of district nurses" and she had therefore been keen to include GPs on various committees including the QNI's Committee.

23. D/N 08, 22/08/96, Oral History: Mrs. Marjorie Voss. She trained SRN 1941–1944 at West Middlesex, then Part 1 midwifery before becoming a district nurse in Ashford, Middlesex. Her initial training was done on the job but she later (after 17 years) undertook Queen's Nurse's training.

24. "Queen's Nurses' League Conference," *QNM* XXXI, no. 11 (1942): 83–95.

25. V. H. Giles, "To the Hospital Nurse From a Queen's Nurse," *QNM* XXVIII, no. 10 (1940): 30.

26. Williams, "Recollections of the RCN and District Nursing," 25–27.
27. White, *The Effects of the NHS*, 143–160; Baly, *A History of the Queen's Nursing Institute*.
28. Ministry of Health and Armer (Chair) et al., *Report of the Working Party*.
29. "Editorial: Training the District Nurses," *The Lancet* (September 10, 1955): 543–544, quoted from the Minority Report that "in one populous county, . . . there are still more than 20,000 pail closets, more than 10,000 privy closets, more than 8,500 privy middens, more than 3,500 houses depending for water on springs and wells, and a further 700-odd relying on standpipes."
30. Ibid.
31. Ibid.
32. Ministry of Health and Armer (Chair) et al., *Report of the Working Party*.
33. This was a valuable if short-lived contribution to postregistration professional development, closing in 1975 after just fifteen years because the QNI was experiencing considerable financial difficulties.
34. G. Hardy and Brian Lemin, "William Rathbone Staff College: Past, Present and Future," *DN* (September 1972): 120–121.
35. L. Hockey, *Feeling the Pulse* (London: QNI, 1966).; Hockey, *Care in the Balance* (London: QNI, 1968).
36. See, for example, L. Hockey and A. Buttimore, eds., *Co-operation in Patient Care: Studies of District Nurses Attached to Hospital and General Medical Practice* (London: QNI, 1970); L. Hockey, "The Family Care Team: Philosophy, Problems, Possibilities," in *Ciba Foundation Symposium on Teamwork for World Health*, eds. G. Wolstenholme and M. O'Connor (London: Churchill, 1971): 103–115; M. H. Skeet, *Home From Hospital* (London: Dan Mason Research Committee, 1970); J. Carre, "Health Care in the Community," *Nursing Mirror* (May 24, 1974): 32, reported, "In one area in Essex the number of visits by district nurses has increased by 6,000 in one year following the appointment of a district nurse liaison officer to her local group of hospitals."
37. A. Carr et al., *The Education and Training of District Nurses* (Bolton: Bolton College of Education, 1977).
38. SA/QNI Box 62 F7/3: Correspondence With Outside Bodies: Briggs Committee on Nursing, 1971–1972.
39. Department of Health and Social Security and P. A. Briggs (Chair), et al., Cmnd. 5115: *Report of the Committee on Nursing* (1972).
40. "Queen's Nurses' League Conference," *QNM* XXXI, no. 11 (1942): 83–95.
41. Ibid.
42. Baly *A History of the Queen's* Institute, 84–85.
43. D. Walker, "The Future Public Health Nurse and Her Team," *DN* 8, no. 11 (1965): 200–203, suggested this was to some extent lessened by the setting-up of the Councils for the Training of Health Visitors and for Training in Social Work in 1962.
44. 2002, Personal Testimony: Miss M. I. Sankey MBE.
45. Sankey, *Thank You Miss Hunter*, 58–59.
46. D/N 11, 01/10/96, Oral History: Mrs. Betty Reid. She trained SRN 1950–1953 in Aberdare, where she worked for a while before taking Queen's Nurse's training in Bristol prior to working in the district in Hirwaun, South Wales.
47. "Pay Settlement for District Nurses," *QNM* XXXLVI, no. 12 (1957): 180.
48. SA/QNI Box 62 F/7/9: Correspondence with Department of Health and Social Security (1965–1975).
49. D/N 25, 17/05/00, Oral History: Mrs. Connie Pennington. She trained 1944 to 1947 at the London Hospital, followed by SCM at Liverpool and HV Cert. at Liverpool and St. Helen's, working there as an HV.

50. D/N 13, 02/10/96, Oral History: Mrs. Dorothy Mitchell. After fever nursing training she did general nurse training from 1939 to 1942 (Birmingham) before returning to Cardiff as a district nurse, learning on the job and becoming a district nursing officer.
51. CMAC/GP29/08, c. 1980, Oral History: Frank W. Bonb.
52. CMAC/GP29/38, c. 1980, Oral History: John J. Hopkinson.
53. D/N 26, 18/05/00, Oral History: Mrs. Elaine Parr (see n.5).
54. R. Ferguson, "Autonomy, Tension and Trade-Off: Attitudes to Doctors in the History of District Nursing," *International History of Nursing Journal* 6 (2001): 10–17.
55. L. Stein, "The Doctor/Nurse Game," in *Readings in the Sociology of Nursing*, eds. R. Dingwall and J. McIntosh (Edinburgh: Churchill Livingstone, 1978), 109.
56. Oral testimony: QNIT 44/1.
57. Ferguson, "Autonomy, Tension and Trade-Off," 10–17.
58. E. J. Merry, "The Role of the District Nurse in Home Care," *The Practitioner*, 177 (July 1956): 54–58.
59. J. A. S. Forman, "What the GP Expects of the District Nurse and Midwife," *DN* 6 (July–August 1963): 74–77, 102–104.
60. D/N 38, 01/03/01, Oral History: Mr. Arthur Brompton. He was trained 1953 to 1956 at Nottingham then Queen's Nurse's training in 1956.
61. Consultative Council on Medical and Allied Services, *Dawson Report* (1920).
62. I. Fisher, "A Personal Review of the N.H.S," *Midwife, Health Visitor and Community Nurse*, 4 (August 1968), 329–331; Hardy, *Health and Medicine*, 143–147 noted the enormous demand for false teeth and spectacles and a dramatic increase in GP-prescribed drugs.
63. G. O. Barber, "The Link to Health," *South African Nursing Journal* (February 1960): 16–17. This article, although published in South Africa, was written by a British GP working in the United Kingdom.
64. CMAC/GP29/16, c. 1980, Oral History: Frederick Barber.
65. CMAC/GP29/21, c. 1980, Oral History: John A. Hallinham.
66. CMAC/GP29/12, c. 1980, Oral History: Alec S. Bookless.
67. CMAC/GP29/02, c. 1980, Oral History: John Scott Makepeace.
68. CMAC/GP29/06, c. 1980, Oral History: Margaret A. Norton.
69. M. Baly, *Nursing and Social Change* (1980), 121.
70. S. Walby et al., *Medicine and Nursing*, 57.
71. Hardy, *Health and Medicine*, 142.
72. S. J. L. Taylor and Nuffield Provincial Hospitals Trust for Research and Policy Studies in Health Services, *Good General Practice: A Report of a Survey* (1954), 369–380.
73. Ibid., 372.
74. Central Health Services Council, *The Field of Work of the Family Doctor: Report of the Sub-Committee of the Standing Medical Advisory Committee (The Gillie Report)* (1963). See also J. M. Griffiths and K.A Luker, "Intraprofessional Teamwork in District Nursing: In Whose Interest?" *Journal of Advanced Nursing* 20, no. 6 (1994): 1038–1045; Hockey, "The Family Care Team," 103–115.
75. Central Health Services Council, *The Field of Work of the Family Doctor*.
76. Forman, "What the GP Expects," 74–77, 102–104.
77. Walker, "The Future Public Health Nurse," 200–203.
78. RCN Executive Committee, "Occasional Papers: The Future of District Nursing," *NT* (March 20, 1969): 45–48.

79. D/N 10, 27/09/96, Oral History: Mrs. Elaine Ryder: She trained SRN St. George's Hospital, London from 1969 to 1972, and later moved from hospital to district with minimal training in Chiswick working in several districts in London and Chester.
80. D/N 24, 17/05/00, Oral History: Mrs. Jean Fairclough. She trained SEN, then SRN in 1965 and Part 1 Midwifery at St. Helen's, working as a district nurse there before taking HV cert.
81. DHSS, *Nursing in Primary Health Care* (London: HMSO, 1977): Circular CNO(77) 8.
82. Digby, *The Evolution of British General Practice*, 338–339, described a decline in numbers of hospital, public health, and other public appointments held by GPs and a restriction in the range of clinical work entailed in those remaining open to them as generalists.
83. J. Bliss and Alison While, "Team Work and Collaboration: The Position of District Nursing 1948–1974," *IHNJ* 5, no. 3 (2000): 22–29.
84. Stocks, *A Hundred Years*, 181–182.
85. D/N 07, 13/08/96, Oral History: Dr. Lisbeth Hockey.
86. From interview QNIT 13/2, p. 12: 1917–1978.
87. Ibid.
88. D/N 18, 13/02/97, Oral History: Mrs. Sylvia Diamond (see earlier).
89. A. Mc Master, "'Are We to Lose Our Nurse?' Implications of the National Health Service Act 1948 in the Village," *Journal of the National Council of Social Services* (Autumn 1948): 15–17.
90. D/N 26, 18/05/00, Oral History: Mrs. Elaine Parr.
91. CMAC/GP29/32, c. 1980, Oral History: Robert Hugh Clarke.
92. G. F. Petty, "Patients, Nurses and Doctors," *DN* 4, no. 4 (1961): 76–78.
93. E. Roberts, *Women and Families: An Oral History, 1940–1970* (1995), 175–198.
94. D/N 27, 18/05/00, Oral History: Mr. Alwen Friar (see earlier).
95. P. Abbott, "Conflict Over Grey Areas: District Nurses and Home Helps Providing Community Care," in *The Sociology of the Caring Professions*, eds. P. Abbott and Liz Meerabeau (London: The UCL Press, 1998), 199–209.
96. Ibid.
97. D/N 26, 18/05/00, Oral History: Mrs. Elaine Parr (see earlier).
98. Roberts, *Women and Families*, 7. However, Hardy, *Health and Medicine*, 152–165, saw the impact of the therapeutic revolution since 1945 as "variable."
99. Ibid., 146–147.

CHAPTER 5 TOWN NURSE, COUNTRY NURSE

1. From interview, QNIT 50/3, p. 10: 1922–c .1980.
2. QNI Archives (CMAC), c. 1913–1939, SA/QNI Box 115 Q6/11-22: Rolls of Affiliated Branches, England and Wales.
3. CMAC/GP29/59, c. 1980, Oral History: Samuel L. Isaacs.
4. R. McKenzie, *Lifting Every Voice: A Report and Action Programme to Address Institutional Racism at the National Assembly of Wales* (London: Public and Commercial Services Union, 2001), 17–18.
5. Ibid.
6. D/N 33, 29/03/01, Oral History: Mrs. Marion Hurst: She trained SRN c. 1950 to 1953 (Swansea) and later worked as a district nurse learning on the job only training after a career break in late 1960s.
7. SA/QNI Box 115 Q6/11-22: Rolls of Affiliated Branches, England and Wales.

8. "Institute News: Wales," *QNM* XIX, no. 1 (1922): 17.
9. SA/QNI Box 115 Q6/11-22: Rolls of Affiliated Branches, England and Wales.
10. The local Miners' Federations in the early postwar period provided financial support to local hospitals and libraries; therefore it is reasonable to suggest they might have contributed toward the cost of a district nurse. I am most grateful to Mr. G. G. Lloyd for this information.
11. D/N 13, 02/10/96, Oral History: Mrs. Dorothy Mitchell.
12. From interview QNIT 40/2, Summary, p. 2: 1934–1994.
13. From interview QNIT 19/2, p. 19: 1915–1975.
14. In 1922 it was reported as having Lady Blythswood as "an active President and chairperson." "Institute News: Wales," *QNM* XIXl, no. 1 (1922): 17.
15. D/N 29, 24/05/01, Oral History: Mrs. E. Morris (see earlier).
16. RCN/T/33 Oral testimony: Mrs. Lillian Miller, Brecon.
17. D/N 32, 01/02/01, Oral History: Mrs. Lillian Miller (see earlier).
18. RCN/T/12 Oral Testimony: Mrs. Betty Reid, Hiruian.
19. D/N 39, 11/04/01, Oral History: Mrs. Jean Frost. She trained SRN partly at Weymouth and partly in the army (Queen Alexandra's) from 1952 to 1955, then SCM in London followed by Queen's Nurse in 1958 working in London and Weymouth as a district nurse.
20. "Experience of a Nurse in Rural Wales," *QNM* XXX, no. 3 (1941): 5–6.
21. D/N 11, 01/10/96, Oral History: Mrs. Betty Reid (see earlier).
22. D/N 26, 18/05/00, Oral History: Mrs. Elaine Parr (see earlier).
23. D/N 09, 29/08/96, Oral History: Miss Audrey Smith. She trained SRN in Weymouth from 1946ro 1949 and did SCM in Southampton before returning to Weymouth as a district nurse, learning on the job and later becoming a district nursing officer there.
24. SA/QNI Box 115 Q6/11-22: Rolls of Affiliated Branches, England and Wales.
25. A. M. Peterkin, "The Scope and Conditions of District Nursing," *QNM* XXIV, no. 5 (1931): 128–132.
26. "Editorial," *QNM* XXVIII, no. 9 (1939): 252–253. The extension of this public health and preventative role was felt to be a major factor contributing to the inadequate numbers of district nursing staff by 1939.
27. "From the Districts: Annual Meetings," *QNM* XXV (1932): 277–282.
28. P. Gibb, "District Nursing in the Highlands and Islands of Scotland: 1890–1940," *History of Nursing Journal* 4 (1992–1993): 319.
29. Ibid., 329.
30. J. Curnow, "The Provision of Healthcare in Remote Communities," in *The NHS in Scotland: The Legacy of the Past and the Prospect of the Future*, ed. C. Nottingham (Aldershot: Ashgate, 2000), 125.
31. QNIT 48/2, Summary, p. 5: 1933–1986.
32. From interview QNIT 55/1, p. 3: 1915–1975.
33. From interview QNIT 50/3, p. 7: 1922–c. 1980.
34. For a history of the Scottish air ambulance service, see Iain Hutchison, *Air Ambulance: Six Decades of the Scottish Air Ambulance Service* (Erskine: Kea Publishing, 1996). See also Capt. Alan Whitfield, *Island Pilot* (Shetland: The Shetland Times, 1995).
35. From interview QNIT 48/2, p. 6: 1933–1986.
36. From interview QNIT 29/1, p. 7: 1942–int.
37. National Archives: FD1/5519, *Memorandum on District Nursing in Relation to the Welfare of Munition Workers Submitted by the Public Health Section of the Royal College of Nursing* (13/08/1940).

38. D/N 19, 13/02/97, Oral History: Miss K. Larder. She trained SRN in Oldham, Lancsashire, and SCM in Edinburgh some time before taking a district nursing post in Wiltshire, for which she received no official training.
39. W. Temple, *Men Without Work: A Report Made to the Pilgrim Trust* (Pilgrim Trust, 1938): 82.
40. Ibid., 133–143.
41. "No. 4 'Mustn't Grumble,'" *Out of the Doll's House* (BBC TV Documentary Series: 1989).
42. D/N 25, 17/05/00, Oral History: Mrs. Connie Pennington. She trained SRN at the London Hospital from 1944 to 1947 before moving to Liverpool to complete her midwifery training, later becoming a district nurse and health visitor.
43. Glamorgan Records Office D/D X 287/1-4: Barry District Nursing Association annual report books: March 1891–June 1900, June 1923–Sept. 1926, Oct. 1926–Nov. 1931.
44. Glamorgan Records Office 1912-46, D/D X1 1/1-34: Minutes Glamorganshire Insurance Committee.
45. Temple, *Men Without Work*, 82–83.
46. Ibid., 272–277.
47. Ibid., 65–73.
48. A. Antrobus, "Pioneers Still," *Guardian* (January 29, 1965); Hardy and Lemin, "William Rathbone Staff College," 120–121.
49. Temple, *Men Without Work*, 29.
50. Liverpool Record Office: 352 WOO Woolton District Nursing Society, Liverpool: 352 WOO/1/3-5 Minutes 1925-50.
51. QNI Inspector's reports record populations in 1914 estimated at 2,000, falling to 1,000 in 1923, and back up to 2,559 in 1931.
52. According to QNI Inspectors' reports, rising from 13,000 in 1917 to 16,821 by 1931.
53. This was a relatively common problem during World War I and lasted for a little while afterward.
54. SA/QNI Box 115 Q6/11-22: Rolls of Affiliated Branches, England and Wales.
55. Burdett, *Burdett's Hospitals and Charities Yearbooks*.
56. SA/QNI Box 115 Q6/11-22: Rolls of Affiliated Branches, England and Wales.
57. "The New District Nurses' Home at St. Helen's," *QNM* XXII, no. 9 (1927): 205; "Enlargement of the Home at St. Helen's," *QNM* XXVII, no. 8 (1935): 242–243.
58. SA/QNI Box 81 H/13/7/2: Notes on interview dated 08/07/1942, between representatives of the QNI and the Interdepartmental Committee on Social Insurance and Allied Services.
59. D/N 27, 18/05/00, Oral History: Mr. Alwen Friar (see earlier).
60. Roberts, "The Recipients' View of Welfare," 203–226, noted variations across the county during this period, such as Barrow-in-Furness suffering forty-nine percent unemployment in the Depression of 1922 in which shipbuilding was badly hit, compared with only seven percent in Wigan and ten percent in Bolton, whereas 1931 and 1932 were more uniformly bad years throughout the county, with levels ranging between twenty-seven percent (Barrow) and forty-seven percent (Blackburn).
61. Digby, *The Evolution of British General Practice*, 75–78.
62. For the purposes of this book, this is simply taking "culture" as relating to a system of interrelated values and customs representing the collective experience of a particular group of people.

CHAPTER 6 TECHNOLOGY, TREATMENT, AND TLC

1. Merry and Irven, *District Nursing*, 252.
2. D/N 38, 01/03/01, Oral History: Mr. Arthur Brompton.
3. Ibid.
4. M. Darmady, "Central Sterile Supply Services and Their Application to District Work," *DN* 4, no. 4 (1961): 83–86.
5. Typically operations in the home might have included tonsillectomy, circumcision, incision of an abscess, and "minor" gynaecological conditions such as curettage following spontaneous abortion. The district nurse's duty was to prepare the patient beforehand, to assist the GP during the operation (which might include help with the administration of anaesthetic), and to provide aftercare.
6. Merry and Irven, *District Nursing*, 125–145.
7. D/N 26, 18/05/00, Oral History: Mrs. Elaine Parr.
8. See, for example, Jill A. David, *Wound Management: A Comprehensive Guide to Dressing and Healing, Practical Nursing Handbook* (London: Dunitz, 1986); Brian Gilchrist, "The Effect of an Oxygen Impermeable Occlusive Dressing on Bacterial Flora and Wound Healing in Chronic Venous Ulceration" (M.Sc. diss., King's College London, Department of Nursing Studies, 1986); Sue Bale and Vanessa Jones, *Wound Care Nursing: A Patient-Centred Approach* (London: Bailliere Tindall, 1997); Centre for Evidence-Based Nursing, Royal College of Nursing, University of York, School of Nursing, Midwifery and Health Visiting, and University of Manchester, *The Management of Patients With Venous Leg Ulcers: Technical Report, Clinical Practice Guidelines* (London: RCN, 1998). An early, more reactionary example of this type of study comparing results of CSSD sterilised dressings on wounds with those using gauze sterilised by oven baking was written by Arthur W. Brompton, "Dressings in the Home Today," *DN* 11, no. 9 (1968): 167–168.
9. SA/QNI Box 102 X20/1-2: East London Nursing Society, E. S. Clewes, *Ninth Annual Superintendent's Report* (dated 17/06/68).
10. Ramsay, *The History of a Hundred Years*.
11. From the late 1940s onward, the World Health Organisation launched successive immunization campaigns against diphtheria, tetanus, poliomyelitis, measles, whooping cough, and tuberculosis, focussing particularly on children and young adults.
12. Baly, *A History of the Queen's Institute*, 93, gave a mortality rate from tuberculosis as 992 per million population in 1931, and Merry and Irven, *District Nursing*, devoted five pages to "Home Nursing of Tuberculosis" in their textbook, indicating a high priority at that time.
13. N. M. Dixon, "Changes in District Nursing," *DN* 1, no. 2 (1958): 24.
14. Petty, "Patients, Nurses and Doctors," 76–78.
15. Roberts, *Women and Families*, 22-44; also Hardy, *Health and Medicine*, 139–140, stated that in the period 1945 to 1955, three million houses were built although "demand continued to outstrip supply."
16. Williams, "Recollections of the RCN and District Nursing," 25–27.
17. SD/2, 04/07/98, Oral History: Miss Beckie Saunders. She trained SRN from 1938 to 1941 (UCL London) then SCM (Paisley) and Queen's Nurse in London, working as a district nurse in East Sussex before gaining HV certificate in 1946.
18. Central Council for District Nursing in London, *History of the Central Council for District Nursing in London*, 13.
19. P. Jordan, *District Nurse* (London: Weidenfeld & Nicolson, 1977), 47.
20. Baly, *Nursing, Past Into Present Series* (London: Batsford, 1977), 91.

21. See, for example, "The 'Ivy' Motor Cycle," *QNM* XX, no. 3 (1923): 140; "The McKenzie Motor Cycle," *QNM* XX, no. 3 (1923): 139.
22. "Notes From the Districts: Wales," *QNM* XXIII, no. 1 (1928): 37–38.
23. Stocks, *A Hundred Years*, 163.
24. SA/QNI Box 115 Q6/11-22: Rolls of Affiliated Branches, England and Wales c. 1913–1939.
25. Queen's Institute of District Nursing, *Survey of District Nursing in England and Wales* (London: QNI, 1935).
26. Queen's Institute of District Nursing, *Summary of Evidence Submitted to the Interdepartmental Committee on Nursing Services* (London: QNI, 1938).
27. Until this point the population felt to warrant a Queen's Nurse had been fixed at 3,000, and below this figure affiliated associations were considered justified in employing a village nurse-midwife instead.
28. D/N 32, 01/02/01, Oral History: Mrs. Lillian Miller. She trained SRN from 1931 to 1934 (London) and Queen's Nurse, also in London soon afterward before returning to Neath Valley, South Wales.
29. From interview QNIT 31/1, p. 8: 1918–1979.
30. From interview QNIT 14/2, Summary, p. 8: 1917–1977.
31. From interview QNIT 11/1, p. 7: 1913–1973.
32. Ibid., 10.
33. From interview QNIT 13/2, pp. 15–16: 1917–1978.
34. J. Elise Gordon, "Scottish Journey—6: With the nurses of the Western Isles (III)," *Nursing Mirror* (July 10, 1948): 235.
35. Digby, *The Evolution of British General Practice*, 144.
36. D/N 17, 16/01/97, Oral History: Mrs. Evelyn Whitaker: Mrs. Whitaker worked as a nurse, midwife, HV, and school nurse, training from 1928 to 1931 (London), SCM in 1932 (Watford), and Queen's Nurse (Plumstead) in approximately 1934.
37. I am indebted to District Nursing Sister Wendy Lloyd-Sweet for her contribution to this discussion.
38. SA/QNI Box 81/H18: Correspondence, Questionnaires, Report of delegations to the Postmaster General, 1932–1935.
39. Ibid.
40. Ibid., quoted in report but name and address not given.
41. Central Council for District Nursing in London, *History of the Central Council for District Nursing in London*, 10.
42. Digby, *The Evolution of British General Practice*, 275–279.
43. M. Currie, *Fever Hospitals and Fever Nurses: A British Social History of Fever Nurses: A National Service* (London: Routledge, 2005) provides a detailed description of the rise and fall of this branch of nursing.

CHAPTER 7 DISTRICT NURSING PROFESSIONALISATION

1. H. Perkin, *The Rise of Professional Society: England Since 1880* (London: Routledge, 1989).
2. Digby, *Making a Medical Living*, 37.
3. E. Freidson, *Profession of Medicine: A Study of the Sociology of Applied Knowledge* (Chicago: University of Chicago Press, 1988); and P. Wilding, *Professional Power and Social Welfare* (London: Routledge & Kagan Paul, 1982).
4. For example, M. Crouch, "The Future—Profession or Vocation," *QNM* XXXIX, no. 9 (1950): 130–133, 139, was written in a quasi-religious style with biblical quotations urging a more vocational outlook and self-renunciation in

contrast to the concerns about professional status, pay, and conditions of service that she felt were damaging to the underlying ethos of district nursing. However, similar concerns were expressed by L. Mackay, "Nursing: Will the Idea of a Vocation Survive?" in *The Sociology of the Caring Professions*, eds. P. Abbott and Liz Meerabeau (1998), 54–72, referring to the view of the "new nurse" that "nursing is a job like any other" combined with transfer of patient to customer status and associated "righteous" attitudes.

5. A. Giddens, *Sociology* (3rd ed., Cambridge: Polity Press, 1997).
6. Unlike the professions of clergy, law, and military, medicine and nursing have no heads such as Lord Chief Justice, Archbishop, or Commander in Chief, and were not and are not bound by an oath of loyalty to the monarch, but rather to themselves through the (resurrected) Hippocratic Oath or Professional Code of Conduct.
7. For example, appointments in public health, hospital consultancies, the colonial medical service, or prison service. "Editorial," *QNM* XVIII, no. 4 (1921): 62–63, urged nurses to comply with registration sooner rather than leaving it too late, despite being given "two years of grace" and records the expectation of professionalisation that "The day is not far distant when Public Health and other State appointments will go to nurses who are registered rather than to those who have not registered."
8. G. Larkin, *Occupational Monopoly and Modern Medicine*.
9. M. Foucault, *The Birth of the Clinic: An Archaeology of Medical Perception* (London: Tavistock, 1973).
10. M. S. Larson, *The Rise of Professionalism: A Sociological Analysis* (Berkeley: University of California Press, 1977), 15.
11. S. Sinclair, *Making Doctors: An Institutional Apprenticeship* (Oxford: Berg, 1997), 151.
12. Davies, *Gender and the Professional Predicament in Nursing*; Witz, *Professions and Patriarchy*.
13. M. Stacey, "Social Sciences and the State: Fighting Like a Woman," in *The Public and the Private*, eds. E. Gamarnikow et al. (Aldershot: Gower, 1983).
14. H. Wilensky, "The Professionalisation of Everyone," *American Journal of Sociology* LXX, no. 2 (1964): 143–144.
15. P. Bellaby and P. Oribabor, " 'The History of the Present': Contradiction and Struggle in Nursing," in *Rewriting Nursing History*, ed. C. Davies, 159–161.
16. V. L. Bullough, *The Development of Medicine as a Profession: The Contribution of the Medieval University to Modern Medicine* (Basel, Switzerland: Karger, 1966), quoted in H. C. Burnham, "How the Idea of Profession Changed the Writing of Medical History," *Medical History* Supplement No. 18 (1998): 105.
17. N. D. Jewson, "The Disappearance of the Sick-Man From Medical Cosmology, 1770–1870," *Sociology* (1976): 10.
18. Ibid.
19. S. Marks, *Divided Sisterhood*, 4–7.
20. W. F. Bynum, *Science and the Practice of Medicine in the Nineteenth Century* (Cambridge: Cambridge University Press, 1994), 188.
21. Walby, et al., *Medicine and Nursing*, 52.
22. See also J. Snowball, "Asking Nurses About Advocating for Patients: 'Reactive' and 'Proactive' Accounts," *Journal of Advanced Nursing* 24 (1996): 67–75; A. Digby and H. Sweet, "Nurses as Culture Brokers in Twentieth-Century South Africa," in *Plural Medicine, Tradition and Modernity, 1800–2000*, ed. W. Ernst (London: Routledge, 2002).
23. This concept is discussed in depth in Walby et al., *Medicine and Nursing*, 52.
24. Rafferty, *The Politics of Nursing Knowledge*, 186–187.

25. White, *Social Change and the Development of the Nursing Profession.*
26. QNI Archives, C., 1907, 1910, 1932, SA/QNI/Box 79/H8/2: Correspondence re. a case of friction between doctor and nurse, 1907, and cuttings, 1910, 1932. Correspondence between GPs debating the reasons for reluctance on behalf of some GPs to take advantage of district nurses in reducing workloads.
27. Digby, *Making a Medical Living*, 6.
28. K. Williams, "From Sarah Gamp to Florence Nightingale: A Critical Study of Hospital Nursing Systems from 1840 to 1897," in *Rewriting Nursing History*, ed. C. Davies, 41–75.
29. Margaret Breay was a close colleague of Mrs. Bedford Fenwick. Over a forty-year partnership, she became assistant editor of *Nursing Record* (later, *British Journal of Nursing*) in 1902 and was secretary and treasurer of all the various societies founded by Mrs. Bedford Fenwick, including the ICN as well as being joint author with her of first history of ICN. We are indebted to Susan McGann, Archivist RCN, for this information.
30. Mortimer, "The Nurse in Edinburgh," 271–286.
31. A. M. Carr Saunders and P. A. Wilson, *The Professions* (Oxford: Clarendon, 1933), 120, 321, referred to both the Association of Hospital Matrons and the College of Nursing as "Professional Associations."
32. A. J. Dalzell-Ward, "The Reason and Need for Professional Organisations," *Nursing Mirror* 53 (November 8, 1957): 431–432.
33. M. Wilmshurst, "Fifty Years an Institute," *Nursing Times* XXXIII, no. 1677 (June 19, 1937).
34. Anderson, "Queen's Nurses' League,"51–52.
35. "The Assistant Nurse," *QNM*, XXXII, no. 1 (1943): 1–2, recommended a scheme of training and enrolment for "such work as she will be permitted to undertake" would best "safeguard the Registered Nurse from the unfair competition from which she has suffered in the past." This expression of professional concern is perhaps explained by the concern expressed in the same article that "when the war ends all sorts of women who have been doing nursing work of various kinds will be let loose on the general public and if allowed to practice as 'nurses' with no supervision and no control the lot of the SRN will be pitiable indeed." The question of supervision remained a headache within community nursing for some time; see also "Editorial: The Assistant Nurse," *QNM*, XXXIV, no. 4 (1945): 33.
36. SA/QNI Box 79 H8/1: 1908-19 Correspondence and Minutes of meetings with the BMA re. proposed changes to the rules of County Nursing Associations: Correspondence between QNI and BMA following protests from Penwith Medical Union, Cornwall.
37. C. Hart, *Behind the Mask: Nurses, Their Unions and Nursing Policy* (London: Bailliere Tindall, 1994) 24–26.
38. Maguire, "Report of an Address," *QNM* XXXIV, no. 1 (1945): 2–5.
39. See, for example, issues raised in 1942: "Queen's Nurses' League Conference," *QNM* XXXI, no. 11 (1942): 83–95, relating to relationships with other professional organisations, salaries, interprofessional issues, postwar refresher courses, and the need for State recognition of Queen's training.
40. "The Ministry of Health Superannuation of Nurses and Midwives," *QNM* XXXIV, no. 5 (1945): 43–44.
41. Kratz, "District Nursing," 80–91, referring to Ministry of Health and Armer (Chair) et al., *Report of the Working Party*.
42. "Training of District Nurses," *Royal Society of Health Journal* 11 (November 1957): 728–729.
43. "Editorial," *DN*, 1, no. 8 (1958): 175.

44. D. A. Shadwell, "District Nursing," *The Times* (September 27–29, 1926).
45. R. W. Rave, "Annual Meeting Address to the Queen's Institute of District Nursing," *QNM*, XXXVIII, no. 10 (1949): 129–133, speaking on the necessity for special training in district nursing.
46. Royal College of Nursing, *Specialties in Nursing: A Report of the Working Party Investigating the Development of Specialties Within the Nursing Profession* (1988), differentiated between a specialist (as in expert practitioner with additional qualifications) and someone working in a specialised field or specialty.
47. Burnham, "How the Idea of Profession Changed the Writing of Medical History," 170–171.
48. RCN Executive Committee, "Occasional Papers: The Future of District Nursing," *Nursing Times* (March 20, 1969): 45–48.
49. Ibid.
50. F. H. Haste and L. D. Macdonald, "The Role of the Specialist in Community Nursing: Perceptions of Specialist and District Nurses," *International Journal of Nursing Studies* 29, no. 1 (1992): 37–47.
51. S. Battle, J. Moran-Ellis, and B. Salter, *The District Nurse's Changing Role* (1985), 11
52. D. Gittins, *Madness in Its Place: Narratives of Severalls Hospital, 1913–1997* (London: Routledge, 1998); D. Gittins, "Silences: The Case of a Psychiatric Hospital," in *Narrative and Genre*, eds. M. Chamberlain and P. Thompson (London: Routledge, 1998), 46–62.
53. This is described in L. Stein, "The Doctor-Nurse Game," *Archives of General Psychiatry* 16 (1967): 698–703; Stein, "The Doctor-Nurse Game," particularly in negotiating differences of opinion and professional judgment and later by D. Allen, "Doctor-Nurse Relationships: Accomplishing the Skill Mix in Health Care," in *The Sociology of the Caring Professions*, eds. P. Abbott and Liz Meerabeau (London: UCL Press, 1998), looking at the negotiation of professional boundaries.
54. D/N 21, 15/05/00, Oral History: Mrs. Elizabeth Skepper. She trained SRN from 1954 to 1957 St. Helen's, and later worked in the district, learning on the job until later local authority training in 1973.
55. Walby et al., *Medicine and Nursing*, 68.
56. M. F. Antrobus, *District Nursing: The Nurse, the Patients and the Work* (London: Faber & Faber, 1985).
57. DoH, 1993, Social Services Inspectorate/Regional Health Authority Community Care Monitoring: National Summary; A. Timmins, *Dilemmas of Discharge: The Case of District Nursing* (Nottingham: University of Nottingham Department of Nursing and Midwifery Studies, 1996).
58. Abbott and Wallace, "Health Visiting, Social Work, Nursing and Midwifery: A History," 20–53, explored this idea in greater depth with particular reference to the Briggs Report in 1972 supporting the professional model, whereas the *Griffiths Report* (1983) supported a more managerial system returning to the professional stance with Project 2000.
59. Davies, *Gender and the Professional Predicament in Nursing*, 147.

CHAPTER 8 CARE AND NURSES' LIVES

1. L. Steele, "Long-Term Care for the Elderly: The Issue Explained," *The Guardian*, (March 19, 2001) http://society.guardian.co.uk/longtermcare/story/0,8150,459332,00.html

2. For the lay response to this policy, see Alzheimer's Society, "Is Free Nursing Care 'Unfair and Unworkable'?" (November 2002) http://www.alzheimers. org.uk/pdf/Free%20Nursing%20Care%20Nov%202004.pdf, June 9, 2004.

3. Joseph Rowntree Foundation, Findings Web site, "Lessons From the Funding of Long-Term Care in Scotland" (January 2006). http://www.jrf.org.uk/ knowledge/findings/socialcare/0036.asp, accessed May 6, 2006.

4. Oral testimony: QNIT 08/1.

5. This was discussed in an informal conversation. It is neither documented nor archived.

6. Oral testimony: QNIT 19/2.

7. Oral testimony: QNIT 43/2.

8. Oral testimony: QNIT 25/2.

9. Ibid.

10. Ibid.

11. Oral testimony: QNIT 26/1.

12. J. Savage, *Nurses, Gender and Sexuality* (London: Heinemann Nursing, 1987), cited in I. Marsh, *Sociology* (London: Prentice Hall, 2000), 466.

13. A. Bradshaw, "The Virtue of Nursing: The Covenant of Care," *Journal of Medical Ethics*, 25 (1999): 477–481.

14. Oral testimony: QNIT 20/2.

15. H. Kuhse, *Caring: Nurses, Women and Ethics* (Oxford: Blackwell, 1997): 56–58, 62.

16. Ferguson, "Autonomy, Tension and Trade-Off," 6.

17. Oral testimony: QNIT 21/2.

18. J. Fink, ed., *Care. Personal Lives and Social Policy* (Bristol: Policy Press in association with The Open University, 2004).

19. The name here has been changed, as written permission to use her name was not received from the original interviewee.

20. Oral testimony: QNIT 12/1.

21. Ibid.

22. Ibid.

23. L. Ross, *Nurses' Perceptions of Spiritual Care* (Aldershot: Avebury, 1997), xv.

24. Oral testimony: QNIT 12/1.

25. Ross, *Nurses' Perceptions of Spiritual Care*, 27.

26. Ibid., 33.

27. Oral testimony: QNIT 12/1.

28. Davies, *Gender and the Professional Predicament in Nursing*, 150.

29. In September 2005, the total headcount of nursing and midwifery staff in Scotland was 65,816 (men = 6,664); of these 2,631(men = 47) were district nurses. Figures provided by the Information Statistics Division of the NHS, May 2006.

30. "'M.E.S.' John Beart District Nurse," *DN* (November 1968): 169–170.

31. Midwifery was not open to men until the Sex Discrimination Act (1975) challenged the barriers that stood in their way. They were then allowed to opt for midwifery training with some restrictions. In 1983 the Secretary of State announced that all restrictions of the 1975 Act in this regard should be removed. Men were then free to train and practice as midwives.

32. "Impressions and Experiences of a Male District Nurse," *QNM* XXXVII, no. 12 (1948): 146–147. The anonymous author, as one of the first four male nurses to undergo Queen's training, stated that his average daily travelling distance by bicycle in Leicester was 21 miles.

33. Oral testimony: D/N 18.

34. Digby, *The Evolution of British General Practice*, 154–186, described the controversy over female doctors accepting male patients, and divisions among the

medical elite and the general public alike over "the suitability of women for general practice."

35. Documentation indicating Mr. Orr's agreement to have his name used is held with the tape and transcript of his interview at the RCN Archive.

36. Given the course of the war, Mr. Orr could not have been sent to Italy until 1943. We have to assume that he was stationed in Britain for approximately two years.

37. Oral testimony: QNIT 07/2.

38. Ibid.

39. Although the original conversation was not recorded, it was followed up by e-mail communication at a later date. Hard copy of this is logged with transcripts in the RCN Archive.

40. Due to difficulties in recruiting staff to this remote district, after her retirement in 1986, this nurse stepped in on several occasions to fill the post temporarily until a new nurse was appointed.

41. From e-mail communication with Mr. Peterson. Hard copy of this is logged with transcripts in the RCN Archive.

42. Ibid.

43. Ibid.

44. Davies, *Gender and the Professional Predicament in Nursing*.

45. Oral testimony: QNIT 58/2.

46. Ibid.

47. Oral testimony: QNIT 53/1.

48. Oral testimony: QNIT 26/1.

49. Oral testimony: QNIT 12/1.

50. Oral testimony: QNIT 54/1.

51. A. Worth et al., *Assessment of Need for District Nursing* (Glasgow: Department of Nursing and Community Health, Glasgow Caledonian University, 1995), 77–78.

52. Ibid.

53. Ibid.

54. Kelly and Symonds, *The Social Construction of Community Nursing*, 118.

55. Ibid., 128.

CHAPTER 9 PORTRAITS OF A DISTRICT NURSE

1. Perhaps the most notable exceptions being Summers, "The Mysterious Demise of Sarah Gamp," 365–386; Williams, "From Sarah Gamp to Florence Nightingale," 41–75.; and Fenne, "Every Woman Is a Nurse," although these all concentrate on the nineteenth century.

2. For historical accounts of district nursing see Stocks, *A Hundred Years*; Baly, *A History of the Queen's Nursing Institute*; Dingwall et al., *An Introduction to the Social History of Nursing*; H. Sweet and R. Ferguson, "District Nursing History," in *District Nursing. Providing Care in a Supportive Context*, eds. S. Lawton et al. (Edinburgh: Harcourt, 2000); Fox, "District Nursing and the Work of Nursing Associations in England and Wales"; J. Hawker, "Parish Nursing in Dorset." See also archive material relating to nursing associations and the QNI held in the Contemporary Medical Archives (CMA) collection, The Wellcome Institute Library, London. Records of the QNI Scotland are held at the Royal College of Nursing Archive, Edinburgh.

3. First Principal Nursing Officer and Inspector to the Queen's Institute (1890-91), QNI Council member and Founder-Treasurer of the Midwives Institute, niece of William Rathbone.

4. "Editorial: The Prophetic Vision," *Nursing Notes and Midwives' Chronicle* XXVI, no. 311 (1913): 299, report of speech given by Miss Paget at the unveiling in Liverpool of the first memorial to Florence Nightingale.
5. Department of Health and Social Security and P. A. Briggs (Chair) et al., Cmnd. 5115: Report of the Committee on Nursing (1972).
6. "A New Home at Watford," *QNM* XXVII, no. 6 (June 1935): 179–181.
7. Dickens, *The Life and Adventures of Martin Chuzzlewit*.
8. D. Brindle, "In Gladys's Footsteps," *The Guardian* (Wednesday March 3, 1999): 33.
9. V. Hyde, "Community Nursing: A Unified Discipline?" in *Community Nursing: Dimensions and Dilemmas*, eds. P. Cain, V. Hyde, and E. Howkins (London: Arnold, 1995), 3.
10. Ibid, 2.
11. "A League for Queen's Nurses," *QNM* XXIII, no. 1 (1938): 7–9.
12. L. M. Egerton, "A Paper," *QNM* XXIII, no. 7 (1929): 121–123.
13. Loane, *The Queen's Poor* (reprint of 1st edition with new introduction by Susan Cohen and Clive Fleay; London: Middlesex University Press, 1998) See also, for example, M. Loane, *The Incidental Opportunities of District Nursing* (London: Edward Arnold, 1905); M. Loane, *The Next Street But One* (London: Edward Arnold, 1907); and M. Loane, *Outlines of Routine in District Nursing* (London: Scientific Press, 1905).
14. Loane, *The Queen's Poor*, 111–112.
15. F. Dacre Craven, *A Guide to District Nurses and Home Nursing*.
16. Some Queen's Superintendents, *Handbook for Queen's Nurses* (1924, 1932, 1943 editions)
17. Merry and Irven, *District Nursing*.
18. See, for example, Queen's Institute of District Nursing, *Queen's Nurses at Work in Country Districts* (c. 1930's); *Nurse* (1940); *District Nurse*, Director, John Page (1942). In addition, Stocks' notes (SA/QNI Box 114 P13/1-11: 1956–65 Correspondence and material used by Stocks for preparation of *A Hundred Years of District Nursing*) refer to three motion pictures made for the QNI for the ICN in 1937, the first made in Bloomsbury, Birmingham, Edinburgh, and Hackney about postregistration district nurse training, loans and interhospital cooperation; the second at Huddersfield showing maternity nursing and the routine ante and postnatal care (in two parts); and the third filmed at St. Helen's District Nursing Association showing industrial area district nursing, "Bag day" and staff leaving the home on foot, bicycle, and car.
19. Queen's Institute of District Nursing, Director: Don Higgins, *Town Nurse, Country Nurse* (1965); Director: Trevor Payne, *A New Way of Caring*, (1973); and "No. 4: Mustn't Grumble," *Out of the Doll's House*, BBC TV series (1989).
20. For example, Queen's Institute of District Nursing, *The Training and Work of District Nurses* (1964); Queen's Institute of District Nursing, *The Queen's Institute* (1970); Queen's Institute of District Nursing, *Queen's Institute of District Nursing* (c. 1960).
21. J. Cunningham, "The British District Nurse on the Films," *South African Nursing. Journal* (May 1949): 40–41; E. P. Hubbard, "Film Star for a Fortnight," *QNM* XXXVII, no. 3 (1949), 32–33; E. J. Merry, "The District Nursing Film 'Friend of the Family'," *QNM* XXXVII, no. 7 (1949): 81–82. The cost of £8,000 was provided by the South African Gift Fund.
22. Merry, "The District Nursing Film 'Friend of the Family,' " 81–82.
23. E. J. Merry, "Recruitment of District Nurses," *DN* 1, no. 4 (1958): 87.
24. 1940, *Nurse*.

25. 1942, *District Nurse*, Director: John Page.
26. Merry, "Recruitment of District Nurses," 87.
27. "No. 4: Mustn't Grumble," *Out of the Doll's House*, BBC TV series (1989).
28. Oral testimony: D/N 25.
29. H. Sweet, "Town Nurse and Country Nurse: Viewing an Early C20th District Nursing Landscape Using a Lancashire Case Study," in *Busy Women: A Century of Change in Women's Lives 1840–1940*, eds. H. Sweet et al. (In preparation).
30. J. Hallam, *Nursing the Image: Media, Culture and Professional Identity* (London: Routledge, 2000), 5.
31. A. J. Cronin, *The Citadel* (London: New English Library, 1937).
32. Ibid.
33. See W. Ingram and BBC TV Wales, 1985, NFTVA 8.021 242 AA: *District Nurse* Series, Episode 16/12/85 "Don't Wait Up," pilot programme for the series. The series itself was cowritten by Tony Holland, Harry Duffin, and Julia Smith. Miller also wrote a number of screenplays with a nursing and medical flavour for BBC television dramatisation, including *Ambulance* and *Casualty*, and these all appear to have been similarly well researched, although we have been unable to uncover any medical background to this author.
34. L. Rush, "(9) Health Visitor," *Angels* (1976).
35. P. Milne, "(13) Walkabout," *Angels* (1976).
36. Hallam, *Nursing the Image*, 79–82, noted high audience ratings peaking at 12 million viewers despite placing nurses rather than doctors at the centre of the drama.
37. Ibid.
38. Stocks, *A Hundred Years*, ; and Baly, *A History of the Queen's Institute*. Both consider it sufficiently relevant to their historical studies to carry photographic evidence of the changing uniforms of district nurses in these works.

CHAPTER 10 DISCUSSION AND CONCLUSION

1. Summers, "The Mysterious Demise of Sarah Gamp," 365–386.
2. Hyde, "Community Nursing," 1.
3. Ibid.
4. G. Baker, J. M. Bevan, et al., *Community Nursing: Research and Recent Developments* (London: Croom Helm, 1987), 1.
5. Allen, "Doctor-Nurse Relationships," 226–228.
6. Oral Testimony: D/N 07.
7. J. M. Griffiths and K. A. Luker, "Intraprofessional Teamwork in District Nursing: In Whose Interest?" *Journal of Advanced Nursing* 20, no. 6 (1994): 1038–1045.
8. K. Buhler-Wilkerson, *No Place Like Home: A History of Nursing and Home Care in the United States* (Baltimore: Johns Hopkins University Press, 2001).
9. See Digby and Sweet, "Nurses as Culture Brokers,"; H. Sweet, " 'Wanted: 16 Nurses of the Better Educated Type'—Provision of Nurses to South Africa in the Early C20th," *Nursing Inquiry* (September 2004); Marks, *Divided Sisterhood;* Searle, *The History of the Development of Nursing in South Africa.*
10. This was claimed by Hockey, *Care in the Balance*, and was also the case with most of our oral history interviewees.
11. See www.rcn.org.uk/professional/defining_nursing.html; the current draft definition states that nursing is "the use of clinical judgment and the provision of care to enable people to promote, improve, maintain, or recover health, or when death is inevitable, to die peacefully.".

12. H. Low and Jo Hesketh, *District Nursing: The Invisible Workforce* (London: The English National Board for Nursing, Midwifery and Health Visiting with The Queen's Nursing Institute, 2002).

13. J. M. McGuire, *The Expanded Role of the Nurse*, cited in *Community Nursing: Research and Recent Developments*, eds. G. Baker et al. (London: Croom Helm, 1987), 69.

14. See *An Oral History of General Practice in Paisley: Locality the Diffusion of Knowledge c. 1950–1990*, an oral history project undertaken by Graham Smith and funded by the Wellcome Trust. This work is currently unpublished. All recordings are to be lodged with the Glasgow University Archive.

15. P. D'Antonio, "Revisiting and Rethinking the Rewriting of Nursing History," *Bulletin of the History of Medicine* 73, no. 2 (1999): 272.

Sources and Bibliography

MANUSCRIPTS

Dorset Record Office

D457/5-6: *Alderholt District Nursing Association: Minutes 1918–43 and 1944–1962.*

Glamorgan County Archives and Records Office

D/D X1 1/1-34: *Minutes Glamorganshire Insurance Committee 1912–46.*
D/D X 236: *Private Papers of District Nurse Ann Evans 1928–1958.*
D/D X 287/1-4: *Barry District Nursing Association Annual Report Books: March 1891–June 1900, June 1923–Sept. 1926, Oct. 1926–Nov. 1931.*

Liverpool Record Office

352 WOO/1/3-5: *Woolton District Nursing Society, Liverpool, Minutes 1925–50.*

National Archives, Kew

D.2/1 *Memorandum on Matters . . . September 1926*, notes from WSIHVA taken at Kew.
FD1/5519 *Memorandum on District Nursing in Relation to the Welfare of Munition Workers Submitted by the Public Health Section of the Royal College of Nursing* (13/08/1940)

National Film and Television Archives

District Nurse, Pilot for series, Episode 16/12/85, "Don't Wait up," Written by W. Ingram, BBC TV Wales (1985).
A New Way of Caring, Directed by Trevor Payne (1973).
Ambulance, Written by H. Miller (1975).
Casualty! Written by H. Miller (1982).
"Health Visitor" (Episode 9), *Angels*. Directed by Derek Martinus, written by Len Rush (BBC1 1/11/1976).
"Walkabout" (Episode 13), *Angels*. Directed by Christopher Barry, written by Paula Milne (BBC1 29/9/1976).

Ministry of Information, *Nurse* (1940).
Ministry of Information, *District Nurse*. Directed by John Page (1942).
Queen's Institute of District Nursing, *Queen's Nurses at Work in Country Districts* (c. 1930's).
Queen's Institute of District Nursing, *Town Nurse, Country Nurse*. Directed by Don Higgins (1965).

RCN Archives

QNI/A.15: *Synopsis of Proceedings at the Conference of Delegates From Affiliated Associations Held on Wednesday, 17th May 1933.*
QNI/A.68: *Queen's Institute of District Nursing. Report of the Scottish Council for the Year Ending 31st October 1948.*
QNI/B.2/6: *Minutes of Meeting of the Scottish Council, QNI Scotland* (1948).
QNI/B.1/14: *Minutes of the Executive Council, QNI Scotland 1948–49.*
QNI/B.7: 1934–1949: *Minutes of the Advisory Committee on the Work of the Nurse Commissioners for Tuberculosis in Scotland.*
QNI/D.4/1: *Leith Jubilee Nurses Association Minute Book 1920–1933.*
QNI/D.2: *Papers of the Comrie & Crieff District Nursing Association.*
SD/1: 21/07/98, *Oral History: Miss Alfra Leckie.*
SD/4: 17/08/98, *Oral History: Miss J. Jerratt.*
SD/5: 17/07/98, *Oral History: Miss Sue Aylmer*

Wellcome Trust Library, CMAC

CMAC Queen's Institute Archives

SA/QNI Box 1 B8-37, Box 2 B38-45: *Published Annual Reports 1910–1947.*
SA/QNI Box 62 F7/3: *Correspondence With Outside Bodies: Briggs Committee on Nursing, 1971–72.*
SA/QNI Box 62 F/7/9: *Correspondence With Department of Health and Social Security (1965–75).*
SA/QNI Box 79 H4/1-3: *Fundraising Correspondence.*
SA/QNI Box 79 H8/1: *Correspondence and Minutes of Meetings With the BMA (1908–1910) re. Proposed Changes to the Rules of County Nursing Associations.*
SA/QNI Box 79 H8/2: *Correspondence re. a Case of Friction Between Doctor and Nurse, 1907, and Cuttings, 1910, 1932.*
SA/QNI Box 83 H/23: *Correspondence With Ministry of Health, and Statistics of Cases Treated.*
SA/QNI Box 83 H/27/1-4: *Introduction of the NHS, 1947.*
SA/QNI Box 81 H/13/7/2: *Notes on Interviews Between Representatives of the QNI and the Interdepartmental Committee on Social Insurance and Allied Services.*
SA/QNI Box 81 H18: *Correspondence, Questionnaires, Report of Delegations to the Postmaster General, 1932–1935.*
SA/QNI Box 102 X20/1-2: East London Nursing Society, E. S. Clewes, *Ninth Annual Superintendent's Report* (dated 17/06/68).
SA/QNI Box 111 P6/8: *Recruitment pamphlets, 1931, 1933, 1938;* also 'Queen's Institute of District Nursing' Form T9 (4.31, 5.33, 6.38, respectively).
SA/QNI Box 111 P6/16 Pamphlet: *Queen's Nurses—and What They Do* (QNI: c. 1945).
SA/QNI Box 111 P6/18 1949: *Appeal for Annual Subscriptions to QNI.*

SA/QNI Box 111 P6/20 1951: *"Alphabet of Activities: Q—Queen's Institute of District Nursing"* in: *Union of Girls Schools Record 75(Spring 1951)*: 257-259.
SA/QNI Box 112 P7/69: Ann Mackenzie (on behalf of steering group District Nursing Association (UK)), *Key Issues in District Nursing: Paper 1: The District Nurse Within the Community Context* (1989): 15–16.
SA/QNI Box 113: Extract from an article by F. M. Roberts, *King Edward VII Order of Nurses* (c. 1950).
SA/QNI Box 114 P13/1-11: Correspondence and Material Used by M. Stocks for Preparation of *"A Hundred Years of District Nursing"* (1956–1965).
SA/QNI Box 114 Q1/6: QVJIN, *Agreement of Affiliation Approval (dated 24/03/1908) for Coedpoeth and Minerva District Nursing Association and Inspector's Report (1909)*.
SA/QNI Box 115 Q6/11-22: *Rolls of Affiliated Branches, England and Wales, Including Queen's Institute's Registers c. 1913–1939*.
QNI, *Summary of Evidence Submitted to the Interdepartmental Committee on Nursing Services* (1938).

CMAC Moving Image and Sound Collections

1458B, Episode No. 4 'Mustn't Grumble,' *Out of the Doll's House* (BBC TV Documentary Series: 1989).

CMAC General Practitioners Oral History Collection

GP29/02, c. 1980, Oral History: John Scott Makepeace.
GP29/06, c. 1980, Oral History: Margaret A. Norton.
GP29/08, c. 1980, Oral History: Frank W. Bonb.
GP29/12, c. 1980, Oral History: Alec S. Bookless.
GP29/16, c. 1980, Oral History: Frederick Barber.
GP29/21, c. 1980, Oral History: John A. Hallinham.
GP29/32, c. 1980, Oral History: Robert Hugh Clarke.
GP29/38, c. 1980, Oral History: John J. Hopkinson.
GP29/59, c. 1980, Oral History: Samuel L. Isaacs.

OFFICIAL PAPERS AND REPORTS

Consultative Council on Medical and Allied Services, *Report of the Future Provision on Medical and Allied Services* (otherwise referred to as "Dawson Report") (London: HMSO, 1920).
The Rt Hon The Earl of Athlone (Chair of Enquiry), *Ministry of Health, Board of Education: Interdepartmental Committee on Nursing Services, Interim Report* (1939).
Lord Rushcliffe (Chair) MOH Cmd 6487, *Second Report of Nurses' Salaries Committee: Salaries and Emoluments of Male Nurses, Public Health Nurses, District Nurses and State Registered Nurses in Nurseries* (1943).
S. J. L. Taylor and Nuffield Provincial Hospitals Trust for Research and Policy Studies in Health Services, *Good General Practice: A Report of a Survey* (1954).
Ministry of Health and S. F. Armer (Chair) et al., *Report of the Working Party on the Training of District Nurses* (1955).

Robert Carr and National Joint Advisory Council Training for Skill, *Recruitment and Training of Young Workers in Industry* (otherwise referred to as the "Carr Report" (London: Ministry of Labour and National Service by HMSO, 1958).

Baron Geoffrey Crowther and Central Advisory Council for Education. *15 to 18* (otherwise referred to as the "Crowther Report") (London: HMSO, 1959).

Central Health Services Council, *The Field of Work of the Family Doctor: Report of the Sub-Committee of the Standing Medical Advisory Committee (The Gillie Report)* (1963).

Department of Health and Social Security, *The State of the Public Health: Report of the Chief Medical Officer* (1970).

Department of Health and Social Security (Cmnd. 5055), *National Health Service Reorganisation* (1972).

Department of Health and Social Security and P. A. Briggs (Chair) et al. (Cmnd. 5115), *Report of the Committee on Nursing* (1972).

General Nursing Council, *Educational Policy 1977 Annual Report* (1977).

Department of Health and Social Security, *Nursing in Primary Health Care* (London: HMSO, 1977), Circular CNO(77) 8.

Royal College of Nursing, *Specialties in Nursing: A Report of the Working Party Investigating the Development of Specialties Within the Nursing Profession* (1988).

Department of Health, *Social Services Inspectorate/Regional Health Authority Community Care Monitoring: National Summary* (London: Department of Health, 1993).

JOURNAL ARTICLES

"A Call to Women: The Dearth of Nurses." *QNM* XXXIV, no. 5 (1945): 43–45.

Anderson, E. "Queen's Nurses' League—Leeds and District Branch Report of Lecture by Dr. A. Antrobus entitled 'Pioneers Still.'" *Guardian* (January 29, 1965).

Anderson, G. "An Oversight in Nursing History." *Journal of History of Medicine* (Summer 1948): 417–426.

"Annual Meeting at Blackburn." *QNM* XXV (1932): 209–210.

'Another Devonshire GP:' "Letters, Notes and Answers: Doctors and District Nurses." *BMJ* 1 (April 2, 1932): 642.

"The Assistant Nurse." *QNM*, XXXII, no. 1 (1943): 1–2.

"Association of Queen's Superintendents in the Northern Counties." *QNM* XIX, no. 2 (1922): 25–29.

"At a Rest Centre." *QNM* XXX, no. 3 (1941): 25.

Balme, H. "Post-War Reconstruction." *QNM*, XXXII, no. 4 (1943): 51–52.

Barber, G. O. "The Link to Health." *South African Nursing Journal* (February 1960): 16–17.

Barford, A. M. "Letters, Notes and Answers: Doctors and District Nurses." *BMJ* 1 (April 23, 1832): 784.

Barlow, K. E. "The Evolution of the Queen's Nurse in Regard to the Ministry of Health." *QNM* (1919): 49–50.

Bartlett, S. "Letters, Notes and Answers: Doctors and District Nurses." *BMJ* 1 (April 16, 1932): 738.

Bliss, J., and Alison While. "Team Work and Collaboration: The Position of District Nursing 1948–1974." *IHNJ* 5, no. 3 (2000): 22–29.

Bradshaw, A. "The Virtue of Nursing: The Covenant of Care." *Journal of Medical Ethics*, 25 (1999): 477–481.

Brindle, D. "In Gladys's Footsteps." *The Guardian* (March 3, 1999): 33.

Burnham, H. C. "How the Idea of Profession Changed the Writing of Medical History." *Medical History* Supplement No. 18 (1998): 105.

"Cardiff." *QNM* XXII, no. 6 (1926): 135.

Carre, J. "Health Care in the Community." *Nursing Mirror* (May 24, 1974): 32.

Challis, "On Starting a District Nursing Association." *QNM* XIX, nos. 1 & 2 (1922): 3–4, 34–35.

"Community Care: The Ten Year Plan." *DN* 6 (May 1963): 31.

"Conference on District Nursing at Mortimer Hall." *QNM* XVII (1919): 33–34.

"Correspondence: Twenty Years a Queen's Nurse." *Nursing Mirror* (29 November 1941).

'A Country Practitioner': "Correspondence." *BMJ* 25, no. 3 (1899): 762.

'Country Practitioner': "Letters, Notes and Answers: Doctors and District Nurses." *BMJ* 1 (May 7, 1932): 872.

Crouch, M. "The Future—Profession or Vocation." *QNM* XXXIX, no. 9 (1950): 130–133, 139.

Crowther, M. A. "Medicine and the End of the Poor Law." *SHM*, 38 (1986): 74–76.

Cunningham, J. "The British District Nurse on the Films." *South African Nursing Journal* (May 1949): 40–41.

Dalzell-Ward, A. J. "The Reason and Need for Professional Organisations." *Nursing Mirror* 53 (November 8, 1957): 431–432.

D'Antonio, P. "Revisiting and Rethinking the Rewriting of Nursing History." *Bulletin of the History of Medicine* 73, no. 2 (1999): 272.

Darmady, M. "Central Sterile Supply Services and Their Application to District Work." *DN* 4, no. 4 (1961): 83–86.

Davies, C. "The Health Visitor as Mother's Friend: A Woman's Place in Public Health 1900–14." *SHM* 1 (1988): 39–59.

Dill, G. "Letters, Notes and Answers: Doctors and District Nurses." *BMJ* 1 (March 19, 1932): 550.

"Districts Give Cars to County." *The Shetland Times* (October 1, 1948): 2.

Dixon, N. M. "Changes in District Nursing." *DN*, 1, no. 2 (1958): 24.

Dixon, S. "The Archive of the Queen's Nursing Institute in the Contemporary Medical Archives Centre." *Medical History* 45 (2000): 251–266.

du Sautoy, C. "Glimpses From the Past." *DN* 5, no. 11 (1963): 260.

"East London Nursing Society." *QNM* XXVI, no. 2 (1933): 68–69.

"Editorial." *QNM* XVII, no. 4 (1920): 65–66.

"Editorial." *QNM* XVIII, no. 4 (1921): 62–63.

"Editorial." *QNM* XXI, no. 1 (1924): 176–177.

"Editorial." *QNM* XXIII, no. 5 (1929): 89–91.

"Editorial." *QNM* XXVII, no. 3 (1934): 93–94.

"Editorial." *QNM* XXVII, no. 8 (1935): 232–233.

"Editorial." *QNM* XXVIII, no. 9 (1939): 252–253.

"Editorial." *QNM* XXXI, no. 5 (1942).

"Editorial." *QNM*, XXXII, no. 8 (1943): 91–92.

"Editorial." *DN*, 1, no. 8 (1958): 175.

"Editorial." *DN* 2, no. 8 (1959): 177.

"Editorial: The Assistant Nurse." *QNM*, XXXIV, no. 4 (1945): 33.

"Editorial: A Message to Queen's Nurses." *QNM*, XXVIII, no. 11 (1939): 312.

"Editorial: The Prophetic Vision." *Nursing Notes and Midwives' Chronicle* XXVI, no. 311 (1913): 299.

"Editorial: State Registration." *QNM* XVII, no. 1 (1920): 1–2.

"Editorial: 'This was their finest hour'—Mr. Churchill." *QNM* XXIX, no. 3 (1940): 45–46.

"Editorial: Training the District Nurses." *The Lancet* (September 10, 1955): 543–544.

Egerton, L. M. "A Paper." *QNM* XXIII, no. 7 (1929): 121–123.

Ellice, G. "A Century of District Nursing." *The Countryman* 94, no. 2 (1989).

"Enlargement of the Home at St. Helen's." *QNM* XXVII, no. 8 (1935): 242–243.

"Experience of a Nurse in Rural Wales." *QNM* XXX, no. 3 (1941): 5–6.

"Experiences of a Queen's Nurse Serving in QAIMNS." *QNM* XXIX, no. 3 (1940): 46–47.

Ferguson, R. "Autonomy, Tension and Trade-Off: Attitudes to Doctors in the History of District Nursing." *International History of Nursing Journal* 6 (2001): 10–17.

Fisher, I. "A Personal Review of the N.H.S." *Midwife, Health Visitor and Community Nurse*, 4 (August 1968): 329–331.

Forman, J. A. S. "What the GP Expects of the District Nurse and Midwife." *DN* 6 (July–August 1963): 74–77, 102–104.

Fox, E. "District Nursing in England and Wales Before the National Health Service: The Neglected Evidence." *Medical History* 38 (1994): 303–321.

Fox, E. "An Honourable Calling or a Despised Occupation: Licensed Midwifery." *SHM* 6, no. 2 (1993): 237–259.

Fox, E. "Universal Health Care and Self-Help: Paying for District Nursing Before the National Health Service." *Twentieth Century British History* 7, no. 1 (1996): 83–109.

"From the Districts." *QNM* XXIV, no. 3 (1930): 38–44.

"From the Districts: Annual Meetings." *QNM* XXV (1932): 277–282.

Gente, M. "The Expansion of the Nuclear Family Unit in Great Britain Between 1910 and 1920." *History of the Family* 6, no. 1 (2001): 125–142.

Gibb, P. "District Nursing in the Highlands and Islands of Scotland: 1890–1940." *History of Nursing Journal* 4 (1992): 319.

Giles, V. H. "To the Hospital Nurse From a Queen's Nurse." *QNM* XXVIII, no. 10 (1940): 30.

Godden, J., et al. "The Decline of Myths and Myopia? The Use and Abuse of Nursing History," *The Australian Journal of Advanced Nursing*, 10, no. 2 (1992–1993): 27.

Gordon, J. Elise. "Scottish Journey—6. With the Nurses of the Western Isles (III)." *Nursing Mirror* (July 10, 1948): 235.

"G.P.: Letters, Notes and Answers: Doctors and District Nurses." *BMJ* 1 (March 26, 1932): 598.

Griffiths, J. M., and K. A. Luker. "Intraprofessional Teamwork in District Nursing: In Whose Interest?" *Journal of Advanced Nursing* 20, no. 6 (1994): 1038–1045.

Haddon, C. "Nursing as a Profession for Ladies." *St. Paul's Monthly Magazine* (August 1871): 458.

Hallowes, R. M. "Distinguished British Nurses: 8. Mrs. Dacre Craven (Florence Lees): An Organiser of District Nursing." *Nursing Mirror* (23 December 1955).

Hancox, E. "How We Tackled the Influenza Epidemics: Sheffield." *QNM* (1919): 31–32.

Hardy, G., and Brian Lemin. "William Rathbone Staff College: Past, Present and Future." *DN* (September 1972): 120–121.

Haste, F. H., and L. D. Macdonald. "The Role of the Specialist in Community Nursing: Perceptions of Specialist and District Nurses." *International Journal of Nursing Studies* 29, no. 1 (1992): 37–47.

"How the Work of District Nursing in London Began—and Continues." *QNM* XIX, no. 3 (1922): 49–52.

Hubbard, E. P. "Film Star for a Fortnight." *QNM* XXXVII, no. 3 (1949): 32–33.

Hughes, A. "Answers to Correspondents." *QNM* 1, no. 3 (1904).

Hughes, A. "District Nursing on Provident Lines." *Charity Organisation Review* (July 1910).

Huntman, R. G., et al. "Twixt Candle and Lamp: The Contribution of Elizabeth Fry and the Institution of Nursing Sisters to Nursing Reform." *Medical History*, 43, no. 3 (2002): 351–380.

"Impressions and Experiences of a Male District Nurse." *QNM* XXXVII, no. 12 (1948): 146–147.

"In the Rhondda Valley." *QNM* XXVI, no. 1 (1933): 12–17.

"Institute News: Resignations." *QNM* XXVII, no. 1 (1934): 54.

"Institute News: Wales." *QNM* XVII, no. 3 (1920): 58.

"Institute News: Wales." *QNM* XVII, no. 4 (1920): 79.

"Institute News: Wales." *QNM* XVIII, nos. 2 & 4 (1921): 38, 74.

"Institute News: Wales." *QNM* XIX, no. 1 (1922): 17.

Irven, I. "District Nursing, Its Scope and Opportunities." *Nursing Times* 38 (1942): 469–471.

"The 'Ivy' Motor Cycle." *QNM* XX, no. 3 (1923): 140.

Jewson, N. D. "The Disappearance of the Sick-Man From Medical Cosmology, 1770–1870." *Sociology* (1976): 10.

Johnson, B. M. "Status and Future of the Village Nurse." *QNM* XIX, no. 2 (1922): 29–30.

Jones, C. "Sisters of Charity and the Ailing Poor." *SHM* 2, no. 3 (1989): 339–348.

Kelsey, A. "The Making of Health Visitors: An Historical Perspective, Part 1." *IHNJ* 5, no. 3 (2000): 44–50.

Kelsey, A. "The Making of Health Visitors: An Historical Perspective, Part 2." *IHNJ* 6, no. 2 (2000): 66–70.

Knox-Mearns, M. "How We Tackled the Influenza Epidemics: Leicester." *QNM* (1919): 32–33.

"A League for Queen's Nurses." *QNM* XXIII, no. 1 (1938): 7–9.

"Lethe: A Page From an Assistant Superintendent's Diary." *QNM* XVII, no. 3 (1920): 48–49.

"London's Public Health." *QNM* XXIV, no. 5 (1931): 104–105.

"Long Service Fund." *QNM* XXII, no. 3 (1925): 55–56.

Loudon, I. "Medical Care and the Family Doctor." *Bulletin of the History of Medicine* 58 (1984).

Maggs, C. "A History of Nursing: A History of Caring?" *Journal of Advanced Nursing* 23, no. 3 (1996).

Maguire. "Report of an Address." *QNM* XXXIV, no. 1 (1945): 2–5.

"The McKenzie Motor Cycle." *QNM* XX, no. 3 (1923): 139.

Mc Master, A. "'Are we to lose our nurse?' Implications of the National Health Service Act 1948 in the Village." *Journal of the National Council of Social Services* (Autumn 1948): 15–17.

"Memorandum on History and Work of the Q.I.D.N." *QNM* XXXX, no. 12 (1951): 192–193.

Merry, E. J. "The District Nursing Film 'Friend of the Family'." *QNM* XXXVII, no. 7 (1949): 81–82.

Merry, E. J. "Recruitment of District Nurses." *DN* 1, no. 4 (1958): 87.

Merry E. J. "The Role of the District Nurse in Home Care." *The Practitioner* 177 (July 1956): 54–58.

"M.E.S.: John Beart District Nurse." *DN* (November 1968): 169–170.

"Metropolitan and Southern Counties Association of Queen's Superintendents." *QNM* XIX, no. 2 (1922): 25–29.

"The Ministry of Health Superannuation of Nurses and Midwives." *QNM* XXXIV, no. 5 (1945): 43–44.

"More Nurses for Lancashire." *QNM* XXVIII, no. 10 (1939): 309.

"The Morning Round of a Liverpool 'Queen's' Nurse." *Delegates Local Handbook of Jubilee Congress* (1909): 31–35.

"Mrs. Dacre Craven." *The Nurses' Journal* (February 1898): 16–18.

Nelson, S. "The Fork in the Road: Nursing History Versus the History of Nursing?" *Nursing History Review* 10 (2002): 177.

"Nest: Letters, Notes and Answers: Doctors and Nurses in Industrial Areas." *BMJ* 1 (March 5, 1932): 456.

"The New District Nurses' Home at St. Helen's." *QNM* XXII, no. 9 (1927): 205.

"A New Home at Watford." *QNM* XXVII, no. 6 (1935): 179–181.

Nightingale, F. "Trained Nursing for the Sick Poor: Extracts From Letter by Miss Florence Nightingale Sent to The Times, April 1876." *QNM*, XX, no. 4 (1923): 165–166.

"The 1930 Fund for the Benefit of Trained District Nurses: Report for Year Ending June 30th 1933." *QNM*, XXVI, no. 2 (1933): 77.

"1940 and All That." *QNM* XXIX, no. 4 (1940): 70–71.

"Notes From the Districts: Coedpoeth, Glamorgan, Neath, Pontardawe." *QNM* XXI, no. 4 (1924): 273–274.

"Notes From the Districts: Wales." *QNM* XXIII, no. 1 (1928): 37–38.

"Nurse Receives Honour." *QNM* XXX, no. 3 (1941): 6.

"Pay Settlement for District Nurses." *QNM* XXXLVI, no. 12 (1957): 180.

Peterkin, A. M. "The Scope and Conditions of District Nursing." *QNM* XXIV, no. 5 (1931): 128–132.

Petty, G. F. "Patients, Nurses and Doctors." *DN* 4, no. 4 (1961): 76–78.

"Plymouth Nurses Carry On." *QNM* XXX, no. 9 (1941): 47.

Prochaska, F. K. "Body and Soul: Bible Nurses and The Poor in Victorian London." *Historical Research* 60, no. 143 (1987): 336–348.

"Queen's Institute of District Nursing: Statistics for 1933." *QNM* XXVII, no. 3 (1934): 103–107.

"A Queen's Nurse, a Country District." *QNM* (1919): 53.

"Queen's Nurses' League Conference." *QNM* XXXI, no. 11 (1942): 83–95.

Rave, R. W. "Annual Meeting Address to the Queen's Institute of District Nursing." *QNM* XXXVIII, no. 10 (1949): 129–133.

RCN Executive Committee. "Occasional Papers: The Future of District Nursing" *NT* (March 20, 1969): 45–48.

"Report on the Nursing of Patients in Connection With Local Authorities." *QNM* XXVI, no. 2 (1933): 77.

Shadwell, D. A. "District Nursing." *The Times* (September 27–29, 1926).

Snowball, J. "Asking Nurses About Advocating for Patients: 'Reactive' and 'Proactive' Accounts." *Journal of Advanced Nursing* 24 (1996): 67–75.

"Somerset GP: Letters, Notes and Answers: Doctors and District Nurses." *BMJ* 1 (April 16, 1932): 738.

Summers, A. "The Mysterious Demise of Sarah Gamp: The Domiciliary Nurse and Her Detractors: 1830–60." *Journal of Victorian Studies* 32, no. 3 (1989): 365–386.

"Swanscombe District Nursing Society." *QNM* XVII, no. 3 (1920): 49.

Sweet, H. " 'Wanted: 16 Nurses of the Better Educated Type'—Provision of Nurses to South Africa in the Early C20th." *Nursing Inquiry* (September 2004).

"Training of District Nurses." *Royal Society of Health Journal* 11 (1957): 728–729.

"Transferred Workers." *QNM* XXX, no. 9 (1941): 45.

Walker, D. "The Future Public Health Nurse and Her Team." *DN* 8, no. 11 (1965): 200–203.

"Wartime Experiences and Opportunities." *QNM* XXIX, no. 4 (1940): 69.

Welshman, J. "Family Visitors or Social Workers? Health Visiting and Public Health in England and Wales 1890–1974." *IHNJ* 3, no. 2 (1997): 5–21.

Wilensky, W. "The Professionalisation of Everyone." *American Journal of Sociology* LXX, no. 2 (1964): 143–144.

Williams, D. "Recollections of the RCN and District Nursing." *IHNJ* 4 (1992–1993): 25–27.

Williamson, L. "Soul Sisters: The St. John and Ranyard Nurses in Nineteenth Century London." *IHNJ* 2, no. 2 (1996): 33–49.

Wilmshurst, M. "Fifty Years an Institute." *Nursing Times* XXXIII, no. 1677 (June 19, 1937).

"The Workhouse Mrs. Gamp." *FUN* (March 31, 1866).

BOOKS AND CHAPTERS WITHIN BOOKS

Abbott, P. "Conflict Over Grey Areas: District Nurses and Home Helps Providing Community Care." In *The Sociology of the Caring Professions*, edited by P. Abbott and Liz Meerabeau, 199–209. London: The UCL Press, 1998.

Abbott, P., and Claire Wallace. "Health Visiting, Social Work, Nursing and Midwifery: A History." In *The Sociology of the Caring Professions*, edited by P. Abbott and Liz Meerabeau, 20–53. London: The UCL Press, 1998.

Abel-Smith, B. *A History of the Nursing Profession.* London: Heinemann, 1960.

Ackland, H. W. *Memoirs of the Cholera Epidemic in Oxford 1854.* London: Churchill, 1856.

Allen, D. "Doctor–Nurse Relationships: Accomplishing the Skill Mix in Health Care." In *The Sociology of the Caring Professions*, edited by P. Abbott and Liz Meerabeau. London: UCL Press, 1998.

Allan, P., and M. Jolley. *Nursing, Midwifery and Health Visiting Since 1900.* London: Faber & Faber, 1982.

Antrobus, M. F. *District Nursing: The Nurse, the Patients and the Work.* London: Faber & Faber, 1985.

Baker, G., J. M. Bevan, et al. *Community Nursing: Research and Recent Developments.* London: Croom Helm, 1987.

Baly, M. *Florence Nightingale and the Nursing Legacy.* London: Croom Helm, 1986.

Baly, M. *A History of the Queen's Nursing Institute: 100 Years 1887–1987.* Kent: Croom Helm, 1987.

Baly, M. *As Miss Nightingale Said: Florence Nightingale Through Her Sayings.* London: Scutari Press, 1991.

Battle, S., J. Moran-Ellis, and B. Salter. *The District Nurse's Changing Role.* 1985.

Bellaby, P., and P. Oribabor. "The History of the Present: Contradiction and Struggle in Nursing." In *Rewriting Nursing History*, edited by C. Davies, 159–161. London: Croom Helm, 1982.

Berridge, V. *Health and Society in Britain Since 1939.* Cambridge: Cambridge University Press, 1999.

Bradley, K. *Friends and Visitors: A First History of the Women's Suffrage Movement in Cornwall 1870–1914.* Newmill: The Pattern Press for the Hypatia Trust, 2000.

Braybon, G., and Penny Summerfield. *Out of the Cage: Women's Experiences in Two World Wars.* London: Pandora, 1987.

Buhler-Wilkerson, K. *No Place Like Home: A History of Nursing and Home Care in the United States.* Baltimore: John Hopkins University Press, 2001.

Bullough, V. L. *The Development of Medicine as a Profession: The Contribution of the Medieval University to Modern Medicine.* Basel, Switzerland: S. Karger, 1966.

Burdett, H. *Burdett's Hospitals and Charities Yearbooks*. 1900–1931.
Butterfield, H. *The Whig Interpretation of History*. London: G. Ell & Sons, 1963.
Bynum, W. F. *Science and the Practice of Medicine in the Nineteenth Century*. Cambridge: Cambridge University Press, 1994.
Caine, B. *English Feminism 1780–1980*. Oxford: Oxford University Press, 1997.
Carr Saunders, A. M., and P. A. Wilson. *The Professions*. Oxford: Clarendon, 1933.
Carr, A., et al. *The Education and Training of District Nurses*. Bolton: Bolton College of Education, 1977.
Central Council for District Nursing in London. *History of the Central Council for District Nursing in London, 1914–1966*. London: Central Council for District Nursing in London, 1966.
Central Health Services Council. *The Field of Work of the Family Doctor*. London: Central Health Services Council, 1963.
Chamberlain, M. *Old Wives Tales: Their History, Remedies and Spells*. London: Virago, 1981.
Cormack, A. A. *District Nursing in Scotland: Voluntary and Statutory*. Parish of Peterculter. Aberdeenshire: Banff, 1965.
Craven, F. Dacre. *A Guide to District Nurses and Home Nursing*. London: Macmillan, 1889.
Cronin, A. J. *The Citadel*. London: New English Library, 1937.
Curnow, J. "The Provision of Healthcare in Remote Communities." In *The NHS in Scotland: The Legacy of the Past and the Prospect of the Future*, edited by C. Nottingham. Aldershot: Ashgate, 2000.
Currie, M. *Fever Hospitals and Fever Nurses: A British Social History of Fever Nurses: A National Service*. London: Routledge, 2005.
Davies, C. *Gender and the Professional Predicament in Nursing*. Buckingham: Open University Press, 1995.
Davies, C., ed. *Rewriting Nursing History*. London: Croom Helm, 1980.
Day, E. M., ed. *Cassell's Modern Dictionary of Nursing and Medical Terms*. London: Cassell & Co., 1939.
Dickens, C. *The Life and Adventures of Martin Chuzzlewit*. London: Hazell, Watson and Viney.
Digby, A. *The Evolution of British General Practice 1850–1948*. Oxford: Oxford University Press, 1999.
Digby, A. *Making a Medical Living: Doctors and Patients in the English Market for Medicine 1720–1911*. Cambridge: Cambridge University Press, 1994.
Digby, A., and H. Sweet. "Nurses as Culture Brokers in Twentieth-Century South Africa." In *Plural Medicine, Tradition and Modernity, 1800–2000*, edited by W. Ernst. London: Routledge, 2002.
Dingwall, R. "Problems of Teamwork in Primary Care." In *Teamwork in Personal Social Services and Health Care*, edited by S. Lonsdale, A. Webb, and T. Briggs. London: Croom Helm, 1980.
Dingwall, R., et al. *An Introduction to the Social History of Nursing*. London: Routledge, 1988.
Donnison, J. *Midwives and Medical Men: History of Interprofessional Rivalries and Women's Rights*. London: Heinemann Educational, 1977.
Dunell, M. H., et al. *The Domiciliary Nursing Services*. Leicester: Taylor & Bloxham, 1943.
Ferguson, S., and H. Fitzgerald. *Studies in the Social Services*. London: HMSO/Longmans Green, 1954.
Fink, J., ed. *Care: Personal Lives and Social Policy*. Bristol: Policy Press in association with The Open University, 2004.

Foucault, M. *The Birth of the Clinic: An Archaeology of Medical Perception.* London: Tavistock, 1973.

Freidson, E. *Profession of Medicine: A Study of the Sociology of Applied Knowledge.* Chicago: University of Chicago Press, 1988.

Gamarnikow, E. "Sexual Division of Labour: The Case of Nursing." In *Feminism and Materialism. Women and Modes of Production*, edited by A. Kuhn and A.M. Wolpe, 96–123. London: Routledge & Kegan Paul, 1978.

Giddens, A. *Sociology.* Cambridge: Polity Press, 1997.

Gill, M. F. *District Nursing in Brighton 1877–1974.* Brighton: Benedict Press, c. 1974.

Gittins, D. *Madness in Its Place: Narratives of Severalls Hospital, 1913–1997.* London: Routledge, 1998.

Gittins, D. "Silences: The Case of a Psychiatric Hospital." In *Narrative and Genre*, edited by M. Chamberlain and P. Thompson, 46–62. London: Routledge, 1998.

Grey, M. "Idols of Society; or Gentility and Femininity." In *Victorian Feminism 1850–1900*, edited by P. Levine, 97–98. London: Hutchinson, 1874).

Hallam, J. *Nursing the Image: Media, Culture and Professional Identity.* London: Routledge, 2000.

Hardy, A. *Health and Medicine in Britain Since 1860.* London: Palgrave, 2001.

Hardy, G. *William Rathbone and the Early History of District Nursing.* Ormskirk: G. W. and A. Hesketh, 1981.

Hart, C. *Behind the Mask: Nurses, Their Unions and Nursing Policy.* London: Bailliere Tindall, 1994.

Hockey, L. *Care in the Balance.* London: QNI, 1968.

Hockey, L. "The Family Care Team: Philosophy, Problems, Possibilities." In *Ciba Foundation Symposium on Teamwork for World Health*, edited by G. Wolstenholme and M. O'Connor, 103–115. London: Churchill, 1971.

Hockey, L. *Feeling the Pulse.* London: QNI, 1966.

Hockey, L., and A. Buttimore (eds.). *Co-operation in Patient Care: Studies of District Nurses Attached to Hospital and General Medical Practice.* London: QNI, 1970.

Hogarth, M., and London City Council. *A Survey of District Nursing in the Administrative County of London.* London: London City Council, 1931.

Hurry, J. B. *District Nursing on a Provident Basis.* London, 1898.

Hutchison, Iain. *Air Ambulance: Six Decades of the Scottish Air Ambulance Service.* Erskine: Kea Publishing, 1996.

Hutton, R. *The Pagan Religions of the Ancient British Isles: Their Nature and Legacy.* Oxford: Basil Blackwell, 1991.

Hyde, V. "Community Nursing: A Unified Discipline?" In *Community Nursing: Dimensions and Dilemmas*, edited by P. Cain, V. Hyde, and E. Howkins. London: Arnold, 1995.

Jones, H. *Health and Society in Twentieth Century Britain.* New York: Longman, 1994.

Jordan, P. *District Nurse.* London: Weidenfeld & Nicolson, 1977.

Kelly, A., and A. Symonds. *The Social Construction of Community Nursing.* Basingstoke: Palgrave Macmillan, 2003.

Kratz, C. R. "District Nursing." In *Nursing, Midwifery and Health Visiting Since 1900*, edited by P. Allan and M. Jolley. (London: Faber & Faber, 1982.

Kuhse, H. *Caring: Nurses, Women and Ethics.* Oxford: Blackwell, 1997.

Larkin, G. *Occupational Monopoly and Modern Medicine.* London: Tavistock, 1983.

Larson, M. S. *The Rise of Professionalism: A Sociological Analysis.* Berkeley: University of California Press, 1977.

Lawton, S., et al. *District Nursing: Providing Care in a Supportive Context.* Edinburgh: Churchill Livingstone, 2000.

Leap, N., and B. Hunter. *The Midwife's Tale: An Oral History From Handywoman to Professional Midwife.* London: Scarlet Press, 1993.

Levine, P. *Feminist Lives in Victorian England.* Oxford: Basil Blackwell, 1990.

Lewis, J. *Women and Social Action in Victorian and Edwardian England.* London: Edward Elgar, 1991.

Lewis, J. *Women in Britain Since 1945.* London: Tavistock, 1992.

Littlewood, J., ed. *Current Issues in Community Nursing.* New York: Churchill Livingstone, 1995.

Loane, M. *The Incidental Opportunities of District Nursing.* London: Edward Arnold, 1905.

Loane, M. *The Next Street But One.* London: Edward Arnold, 1907.

Loane, M. *Outlines of Routine in District Nursing.* London: Scientific Press, 1905.

Loane, M. *The Queen's Poor: Life as They Find It in Town and Country.* London: Edward Arnold, 1905.

Loane, M. *Simple Sanitation: The Practical Application of the Laws of Health to Small Dwellings.* London: Scientific Press, 1905.

Loane, M. E. *An Englishman's Castle.* London: Edward Arnold, 1909.

Loudon, I. *Medical Care and the General Practitioner, 1750–1850.* Oxford: Oxford University Press, 1986.

Low, H., and Jo Hesketh. *District Nursing: The Invisible Workforce.* London: The English National Board for Nursing, Midwifery and Health Visiting with The Queen's Nursing Institute, 2002.

Mackay, L. "Nursing: Will the Idea of a Vocation Survive?" In *The Sociology of the Caring Professions*, edited by P. Abbott and Liz Meerabeau, 54–72. London: The UCL Press, 1998.

Maggs, C. "History of Nursing, History of Nurses: Are the Waters Any Clearer?" In *Defining Nursing History: Proceedings of the Fifth Colloquium for Nursing History Research. Edinburgh, September 1999*, edited by B. Mortimer, 4–7. Edinburgh: Queen Margaret University College Edinburgh, 2000.

Maggs, C. *The Origins of General Nursing.* London: Croom Helm, 1983.

Marks, S. *Divided Sisterhood: Race, Class and Gender in the South African Nursing Profession.* Basingstoke: St Martin's Press, 1994.

Marsh, I. *Sociology.* London: Prentice Hall, 2000.

Marwick, A. *Britain in The Century of Total War: War, Peace and Social Change, 1900–1967.* London: Bodley Head, 1968.

Marwick, A. *The Deluge: British Society and The First World War.* London: Bodley Head, 1965.

McGann, S. *The Battle of the Nurses.* London: Scutari Press, 1992.

McGuire, J. M. "The Expanded Role of the Nurse." In *Community Nursing: Research and Recent Developments*, edited by G. Baker et al., 69. London: Croom Helm, 1987.

McKenzie, R. *Lifting Every Voice: A Report and Action Programme to Address Institutional Racism at the National Assembly of Wales.* London: Public and Commercial Services Union, 2001.

Merry, E. J., and I. D. Irven. *District Nursing: A Handbook for District Nurses and for All Concerned in the Administration of a District Nursing Service.* London: Balliere, 1948.

Midwinter, E., ed. *The Development of Social Welfare in Britain.* Buckingham: The Open University, 1994.

Morten, H. *How to Become a Nurse: And How to Succeed* (3rd edition). London: The Scientific Press, 1895.

Oakley, A. *Essays on Women, Medicine and Health*. Edinburgh: Edinburgh University Press, 1993.

Palmer, J. *Edwardian Truro*. (1994)

Perkin, H. *The Rise of Professional Society: England Since 1880*. London: Routledge, 1989.

Periodical Publications. *Punch Among the Doctors*. London: Methuen, 1933.

Peterkin, A. M. *The Work of the Queen's Nurses: How They Minister to the Needs of the Sick*. London: QNI, c. 1925.

Platt, E. *The Story of the Ranyard Mission 1857–1937*. London: Hodder & Stoughton, 1937.

Prochaska, F. *The Voluntary Impulse: Philanthropy in Modern Britain*. London: Faber & Faber, 1988.

Queen's Institute of District Nursing. *The Queen's Institute*. London: QNI, 1970.

Queen's Institute of District Nursing. *Queen's Institute of District Nursing*. London: QNI, c. 1960.

Queen's Institute of District Nursing. *Summary of Evidence Submitted to the Interdepartmental Committee on Nursing Services*. London: QNI, 1938.

Queen's Institute of District Nursing. *Survey of District Nursing in England and Wales*. London: QNI, 1935.

Queen's Institute of District Nursing. *The Training and Work of District Nurses*. London: QNI, 1964.

Queen's Nursing Institute. *Why Not Become a Queen's Nurse? A Worthwhile Career*. London: QNI, c. 1947.

Queen's Superintendents. *Handbook for Queen's Nurses*. London: The Scientific Press, 1924, 1932, 1943.

Rafferty, A. M. *The Politics of Nursing Knowledge*. London: Routledge, 1996.

Ramsay, E. *East London Nursing Society: The History of a Hundred Years*. London: East London Nursing Society, 1968.

Roberts, E. "The Recipients' View of Welfare." In *Oral History, Health and Welfare*, edited by J. Bornat et al., 203–226. London: Routledge, 2000.

Roberts, E. *A Woman's Place: An Oral History of Working-Class Women 1890–1940*. Oxford: Blackwell, 1984.

Roberts, E. *Women and Families: An Oral History, 1940–1970*. Oxford: Blackwell, 1995.

Ross, L. *Nurses' Perceptions of Spiritual Care*. Aldershot: Avebury, 1997.

Sankey, M. I. *Thank You Miss Hunter*. Devon: Kenmar Press, 2001.

Savage, J. *Nurses, Gender and Sexuality*. London: Heinemann Nursing, 1987.

Searle, C. *The History of the Development of Nursing in South Africa, 1652–1960: A Socio-Historical Survey*. Pretoria: The South African Nursing Association, 1965.

Sinclair, S. *Making Doctors: An Institutional Apprenticeship*. Oxford: Berg, 1997.

Smith, H. *The British Women's Suffrage Campaign, 1866–1928*. London: Longman, 1998.

Stacey, M. "Social Sciences and the State: Fighting Like a Woman." In *The Public and the Private*, edited by E. Gamarnikow et al. Aldershot: Gower, 1983.

Stein, L. "The Doctor/Nurse Game." In *Readings in the Sociology of Nursing*, edited by R. Dingwall & J. McIntosh. Edinburgh: Churchill Livingstone, 1978.

Stocks, M. *A Hundred Years of District Nursing*. London: Allen & Unwin, 1960.

Summers, A. "Nurses and Ancillaries in the Christian Era." In *Western Medicine: An Illustrated History*, edited by I. Loudon, 192–205. Oxford: Oxford University Press, 1997.

Sweet, H. "Town Nurse and Country Nurse: Viewing an Early C20th District Nursing Landscape Using a Lancashire Case Study." In *Busy Women: A Century of*

Change in Women's Lives 1840–1940, edited by K. Bradley, H. Sweet, et al. In preparation.

Sweet, H., and Ferguson, R. "District Nursing History." In *District Nursing: Providing Care in a Supportive Context*, edited by S. Lawton et al. Edinburgh: Harcourt, 2000.

Temple, W. *Men Without Work: A Report Made to the Pilgrim Trust*. Pilgrim Trust, 1938.

Timmins, A. *Dilemmas of Discharge: The Case of District Nursing*. Nottingham: University of Nottingham Department of Nursing and Midwifery Studies, 1996.

Walby, S., J. Greenwell, et al. *Medicine and Nursing: Professions in a Changing Health Service*. London: Sage,1994.

Webster, C. *The NHS: A Political History*. Oxford: Oxford University Press, 1998.

Weir, A. J. *Tuberculosis in the Highlands and Islands*. Edinburgh: QIDN Scottish Branch Brochure, 1941.

White, R. *The Effects of the NHS on the Nursing Profession 1948–1961*. London: King's Fund, 1985.

White, R. *Social Change and the Development of the Nursing Profession: A Study of the Poor Law Nursing Service 1848–1948*. London: Henry Kimpton, 1978.

Whitfield, Alan. *Island Pilot*. Shetland: The Shetland Times, 1995.

Wilding, P. *Professional Power and Social Welfare*. London: Routledge & Kegan Paul, 1982.

Wickham, A. "The State and Training Programmes for Women." In *The Changing Experience of Women*, edited by E. Whitelegg et al., 149–151. Oxford: Martin Robinson, 1982.

Wicks, D. *Doctors and Nurses at Work: Rethinking Professional Boundaries*. Buckingham: Open University Press, 1998.

Williams, K. "From Sarah Gamp to Florence Nightingale: A Critical Study of Hospital Nursing Systems from 1840 to 1897." In *Rewriting Nursing History*, edited by C. Davies, 41–75. London: Croom Helm, 1982.

Wilmshurst, M. *A Record of the Work of the Queen's Nurses During the Second World War 1939–1945*. London: QNI, c. 1946.

Witz, A. *Professions and Patriarchy*. London: Routledge, 1992.

Worth, A., et al. *Assessment of Need for District Nursing*. Glasgow: Glasgow Caledonian University, Department of Nursing and Community Health, 1995.

UNPUBLISHED PAPERS AND UNPUBLISHED PROJECTS

Hawker, J. "Parish Nursing in Dorset 1700–1914." Paper presented at the Ailments and Archives conference, Dorset County Records Office, 1995.

McGann, S. "Nurses Are Citizens: The Politics of the College of Nursing (UK) as a Non-Feminist Organisation in the Interwar Period." Paper presented at the European Social Science History Conference, Amsterdam, 2006.

Smith, G. *An Oral History of General Practice in Paisley: Locality the Diffusion of Knowledge c. 1950–1990*. Unpublished project, Wellcome Trust.

UNPUBLISHED THESES

Dougall, R. "Perceptions of Change: An Oral History of District Nursing in Scotland, 1940–1990." Ph.D. thesis, Glasgow Caledonian University 2002.

Fenne, J. J. "'Every Woman Is a Nurse': Domestic Nurses in Nineteenth-Century English Popular Literature (Charles Dickens, Mary Augusta Ward)." Ph.D. thesis, University of Wisconsin-Madison, 2000.

Fox, E. N. "District Nursing and the Work of District Nursing Associations in England and Wales, 1900–48." Ph.D. thesis, London University, 1993.

Jones, H. "The Conservative Party and the Welfare State, 1942–55." Ph.D. thesis, University of London, 1992.

McIntosh, J. B. "An Observation and Time Study of the Work of Domiciliary Nurses." Ph.D. thesis, University of Aberdeen, 1975.

Mortimer, B. "The Nurse in Edinburgh c. 1760–1890: The Impact of Commerce and Professionalisation." Ph.D. thesis, University of Edinburgh, 2002.

Pitt, S. "Midwifery and Medicine: Discourses in Childbirth 1945–1975." Ph.D. thesis, University of Wales, 1996.

Reid, L. "The History of Midwifery in Scotland in the Twentieth Century." Ph.D. thesis, University of Glasgow, 2003.

Sweet, H. M. "District Nursing in England and Wales c. 1919–1979, in the Context of the Development of a Community Health Team." Ph.D. thesis, Oxford Brookes University, 2003.

ORAL AND PERSONAL TESTIMONY

Note: D/N refers to interviews with nurses from England or Wales. QNIT refers to interviews with nurses from Scotland. Recordings of all interviews are held in the RCN Archives, Edinburgh.

D/N 02, 29/08/96, Mrs. Jennifer Hawker.
D/N 03, 18/07/96, Mrs. Gladys Cruttenden.
D/N 07, 13/08/96, Dr. Lisbeth Hockey.
D/N 09, 29/08/96, Miss Audrey Smith.
D/N 10, 27/09/96, Mrs. Elaine Ryder.
D/N 11, 01/10/96, Mrs. Betty Reid.
D/N 13, 02/10/96, Mrs. Dorothy Mitchell.
D/N 17, 16/01/97, Mrs. Evelyn Whitaker.
D/N 18, 13/02/97, Mrs. Sylvia Diamond.
D/N 19, 13/02/97, Miss K. Larder
D/N 20, 12/06/99, Mrs. M. E. Kay.
D/N 21, 15/05/00, Mrs. Elizabeth Skepper.
D/N 24, 17/05/00, Mrs. Jean Fairclough.
D/N 25, 17/05/00, Mrs. Connie Pennington.
D/N 26, 18/05/00, Mrs. Elaine Parr.
D/N 27, 18/05/00, Mr. Alwen Friar.
D/N 29, 24/05/01, Mrs. E. Morris.
D/N 32, 01/02/01, Mrs. Lillian Miller.
D/N 33, 29/03/01, Mrs. Marion Hurst.
D/N 38, 01/03/01, Mr. Arthur Brompton.
D/N 39, 11/04/01, Mrs. Jean Frost.
QNIT 07/2
QNIT 08/1
QNIT 11/1
QNIT 12/1
QNIT 14/1

QNIT 14/2
QNIT 13/2
QNIT 18/2
QNIT 19/2
QNIT 20/2
QNIT 21/2
QNIT 22/2
QNIT 25/2
QNIT 26/1
QNIT 29/1
QNIT 31/1
QNIT 40/2
QNIT 43/2
QNIT 44/1
QNIT 48/2
QNIT 50/3
QNIT 53/1
QNIT 54/1
QNIT 55/1
QNIT 58/2
Personal Testimony: Miss M. I. Sankey MBE (2002).

ELECTRONIC SOURCES

Alzheimer's Society. "Is Free Nursing Care 'Unfair and Unworkable'?" http://www.alzheimers.org.uk/pdf/Free%20Nursing%20Care%20Nov%202004.pdf (accessed June 9, 2004).

Joseph Rowntree Foundation. Findings Web site. "Lessons From the Funding of Long-Term Care in Scotland" (January 2006). http://www.jrf.org.uk/knowledge/findings/socialcare/0036.asp (accessed May 6, 2006).

Steele, L. "Long-Term Care for the Elderly: The Issue Explained." *The Guardian* (March 19, 2001), http://society.guardian.co.uk/longtermcare/story/0,8150,459332,00.html

www.rcn.org.uk/professional/defining_nursing.html

www.cdna.tvu.ac.uk/pnc/Oct (accessed May 14, 2002).

Index

Ackland, Sir Henry 19.
Acts of Parliament:
  Community Care (1993) 3.
  Local Government (1929 & 1963)
    39, 55, 84.
  Maternity and Child Welfare (1918)
    35.
  Midwives (1902 and 1936) 40.
  Nurses' (1949) 88.
  Nurses, Midwives and Health Visi-
    tors (1979) 91, 159
  Nurses' Registration Act (1919) 35,
    36–37, 48
  National Health Insurance (1911) 2,
    27, 28, 30, 33, 42, 121.
  National Health (1948) 2, 3, 5, 10,
    30, 63, 78, 83, 91, 93, 96, 98,
    101, 132, 136, 151, 158–159,
    202.
  Poor Laws 19, 26.
  Representation of the People (1918)
    36.
Affiliation (to QNI) 30, 33, 38–40, 51,
    57, 61, 64, 77, 116, 120, 127,
    207
Advisory Committee on District
    Nurse Training (see: District
    Nursing)
Air ambulance 124–6.
Alexandra, Queen 48, 50.
Alternative medicine 18, 161.
Antibiotics 135, 141, 149, 209.
Armer Report (1953) 6, 88–89, 159.
Athlone, Lord (1939 Report) 64, 79.
Australia 4, 26.

Benevolent Fund (see: Funding; Queen's
    Institute)

Beveridge Report 73, 75, 131.
Bible Nurses (see Mission nurses; Ran-
    yard district nurses)
Breay, Margaret 156
Briggs Report 90, 188, 195–6
British Medical Association (BMA) 27,
    44, 98, 158.
British Red Cross Society 54, 158,
    159.
Bryn-y-Menai 57.
Burdett's Hospital Directories and
    Yearbooks 9.

Canada 25, 64.
Cardiff 101 109, 111, 113, 128–9,
    190.
Central Council for District Nursing in
    London 31, 75, 142.
Central Midwives' Board (CMB) 59
Central Sterile Supplies (CSSD) 12,
    135–9.
Chemist 43, 85, 94, 147.
Childbirth 67, 117, 194.
Children and children's nursing 29, 30,
    35, 43–44, 53–5, 68, 82, 103,
    115, 127, 158, 172, 173, 191,
    197.
Class 6–7, 18–22, 31, 47–50, 53, 130,
    151, 154, 188, 194, 206–207.
College of Nursing (see: Royal College
    of Nursing)
Comforts Guilds 79, 86.
Conditions of Service 3, 6, 7, 11–13,
    26, 30–2, 36–8, 46, 48,
    56–60, 63–4, 74–9, 84–5,
    104, 107, 113–7, 121, 125–6,
    131–2, 135, 158, 193.
Contracts (see: conditions of service)

Communication
Inter-personal/inter-professional
45–6, 49, 60, 89, 92–9, 104,
162, 190, 198, 205
Technology 12, 94–6, 121, 147–9,
203.
Community-Care Team (see also Pri-
mary care team) ix, 3,6, 13,
81, 94, 99, 151.
Community Nursing (see: District
Nursing)
Cornwall 27–8, 32, 44, 120.
Cottage Nurses 26, 46–7, 60.
Council for Nursing, Midwifery and
Health Visiting (see: UKCC)
Craven, Mrs Dacre (née Florence Lees)
24, 28, 48, 192.

Dawson Report 60, 95, 211.
Diabetes (see also: Insulin) 66, 108,
135, 181.
Diamond Jubilee (see: Victoria,
Queen)
Dickens, Charles 3, 17, 188–9.
District Midwifery 3–4, 18, 25–31,
40–47, 51, 58, 69–70, 77, 89,
114–21, 127, 130–1, 148,
163, 168, 174, 180, 191, 194,
204, 209, 211.
District Nursing
Advisory Committee 37.
Associations (see also: named associations and regions; Queen's
Institute)
Administrative Organisation of,
20, 24, 26, 29–31, 38–40,
48–51, 55, 57, 73–8, 110,
116, 127–132.
Role and Responsibilities of, 20,
27–28, 40, 53, 55, 60–61,
119–20, 127, 148.
in Dorset 39, 40, 110, 119–20
in Lancashire 32, 38, 39, 51–3,
74, 120–1, 129–32
in London 18, 20. 24, 31, 55,
78
in Scotland 39, 86, 115–16.
in South Wales 32, 39, 53–7,
114–6, 131, 143
County/Rural Nursing Associations
25, 27, 50, 51, 55, 83, 86,
110–13, 119–20, 129.

Hospitals, Relationships with 4–7,
10–11, 30, 33, 43–44, 45–47,
57–58, 60, 82, 87–8, 89–90,
98–9, 123–24, 125–26, 148–
49, 151, 154–58, 161–163,
199–200, 209–10.
Pay and Conditions of Employment
(see: conditions of service)
Queen's Institute for, (see: Queen's
Institute)
Recruitment 13, 37, 45–7, 58–9, 64,
74, 77–9, 86–8, 92, 107–8,
145, 156, 177, 187–8, 194–5,
200.
Regulation of, (see
Professionalisation)
Training and Curriculum 2, 5–7,
11–26, 31, 33, 37, 38, 40,
44–7, 57–60, 66, 74–7, 81–2,
84–90, 98, 103–4, 111–18,
121, 126–30, 135, 149, 152,
156–64, 177–9, 193–4, 197,
202, 207–8.
UKCC Joint Committee on, (1979)
90.
Workforce (Numbers of Nurses) 18,
38, 40, 49, 57, 64–5, 69, 76,
113–114, 177, 203.
Dorset 18, 39–40, 109–12, 117–20.
Drugs 12, 66, 135, 137, 138, 141–2,
149, 209.
Dual Duty (see: District Midwifery;
Nurse-midwives; Triple Duty)

East London Nursing Association 21–2,
66–7, 78, 140–1, 196.
Edinburgh xi, 9, 100, 116, 122, 178–9.
Education (see: District Nursing: Train-
ing and Curriculum)
Emoluments (see: conditions of service)
Employment (see: conditions of service)
Epidemic 19, 20, 40, 44, 122.
Epidemiology 55.
Equipment (see also: Technology) 49,
51, 79, 104, 112. 135–50,
187, 193.

Federated Superannuation Scheme for
Nurses 57, 113.
Fever Nursing 19–20, 32, 54, 135, 149.
Film and Television 55, 187, 191–200.
Fry, Mrs Elizabeth 18.

Gamp, Mrs Sarah 3, 12, 17, 43, 46–7, 188–9, 198,

Gardens Schemes and fêtes 40, 51, 75.

Gender ix, 7, 11 13, 20–36, 47, 154–8, 165, 170–85, 213.
  gendered values of care 170–3, 176–7.
  and male nurses 7, 13, 163, 177–82.
  and patients 30, 178.

Generalists (see also: Specialists) ix, 7, 17–18, 42, 98, 151–64, 204–6.

General Medical Council 152.

General Nursing Council 36, 37, 42, 88, 90, 152.

General Practitioners (GP)
  As D/N Attachments and fund-holders 2, 3, 12, 83, 92, 94–9, 104, 122, 162, 203, 205, 207, 211.
  Relationships with D/Ns, 6, 12, 27, 33, 42–7, 60, 75, 89, 93–9, 101, 113, 117–8, 123, 140, 151, 153–5, 158, 162, 172, 179–80, 196, 198–9, 204, 210–11.
  Royal College of, 89, 96.
  Surgical practice (domiciliary) 46, 135, 161, 194.
  Wartime work 68–9

Gillie Report 97.

Glasgow 20, 125, 179.

Greenock 179–80.

Health Visitors (see also: Acts of Parliament; Community-care team; Triple duty nurses) 2, 3, 6, 12, 13, 20–21 35–38, 41–2, 53–4, 58–61, 69, 74, 84, 86, 90–103, 107–8, 118, 121–3, 126–7, 129, 151, 158–61, 199, 212

Highlands and Islands (of Scotland) 1, 54–5, 85, 116,121–125, 146–47, 149, 168,180–82, 209.

Hockey, Dr. Lisbeth 6, 89, 204–205.

Hospital Nursing (see also: District Nursing: Hospitals, Relationships with) 3,4,11, 17, 21, 70–74, 87, 93, 104, 135, 150, 143, 153 172, 204.

Emergency Hospital Scheme 67–9, 72.

Hughes, Miss Amy 24, 206.

Hygiene 19, 21, 22, 36, 55, 68, 142.

Image (see also: Status) 3, 6, 8, 13, 17, 22, 28–9, 38, 60–61, 63, 77–9, 81–3, 91, 103–4, 107–9, 115, 132–3, 139, 151, 158, 163, 165, 172, 187–200, 204, 206.

Industrialisation 3, 18, 42, 51–52, 57, 101, 107, 113–118, 125–132, 179, 199, 200

Injuries (see also industrialisation) 68, 70, 108, 118, 132, 199.

Insulin 66, 135, 137, 138, 141.

Islands of Scotland (see Highlands and Islands)

Lady Superintendents 7, 10, 18–22, 28, 48, 60, 128.

Lancashire 5, 38–9, 51–3, 70, 73, 76, 82, 84, 97, 101–2, 109–10, 118, 120, 125–32, 142.

Lees, Florence (see Craven, Mrs Dacre)

Legislation (see: Acts of Parliament)

Lewis, Isle of (see: Islands of Scotland)

Liverpool District Nursing Association (see also: Lancashire; Rathbone) 3–4, 20–21, 31, 48, 67, 83–4, 89, 118, 126–30, 196–7.

Loane, M. 29, 191–2.

Local Government Act (1929) (see: Acts of Parliament)

Local Health Authorities (see also: Medical Officer of Health) 77, 83–7, 261.

London County Council 68, 142.

Long Service Fund 56–7.

Manchester 3, 20, 73, 129, 131.
  and Salford, Ladies' Sanitary Reform Association of, 20.

Marriage 36, 57–9, 81–2, 127, 165, 173, 175–8. Medical Officer of Health (MOH) 37, 54, 87, 159, 169.

Medicines (see: Antibiotics; Drugs; Insulin; Technology)

Merry, Miss E.J. 88, 94, 193.

Metropolitan
  and National Nursing Association
    21, 23, 24.
  and Southern Counties Association
    (of the QNI) 37, 46.
Midwifery (see: District midwifery;
    Puerperal sepsis; Triple duty
    nurses)
Mining 100, 109, 114, 117–8, 125,
    132, 198.
Ministry of Health 10, 35, 38, 40, 51,
    68–83, 88–90, 158
Ministry of Information 195.
Missions, mission nurses and missioners
    2, 3, 17, 18, 20–2, 28–9, 91,
    187–8, 196.
Mobility (of practice) 7, 121, 132, 206.

National Health Service Act (1946) (see
    Acts of Parliament)
National Health Insurance Act (1911)
    (see Acts of Parliament)
Nightingale, Florence 3, 17, 21–4, 48,
    187–8, 195.
  Iconic image of, 171, 188, 193.
Nurse-midwives (see also: District Mid-
    wifery; Triple-duty)
Nurses' Registration Act (see: Acts of
    Parliament)
Nursing care
  Bathing 26, 28, 41, 93, 98, 102,
    112, 139, 142, 166–7, 175,
    179, 182–4, 199, 205, 210.
  Dressings/wound care 18, 68, 140,
    87, 102, 136–40.
  Palliative care 167, 183.
  Range of duties 18, 28–9, 41, 68,
    102, 136–42, 165–8.

Occupational Imperialism ix, 6, 24,
    152–4.
Oral History 5, 8, 10–13, 44, 63, 81–2,
    99, 118, 158,162, 195–6, 200,
    201–7.

Paget, Dame Rosalind 25, 187.
Parasites 126–7, 197.
Patients 1–2, 19–30, 43, 54, 88–9,
    94–104, 122, 140–7, 156–7,
    162, 166, 172–6, 178.
  Rights and Expectations of, 40–42,
    82–3, 99–103, 122, 140–
    2,147, 162–3, 180–3, 203.

and Social class, 2, 19, 20–23, 26,
    43, 53, 109, 112, 130–1, 168.
  Statistics relating to, 18–19, 27–8,
    31–2 38, 44, 51, 53, 76, 78,
    113, 128.
Pay (see: Conditions of service)
Pension schemes 2, 31, 38, 46, 56, 86,
    209.
Penwith District Nursing Association ,
    Cornwall 27–8.
Peterkin, Miss 120.
Pharmacist (see: Chemist)
Pilgrim Trust 128, 130.
Poor Law (see: Acts of Parliament;
    Royal Commission; Work-
    house nurses)
Practice Nurses 2–3, 13, 83, 161–3,
    183, 187, 204–5.
Preventative medicine (see also: Health
    Visitor, Public Health) 1, 31,
    36–7, 56, 98, 120 (f.n. 26),
    160, 187, 197–99.
Primary care team (see also commu-
    nity-care team) 1, 13, 96, 104,
    149.
Private Nursing 2, 12, 18–20, 23–4,
    27, 30–31, 48, 53, 55–8, 75,
    156–8, 169–70.
Professions:
  Clerical and Legal 153.
  Medical ix, 11, 19, 23, 27, 47, 71,
    97–9, 152–154, 159, 163,
    206.
  Nursing ix, 5–8, 36–7, 63, 87, 153,
    155, 158, 163, 194.
  Para-medical professions 3, 5–7,
    151, 153.
  Teaching 11, 36, 158.
Professional:
  Autonomy ix, 6, 41, 43, 48, 61, 90,
    97–9, 104, 123, 152–7, 161,
    172, 176, 184, 199–200, 203,
    206, 210–211.
  Ethics and conduct (see also:
    Patients; Professional Regula-
    tion; Relatives) 7, 96, 152,
    163, 167, 176, 188, 198–200,
    205.
  Isolation 89, 121–4, 145, 147–8,
    155, 168, 180–182, 207–10.
  Regulation 6–7, 17, 22–4, 33–41,
    48, 76–7, 82, 86–90, 103,
    151–2, 159, 164, 202.

Status 5–7, 22, 35, 37, 46, 60, 77, 81–2, 84, 87, 90–6, 102–3, 149, 151–164, 166, 168, 171–2, 176, 184, 188–90, 194, 202, 206.
Professionalisation 5–13, 21–2, 26, 33, 60, 88–9, 151–164, 165, 171–2, 189, 206.
Provident Schemes (see: funding)
Public Health (see also: preventative medicine, sanitary reform) 1, 21, 31, 36–7, 40, 42, 50–6, 59, 63, 69, 75, 77, 83–91, 111–14, 120, 141, 159–60, 194–9.
Publications (see: Books, Recruitment literature)
Puerperal sepsis 53, 54, 108.

Qualifications (see also: Queen's Institute: Training)11, 18, 22, 37, 44, 49, 55, 87, 89, 91, 107, 113, 152, 157–8, 178, 188.
Queen's Institute for District Nursing Affiliation Agreements 30 33, 38–40, 51, 57, 61, 64, 77, 116, 120, 127, 207–8 Inspectors' Reports 39, 49, 108, 112–6, 130, 206.
Royal Charter 25, 26, 35 (f.n. 5), 50, 158.
Rules (see also Affiliation agreements) 27, 30, 33, 77.
Secular status of, 38–9.
Training 2, 7, 22–6, 32–3, 37–8, 40–1, 46–7, 50, 57–60, 75, 77, 84–90, 111, 116, 118, 121, 128–30, 174, 177–9, 190–1, 193–7, 202, 207–8.
Uniform 31, 37, 51, 59, 115, 121, 190–4, 203,
Women's Jubilee Offering 21, 24,

Ranyard District Nurses 1, 18, 20, 38, 75, 82, 86, 88.
Rathbone, William 3, 20–22, 24–5.
Staff College 89, 129, 194.
Recruitment (see district nursing: recruitment)
Registration (see: Nurses' Registration Act)
Relatives 47, 94, 101, 117, 140–1, 149, 159, 163, 168, 179.

Religion (see also: Queen's Institute: Secular status; Ranyard) 13, 18, 20–22, 31, 38, 39, 174–7, 191.
Richmond, Lady Elena (neé Robinson) 71.
Robinson, Mrs Mary 20.
Royal College of Nursing (RCN) 9, 11, 36, 75–80, 87–8, 90, 126, 161, 200.
Royal Commission on the Poor Law Report (1909) 26.
Royal National Pension Fund for Nurses (see also Pension schemes) 31.
Rushcliffe Committee 74–8, 155, 159.

St John's Ambulance 158, 159.
Sanitary Reform 18–21.
School Nursing 29, 31, 41, 51, 54–5, 58, 68, 69, 74, 77,111, 113, 119–20, 161, 199, 201, 204.
Scotland (see: District Nursing: Scotland; Highlands and Islands; also under individual place names)
State Registration (see: Nurses' Registration Act)
Social Workers 13, 69, 75, 89, 91–7, 158, 167–9.
South African District Nursing 26, 206.
Specialisms (medical and nursing) 5, 89. 98, 153, 160–3, 204–6.
Specialists (see also: Generalists) 2, 4, 13, 35, 42, 77, 98, 111–2, 126, 128, 140, 151–64, 167, 201, 204–6.
Sulpha drugs/sulphonamides (see also antibiotics, drugs) 141, 149.
Swansea 57, 109, 112.

Telephones (see also: Communication) 42, 49, 94–5, 117, 121, 123, 142, 144,147–9, 158.
Transport 12, 56, 73, 85, 101, 104, 113, 114–124,142–7, 149, 203–9.
Triple-duty Nurses 2, 4, 41, 69, 107–9, 113, 118–123, 129, 133, 171, 174, 196, 209.
Tuberculosis (TB) 29, 35, 51, 53–55, 69, 111–12, 119, 122, 141–2, 174, 179, 192,

Urban practice 5–7, 19, 26–7, 30, 56, 69–70, 73, 81, 94, 101–2, 107–34, 141–5, 168, 191, 203–4, 211.
UKCC 90, 152.

Victoria, Queen 21, 24, 25.
Village Nurse-midwives (see: Cottage nurses)

Wales
South 5, 39, 56–7, 91–2, 109–115, 118, 125–9, 143, 198.
Welsh Language 116–8, 199.

Wartime:
Blitz 66–73.
Emergency Medical Service 66, 68.
Payment for extra duties 68–72.
World War One 17, 35, 41–2.
World War Two 4, 63–77, 79–80, 82, 87, 132, 158–9, 174, 177–8, 208–9.
Wilmshurst, Miss M. 49, 70–1, 74, 157.
Women Medical Practitioners 11, 23, 153, 163, 178, 196.
Women's Suffrage 28, 36, 156.
Workhouse Infirmary Nurses 19–20, 189.

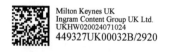